The Unofficial Guide to

Passing OSCEs

THIRD EDITION

Chief Editor: Zeshan Qureshi

ISBN 978-0-957-14990-8

Text, design and illustration © Zeshan Qureshi 2012

Chief Editor Zeshan Qureshi
Published by Zeshan Qureshi. First published 2012

Original design by Zeshan Qureshi and Rob Glenister. Page make-up by Anchorprint Group Limited
Illustrated by Anchorprint Group Limited, Richard Holdsworth (Station 2.25), Reza Jarral (Station 2.16), Nikki Hall (Station 5.7), Camilla Jay Stewart (Drug Charts)
Cover design by Anchorprint Group Limited

A catalogue record for this book is available from the British Library.

Publisher and Chief Editors' Acknowledgements:
I would like to thank all the authors for their hard work, and our distinguished panel of expert reviewers for their specialist input. I am extremely grateful for the support given by medical schools across the UK. I would also like to thank the medical students that have inspired this project, believed in this project, and have helped contribute to, promote, and distribute the book across the UK. Thank you to Caroline Muirhead, James Richard Hamish O 'Kelly, and Emily McCall-Smith for acting as models. Thanks also to Pauline Graham for her invaluable advise.

The authors and publishers would like to thank the following for permission to reproduce their images:

NHS Lothian: Fig 2.1, 2.2 (right), 2.3, 2.4, 2.6-2.10, 2.12-14, 2.16-2.20, 2.21, 2.23-2.49, 2.51, 2.54-2.58, 2.60, 2.62-2.68, 2.71-2, 2.74-75, 2.77-2.79, 2.81, 2.83-84, 2.86, 2.88-91, 2.93, 3.1-10, 3.12-18, 3.20-21, 3.23-53, 3.55-6, 5.1, 5.3, 5.6, 8.1, 8.3-4, 8.6
NHS Fife: Fig 5.2 (bottom), 5.5   Alex Rothman (www.reviseforfinals.co.uk): Fig 2.2 (left), 2.5, 2.11, 2.15, 2.22, 2.50, 2.52-53, 2.59, 2.61, 2.69-70, 2.73, 2.76, 2.80, 2.82, 2.85, 2.87, 2.94, 3.11, 3.19, 3.54, 8.2   Mr David Pothier (www.earatlas.co.uk): Fig 2.92 and 'Common Ear Pathology' (Station 2.24)   Pamela Gulland/Hannah Collinson: ECG 1-6 (Station 5.6)   Dr Ed Friedlander: Fig 5.4   Headshot London (Introduction)

Commissioned photographs by:
Mark Rodrigues: Fig 3.22, 'Assessing Tendons' table and 'Motor Testing' table (Station 3.3)
Reza Jarral: All images: station 5.9   Katrina Mason: All images: station 5.10

Printed and bound by Cambrian Printers in UK

No individual has been paid for authorship, editorial or reviewing contributions. A minimum of £1 from each book sale will be reinvested in medical education, or will go to charities, and we are keen to consider charities of YOUR choosing. So far we have raised money for Heart Research UK, Dreamflight, Bluebells Hospice, Madeleine Steel Charitable Trust, Revise4finals, The Shello Orphanage Fund, Alzheimer's Research Trust, The Magic Wand Appeal, Teenage Cancer Trust, and Southampton MenCap.

Introduction

'The Unofficial Guide to Passing OSCEs' was originally compiled from revision notes made in preparation for Finals Examinations in 2007. It has been evolving ever since to become the success it is today. We believe:

...that fresh graduates have a unique perspective on what works *for students.* We have captured the insight of medical students and recent graduates in the language that they used to make complex material more easily digestible *for students.* This textbook has been written by junior doctors and medical students, but also with the reassurance of review by senior clinicians in their specific specialty

...that medical texts are in *constant* need of being updated. *Every medical student* has the potential to contribute to the education of others by innovative ways of thinking and learning. This book is an open collaboration with you: the readers of the second edition have become the writers of the third edition. You have the power to *contribute* something valuable to medicine. We welcome your suggestions and collaboration on developing this textbook in future, from adding new tips/cases to learn from/stations, to simply making what we have already *even better*

...that medical knowledge should be acquired in a fun and memorable way, which is why in this edition we have published over 300 photographs, included tips from our experts and authors, plus memorable stories of cases that you can learn from

...that medical knowledge should be *spread* and *shared* at a minimal cost to the student. And that we should financially support re-investing in your education as medical students and worthy charities

We appreciate that OSCEs are often the most stressful exams you will take at medical school. This books aims to empower your examination preparation and help you on your way to excelling in the OSCE. We also encourage you to supplement these notes with complementary learning experiences. We wish you all the best in your upcoming examinations and your future medical career.

Please get in touch,
Zeshan

Email: zeshanqureshi@doctors.org.uk
Facebook:_http://www.facebook.com/ groups/213464185413737/
Twitter: @DrZeshanQureshi

This book contains notes on:

11 **History Taking** Stations

25 **Examination** Stations

7 **Orthopaedic** Stations

10 **Communication Skills** Stations

10 **Practical Skills** Stations

3 **Radiology** Stations

9 **Obstetrics and Gynaecology** Stations

10 **Paediatric** Stations

8 **Psychiatry** Stations

11 **Prescribing** Stations

Writing Hospital Letters
Appraising Journals

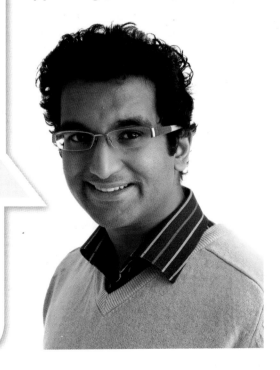

FOREWORD

There are few experiences more daunting for medical students than facing the clinical OSCE. The examiners' faces are often unfamiliar, the pace is out of their control and there is little opportunity to go back and correct mistakes. However, in many ways, those are features of real world practice where junior doctors have to respond to events in real time. For that reason, many medical educators consider the clinical OSCE as the ultimate objective test of readiness to practice.

For many years now I have been in the enviable position of merely having to tick the boxes on the marking form. However, I've not forgotten the stress that the occasion can induce in even the most talented of students. My advice to my own students is that the best way to mitigate the effects of the inevitable stress, and to perform well when the bell sounds, is to be well prepared. *The Unofficial Guide to Passing OSCEs* is intended to support students as they make those preparations. The chapters are clearly written, in simple language that should appeal to students and reflect the fact that the authors themselves have recently been OSCE candidates. It has been my pleasure to work with many of the authors of this book in recent years. They are all part of what I believe is a genuine re-invigoration of the art of teaching amongst junior medical staff that bodes very well for the future of medical education in this country. I am pleased to see that their enthusiasm and talent has culminated in the writing of this book. I hope you will find it valuable as you yourself get ready for the bell to sound.

Simon Maxwell
Professor of Student Learning
University of Edinburgh

The unofficial guide to passing the OSCEs, a book that started off as an idea to collate notes amongst a group of good friends studying for their finals is today venturing into its third edition, getting even better each time! A hearty congratulation to the authors is definitely in order!

OSCEs are a daunting time and sometimes the pressure just gets a little ahead of you at that specific moment of time; the authors realised this very early on whilst pursuing their degrees and hence came up with this fantastic revision tool. The aims of this book are to provide the student with a structure and enable them to apply their magnificent clinical skills learnt after hours of hard work on the wards in an examination setting. It provides the student with simple basic reminders which are important nonetheless at the same time explains and exemplifies how to approach the more intricate and difficult stations. The best bit about this book is that it gives you examples of potential stations hence you can easily use this book with a friend and practise different stations with a guide informing you on your progress.

This book has been revised thoroughly since its conception and now includes even more stations, scenarios and tips to get you the grade you want, not only pass but to do so with flying colours!

Wishing you the very best of luck in your upcoming examinations.

Shamit Shah
Medical Student
University of Southampton

CONTRIBUTORS

Chief Editor

Zeshan Qureshi   Paediatrics Trainee (University of Southampton)

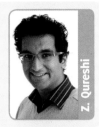

Editors

Seb Gray   Paediatrics Trainee (University of Southampton)

Selina Hennedige-Gray   General Medicine Trainee (University of Southampton)

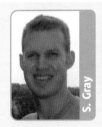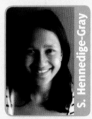

Senior Clinical Editor

Patrick Byrne   GP and Physician in General Medicine
(Belford Hospital, Fort William)

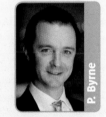

Student and FY1 Editor

Caroline Muirhead   Fourth Year Medical Student (University of Edinburgh)

Kyle Gibson   Academic Foundation Doctor (University of Edinburgh)

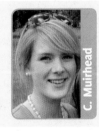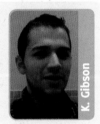

OSCE Station Authors

Moe Alam   Foundation Doctor (University of Southampton)
Blood Transfusion
Warfarin Counselling

Steve Alderson   Academic Foundation Doctor (University of Southampton)
Consent for HIV Testing
Genitourinary Medicine: Sexual History and Vaginal Discharge

James Andrews   General Medicine Trainee (University of Southampton)
Respiratory History (co-author) and Examination

Zoe Clough   Foundation Doctor (University of Southampton)
Cardiovascular Examination

Katie Donaldson   Foundation Doctor (University of Glasgow)
Antenatal Booking
Consent for Endoscopy
Intermittent Claudication
Rectal Examination

Tabera Dionne   Foundation Doctor (Peninsula Medical School)
Haematology History and Examination
Non Accidental Injury

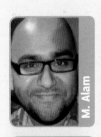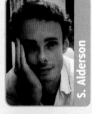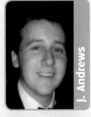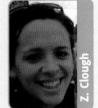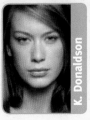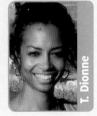

OSCE Station Authors *Continued*

Funglin Foo Foundation Doctor (University of Southampton)
Headache History

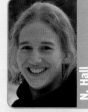
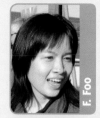

Kyle Gibson Academic Foundation Doctor (University of Edinburgh)
Acromegaly Examination
Cushing's Syndrome Examination
Diarrhoea History (co-author)
ECG Interpretation (co-author)
Respiratory History (co-author)
Thyroid Examination

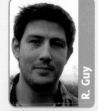
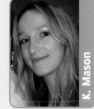

Seb Gray Paediatrics Trainee (University of Southampton)
Paediatrics (Chapter – co-author)
Breast History and Examination (co-author)
Cardiovascular History (co-author)
Dermatological Examination (co-author)
Hernia Repair Consent (co-author)
Gastrointestinal History and Examination (co-author)
Lifestyle Advice Post-Myocardial Infarction (co-author)

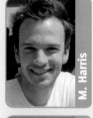
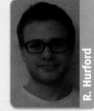

Rob Guy Anaesthetics Trainee (Brighton and Sussex Medical School)
Morphine Counselling

Nikki Hall Foundation Doctor (University of Edinburgh)
Eye Examination
Fundoscopy

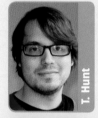
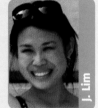

Matthew Harris Foundation Doctor (University of Southampton)
Intermediate Life Support
Discharge Prescribing (co-author)

Selina Hennedige-Gray General Medicine Trainee (University of Southampton)
Breast History and Examination (co-author)
Cardiovascular History (co-author)
Dermatological Examination (co-author)
Hernia Repair Consent (co-author)
Gastrointestinal History and Examination (co-author)
Lifestyle Advice Post-Myocardial Infarction (co-author)

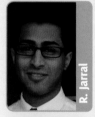
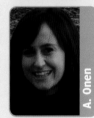

Tobias Hunt Paediatric Trainee (University of Southampton)
Newborn Baby Examination

Rob Hurford Medical Student (University of Nottingham)
Dealing with an Agitated Patient

Reza Jarral Foundation Doctor (Imperial College London)
Hernia Examination
Instruments
Neck Lumps
Stoma Examination
Ulcer Examination

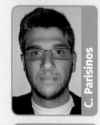
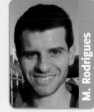

Jade Lim Foundation Doctor (University of Southampton)
Testicular Lump Examination

Katrina Mason Academic Foundation Doctor (University of Bristol)
Ear Examination
Suturing

Alev Onen Foundation Doctor (University of Dundee)
Peripheral Vascular Examination
Varicose Veins Examination

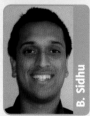

Constantinos Parisinos Academic Foundation Doctor (University of Edinburgh)
Prescribing (Chapter- Coauthor)

Mark Rodrigues Academic Foundation Doctor (University of Edinburgh)
Prescribing (Chapter- Coauthor)
Orthopedics (Chapter)
Radiology (Chapter)

Baldeep Sidhu Foundation Doctor (University of Southampton)
Urinalysis

OSCE Station Authors *Continued*

Matt Sims Foundation Doctor (University of Oxford)
Cerebellar Examination
Cranial Nerves Examination
Lower Limb Neurological Examination
Parkinson's Disease Examination
Upper Limb Neurological Examination

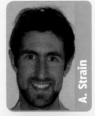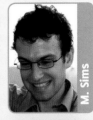

Andrew Strain Foundation Doctor (University of Cambridge)
Urethral Catheterisation

Sabrina Qureshi Medical Student (Kings College London)
Psychiatry (Chapter – co-author)

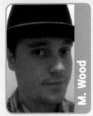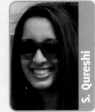

Zeshan Qureshi Paediatrics Trainee (University of Southampton)
Breaking Bad News
Breast History and Examination (co-author)
Cardiovascular History (co-author)
Consent for Post-Mortem Examination
Critical Appraisal (Chapter)
Diarrhoea History (co-author)
Dermatological Examination (co-author)
Death Certification
ECG Interpretation (co-author)
Gastrointestinal History and Examination (co-author)
Hernia Repair Consent (co-author)
Hospital Letters (Chapter)
Intravenous Cannulation and Setting up a Giving Set
Lifestyle Advice Post-Myocardial Infarction
Paediatrics (Chapter – co-author)
Phlebotomy
Psychiatry (Chapter – co-author)
Suicide Risk

Matthew Wood Obstetrics and Gynaecology Trainee
(University of Southampton)
Obstetrics and Gynaecology (Chapter)

Senior Reviewers

Breast Surgery **Mr Kulkarni Dhananjay** (Consultant Breast Surgeon, Western General Hospital, Edinburgh)

Cardiology **Dr Alex Hobson** (Consultant Interventional Cardiologist, Queen Alexandra Hospital, Portsmouth)
Dr Paul Neary (Consultant Cardiologist, Borders General Hospital, Melrose)

Clinical Skills **Jan Heath** (Head of Clinical Skills, University of Southampton)
Sophie Macadie (Clinical Skills Facilitator, University of Southampton)
Ken Arber (Clinical Skills Facilitator, University of Southampton)
Tracey Murphy (Clinical Skills Facilitator, University of Southampton)
Amanda Harper (Clinical Skills Facilitator, University of Southampton)

Communication Skills **Dr Belinda Hacking** (Consultant Clinical Psychologist, Western General Hospital, Edinburgh. Honorary Fellow of Edinburgh University and Coventry University)

Critical Appraisal **Professor Paul Little** (Professor in Primary Care Research, University of Southampton)

Dermatology **Professor Jonathan Rees** (Grant Chair of Dermatology, Western General Hospital, Edinburgh)

Ear, Nose and Throat **Mr David Pottier** (Consultant Otolaryngologist, Toronto General Hospital, Toronto, Canada)

Endocrinology **Dr Mark Strachan** (Consultant Endocrinologist, Western General Hospital, Edinburgh)

Gastroenterology **Dr John Plevris** (Consultant Gastroenterologist, Royal Infirmary of Edinburgh, Edinburgh)

General Practice **Dr Mark Aley** (General Practioner, The Fryern Surgery, Chandlers Ford, Hampshire)
Dr Guy Dixon (General Practice Trainee, University of Liverpool)

General Surgery **Mr Peter Faganholz MD** (Attending Surgeon, Massachusetts General Hospital, Boston, USA; Instructor in Surgery, Harvard Medical School)
Mr Bruce Tulloch (Consultant General Surgeon, Royal Infirmary of Edinburgh, Edinburgh)

Haematology **Dr Julia Anderson** (Consultant Haematologist, Royal Infirmary of Edinburgh, Edinburgh)

Neonatology **Dr Ivor Lewis** (Consultant Paediatrician, Director of Medical Education, East Surrey Hospital, Red Hill)

Senior Reviewers *Continued*

Neurology	**Professor Richard Knight** (Professor of Clinical Neurology, Western General Hospital, Edinburgh)
Obstetrics and Gynaecology	**Dr Paul Mills** (Specialist Registrar in Obstetrics and Gynaecology, Royal Infirmary of Edinburgh, Edinburgh)
Oncology	**Dr Ewen Brown** (Consultant Oncologist, Western General Hospital, Edinburgh)
Ophthalmology	**Professor Baljean Dhillon** (Professor of Ophthalmology, Princess Alexandra Eye Pavillion, Edinburgh)
Orthopaedic Surgery	**Professor Margaret McQueen** (Professor of Orthopaedic Trauma, Royal Infirmary of Edinburgh, Edinburgh)
Pathology	**Dr William Wallace** (Consultant Pathologist, Royal Infirmary of Edinburgh, Edinburgh)
Paediatrics	**Dr Catherine Hill** (Honorary Consultant Paediatrician, Solent NHS Trust) **Dr Sarah Clegg** (Consultant Community Paediatrician, Royal Hospital for Sick Children, Edinburgh) **Dr Ian Rodd** (Consultant Paediatrician, Royal Hampshire County Hospital, Winchester) **Dr Raj Rao** (Consultant Paediatrician with Special interest in Allergy and Respiratory Medicine, Poole Hospital NHS Foundation Trust)
Pharmacology	**Professor Simon Maxwell** (Professor of Student Learning, Clinical Pharmacology and Prescribing, Clinical Pharmacology Unit, University of Edinburgh)
Psychiatry	**Professor Eve Johnstone** (Professor of Psychiatry, Royal Edinburgh Hospital, Edinburgh) **Professor David Cunningham-Owens** (Professor of Clinical Psychiatry, Royal Edinburgh Hospital, Edinburgh) **Dr Robby Steel** (Consultant Liaison Psychiatrist, Royal Infirmary of Edinburgh, Edinburgh) **Dr Killian Welch** (Specialist Registrar in Psychiatry, Royal Edinburgh Hospital, Edinburgh)
Radiology	**Dr Simon Jackson** (Consultant Radiologist, Western General Hospital, Edinburgh)
Respiratory	**Dr Simon Watkin** (Consultant Respiratory Physician, Borders General Hospital, Melrose)
Vascular Surgery	**Mr Andrew Tambyraja** (Specialist Registrar in Vascular Surgery, Royal Infirmary of Edinburgh, Edinburgh)

Student Reviewers

Dana Abraham	University of Southampton	**Helen Mcgeown**	University of Edinburgh
Erin Choa	University of Edinburgh	**Herjit Sidhu**	University of Sheffield
Matthew Clarke	Cardiff University	**Shamit Shah**	University of Southampton
Nick Davison	Barts and the London School of Medicine	**Chudy Uzoho**	University of Southampton
Rob Hurford	University of Nottingham		

FURTHER READINGS

This book has developed from knowledge obtained during medical school. This is a product of textbooks, websites, and other teaching materials. Below are some key sources that we have utilised as students to shape our medical knowledge and in turn help develop the ideas behind this book.

- ABC of Eyes: Khaw PT, Shah P, Elkington AR; Wiley-Blackwell; 2004.
- Abdominal X-Rays Made Easy: Begg JD; Churchill Livingstone; 2006.
- Accident and Emergency Radiology: A Survival Guide: Raby N, Berman L, de Lacey G; Saunders Ltd; 2005.
- Apley's Concise Orthopaedics and Trauma: Solomon L, Warwick DJ, Nayagam S; Hodder Arnold; 2005.
- Breech Presentation, Management (Green-top 20b); Royal College of Obstetricians and Gynaecologists Green Top Guidelines; 2006.
- Caesarean Section Consent Advice from the Royal College of Obstetricians and Gynaecologists: http://www.rcog.org.uk/womens-health/clinical-guidance/caesarean-section-consent-advice.
- Chest X-Rays Made Easy: Corne J, Pointon K; Churchill Livingstone; 2009.
- Davidson's Principles and Practice of Medicine: Colledge NR, Walker BR, Ralston SH; Churchill Livingstone; 2010.
- Dermatology: An Illustrated Colour Text: Gawkrodger D; Churchill Livingstone; 2007.
- Ear, Nose and Throat and Head and Neck Surgery: An Illustrated Colour Text: Dhillon RS, East CA; Churchill Livingstone; 2006.
- Shardlow A, Turner MR. Examination of the Cerebellum. The Journal of Clinical Examination 2008; 5: 5-9.
- Zakaria R, Gregory R. Examination of the Patient with Parkinson's Disease. The Journal of Clinical Examination 2007; 2: 15-19.
- Final MB: A Guide to Success in Clinical Medicine: Dalton H, Reynolds N, Noble SIR, McGovern D; Churchill Livingstone; 2011.
- General Medical Council 'Good Medical Practice' Guidelines: http://www.gmc-uk.org/guidance/good_medical_practice.asp.
- General Practice Notebook: www.gpnotebook.co.uk.
- Illustrated Textbook of Paediatrics: Lissauer T, Clayden G; Mosby; 2007.
- Kumar and Clark Clinical Medicine: Kumar P, Clark M; Saunders Ltd; 2009.
- Lecture Notes: General Surgery: Ellis H, Calne R, Watson C; Wiley-Blackwell; 2011.
- Macleod's Clinical Examination: Douglas G, Nicol F, Robertson C; Churchill Livingstone; 2009.
- Master Medicine: Medicine: A Core Text with Self-Assessment: O'Neill P, Dornan T, Denning D; Churchill Livingstone; 2007.
- Neurological Examination Made Easy: Fuller G; Churchill Livingstone; 2008.
- Obstetrics and Gynaecology: Impey L, Child T; Wiley-Blackwell; 2008.
- Oxford Handbook of Clinical Medicine: Longmore M, Wilkinson I, Davidson E, Foulkes A, Mafi A; OUP Oxford; 2010.
- Oxford Handbook of Obstetrics and Gynaecology: Collins S, Arulkumaran S, Hayes K, Jackson S, Impey L; OUP Oxford; 2008.
- Paediatrics and Child Health: Rudolf M, Lee T, Levene M; Wiley-Blackwell; 2011.
- Placenta Praevia, Placenta Praevia Accreta and Vasa Praevia: Diagnosis and Management (Green-top 27); Royal College of Obstetricians and Gynaecologists Green Top Guidelines; 2011.
- Postpartum Haemorrhage, Prevention and Management (Green-top 52); Royal College of Obstetricians and Gynaecologists Green Top Guidelines; 2009.
- Psychiatry: An Illustrated Colour Text: Stevens L, Rodin I; Churchill Livingstone; 2010.
- Psychiatry PRN: Principles, Reality, Next Steps. Stringer S, Church L, Davison S, Lipsedge M;. Oxford University Press; 2009.
- Quick Starting Contraception; Faculty of Sexual and Reproductive Healthcare Clinical Guidance; 2010.
- The Chest X-Ray: A Survival Guide: de Lacey G, Morley S, Berman L; Saunders Ltd; 2008.
- The ECG Made Easy: Adlam D, Hampton J, Hampton JR; Churchill Livingstone; 2008.
- Urine Dipstick Analysis Article on Patient.co.uk: http://www.patient.co.uk/doctor/Urine-Dipstick-Analysis.htm
- Missed Pill Recommendation; Royal College of Obstetrics and Gynaecologists, 2011 http://www.fsrh.org/pdfs/CEUStatementMissedPills.pdf

CONTENTS

1 History Taking

Some topics are more likely to surface than others are, and many history taking scenarios have not been mentioned here. After completing a year of attachments, the hope is that you will have accumulated enough neuronal connections to cope with any situation thrown at you! When in doubt or under stress, go back to the basics. The simple history taking format and SOCRATES should never be forgotten, and always remember the importance of communication. Maintain good eye contact, ask a mixture of open and closed questions, and you are already halfway there.

For every OSCE station in the finals, remember the following tips:

- Introduce yourself and wash your hands
- Ensure that patient dignity is preserved in the context of the task
- Explain what you are going to do and offer information leaflets, particularly when counselling a patient
- Gain consent
- If you don't know the answer to any question, then admit this, and say you will speak to a colleague and find out the answer
- Thank the patient at the end of the consult

Study Action Plan

- Practice history taking in small groups
- Take turns to be the patient, doctor and assessor: ask your colleagues to take the time to get into a character, and to think of a specific disease and how it might present: this is good clinical revision as well
- Ask your assessor to provide constructive feedback and reflect on this feedback
- Work towards being observed by more experienced clinicians whether in role play scenarios or on the wards with real patients
- If possible, go to acute medical admission wards, and after liaising with staff, clerk in patients 'fresh', discuss them with senior staff, and present them on the ward round. This simulates both a real life role, and the role you might expect an actor to take on in an OSCE

This chapter contains notes on the following histories:

Station 1:
CARDIOVASCULAR HISTORY: CHEST PAIN

Mrs Jones is a 60 year-old lady who presented with a two-hour history of shortness of breath, central chest pain and sweating. Please take a history from Mrs Jones and then present your findings.

Pain History
('SOCRATES' mnemonic)

- **Site:** Central/left/right sided chest pain?
- **Onset:** Sudden or gradual? What was the patient doing when it came on?
- **Character:** Gripping? Crushing? Tearing? Burning? Cramping? Heavy? Tight?
- **Radiation:** Up into the jaw and/or down the left arm? Into the right arm? Through to the back?
- **Associated Symptoms:**
  - **Shortness of Breath:** Orthopnoea, paroxysmal nocturnal dyspnoea. How many pillows do they sleep on? Exercise tolerance: what is their current exercise tolerance? What stops them exercising at that point? What is normal for them?
  - **Autonomic Symptoms:** Nausea, vomiting, sweating
  - **Palpitations:** Were they regular or irregular? Did they start and stop suddenly? Did they precede any chest pain or come after it?
  - **Pre Syncope and Syncope:** Did the patient feel dizzy or light headed? Was their level of consciousness affected?
  - **Ankle Swelling:** Unilateral or bilateral?
  - **Calf Swelling:** Any swelling or rashes noticed in the legs? If so, any pain/redness/tenderness?
  - **Haemoptysis:** May be suggestive of a pulmonary embolism or pneumonia. It is also associated with mitral stenosis, lung cancer, and tuberculosis. Pink frothy sputum is associated with pulmonary oedema
  - **Sputum:** Amount, colour, and frequency
  - **Trauma:** Any recent chest trauma?
- **Timing:**
  - How long does it last? If they have had multiple episodes, are they getting longer in duration or more frequent?
- **Exacerbating and Relieving Factors:**
  - **Exercise:** Is the pain associated with exercise? What is the relationship?
  - **Food:** Does the pain come after eating large meals, or certain foods? Is the pain relieved by antacids? Associated water brash (hypersalivation often post reflux)?
  - **Position:** Does the pain vary with lying flat/sitting forward?
  - **GTN:** Is the pain relieved by GTN? (angina or oesophageal spasm may be relieved, though for oesophageal pain typically takes considerably longer; i.e. 10 minutes, so also ask how long it took the pain to subside)
  - **Analgesia:** Is the pain relieved by paracetamol/morphine?

Cardinal Symptoms

Cardinal Symptoms
Chest pain
Breathlessness
Palpitations
Syncope/Presyncope
Oedema

- Is the pain pleuritic?
- Is there any pain on movement or any tenderness on pressing? (suggestive of a musculoskeletal cause)
- **Severity:** Score out of 10 (with 10 being the worst possible pain and 0 being pain-free). How bad is their pain now? How bad was it at its worst?

Has the patient had anything like this before? If the patient has had a previous heart attack/angina, is this the same type of pain?

Past Medical History

Enquire about the following conditions:

- Myocardial infarction (and any previous cardiac procedures)
- Diabetes mellitus
- Hypercholesterolaemia
- Peripheral vascular disease
- Stroke
- Rheumatic fever

Medication History

- Allergy history including reactions to previous contrast agents. Particularly consider cardiovascular medications such as ACE inhibitors and beta-blockers

Social History

- Smoking status (past, present or never): How many? What? For how long? Then calculate number of pack years (1 pack year = 20 cigarettes/day for 1 year)
- Passive smoking
- Diet
- Exercise
- Housing and stairs: to assess effect of any symptoms on day-to-day life
- Alcohol intake and substance misuse e.g. cocaine

Family History

Enquire about 1st degree relatives:

- Coronary artery disease
- Stroke
- Sudden death
- Hypercholesterolaemia
- Diabetes mellitus
- Cardiomyopathy
- Congenital heart disease

If diseases with stronger genetic associations are suspected e.g. Marfan's syndrome, Hypertrophic Obstructive Cardiomyopathy, also take an extended family history (uncle, aunt, cousins)

Risk Factors for Heart Disease

Modifiable	Non Modifiable
Smoking and Alcohol	Age
Hypercholesterolemia	Male Gender
Obesity (particularly abdominal)	Family History
Hypertension	Previous Cardiovascular Disease
Diabetes	
Sedentary Lifestyle	
Poor compliance with medication	
Stress	

Risk Factors for Pulmonary Embolism

Long haul flights, recent surgery, immobility, previous PE/DVT, family history of PE/DVT, malignancy, obesity, pregnancy, oestrogen therapy, genetic/acquired thrombophilia

Risk assessment by calculating the Well's score can help guide clinical decisions:

Factor	Clinically suspected DVT	Alternative diagnosis less likely than PE	Tachycardia >100	Immobilisation/ surgery in previous four weeks	History of DVT or PE	Haemoptysis	Malignancy
Points	3	3	1.5	1.5	1.5	1	1

Interpretation of Well's score in the context of risk of PE:
≥ 7.0 = high probability
2.0-6.0 = intermediate probability
0-1= low probability

Differential Diagnosis

Cardiac Causes

- Acute Coronary Syndrome (ACS):

	Unstable Angina	Non ST Elevation MI (NSTEMI)	ST Elevation MI (STEMI)
History	Angina occurring with increasing frequency, unpredictably or at rest	History of sustained (>20 min) chest pain	History of sustained (>20 min) chest pain
ECG	ECG may be normal or show ST depression or T wave changes	There may be ST depression, or T wave changes	As for NSTEMI, plus ST elevation (>2mm in 2 contiguous (next to each other) chest leads, or >1mm in limb leads)
Troponin	Troponin is normal	Troponin is elevated	Troponin is elevated, usually significantly

- **Pericarditis:** Pleuritic chest pain worse on lying supine. Widespread saddle-shaped ST elevation on ECG (with no reciprocal ST depression), PR depression (which is virtually diagnostic of pericarditis), and it may be possible to hear a pericardial rub on auscultation (sounds like walking on fresh snow)

- **Stable Angina:** Chest pain with cardiac characteristics, usually lasting less than 20 minutes, relieved by GTN Spray. It typically occurs after walking predictable distances, and is stable

Non Cardiac Causes of Chest Pain

Vascular Causes

- **Aortic Dissection:** Typically sudden onset, tearing, excruciating chest pain radiating to the back; more common in those with hypertension

Musculoskeletal Causes

- Chest Wall Injuries
- Rib Fractures
- Costochondritis

Respiratory Causes

- **Pulmonary Embolism:** Shortness of breath, pleuritic chest pain, haemoptysis, dizziness, syncope
- **Pneumonia:** Shortness of breath, temperature, purulent cough, pleuritic chest pain
- **Pneumothorax:** Sudden onset of shortness of breath and pleuritic chest pain, classically in young, tall, thin, cigarette smokers; more prevalent in asthmatics, COPD and Marfan's Syndrome

GI Causes

- **Gastro-Oesophageal Reflux Disease:** Burning retrosternal discomfort related to meals and position; associated water brash; relieved by antacids
- **Peptic Ulcer Disease:** More commonly epigastric pain, but can present as chest pain; haematemesis
- **Stress Ulcers:** Usually in the context of acutely very sick patients in HDU/ITU settings
- **Hiatus Hernia:** Symptoms similar to GORD
- **Oesophageal Spasm:** Often difficult to differentiate from angina since also relieved by GTN (although takes longer to relieve pain – typically 10 minutes)

Management of Suspected Acute Coronary Syndrome

- **Airway** – Ensure that the airway is patent
- **Breathing** – Give high-flow oxygen via a non-rebreathing mask (if hypoxic only), listen to their chest, especially for basal crackles, measure respiratory rate and oxygen saturations
- **Circulation** – Assess the capillary refill time, pulse, JVP, and blood pressure. Attach cardiac monitor/ECG, establish intravenous access, draw blood, and consider ABGs

If the history is suggestive of dissection (sudden onset of tearing chest pain, often radiating to the back), then look for a widened mediastinum on chest X-ray, radiofemoral delay, marked hypotension, and aortic regurgitation. A minimal troponin rise may be seen, but there are usually no obvious ECG changes of MI. The definitive diagnosis is made with a CT aorta, but there may not be time for this as patients often rapidly become extremely unwell

Investigations

- **Blood tests:** Full blood count, urea and electrolytes, thyroid function, glucose, cardiac enzymes (troponin 12 hours from onset of chest pain, and in some centres an additional baseline troponin), lipid profile
- **Chest X-Ray:** A widened mediastinum may increase suspicion of aortic dissection; may show signs of acute left ventricular failure
- **Serial ECGs:** If pain persists, or if new episodes of pain, look for evolving ECG changes

Summary of ECG changes seen in a STEMI (to differentiate from an NSTEMI)

- **Anterior or anteroseptal:** ST elevation in V1-4
- **Inferior:** ST elevation in leads II, III, and aVF
- **Lateral:** ST elevation in V5-6 and/or lead I and aVL (high lateral)
- **Posterior:** anterior ST depression and positive R wave – if suspected ECG with posterior leads can be performed

An echocardiogram post myocardial infarction should be done to assess left ventricular function, and to look for complications such as mitral regurgitation. A coronary angiogram will assess whether any stenotic vessels are amenable to either stenting or bypass surgery. Secondary prevention should be started: ACE inhibitors, statins, beta-blockers, aspirin and clopidogrel, unless contraindicated. Patients should be screened and treated appropriately for hypercholesterolemia and diabetes.

What is the immediate treatment of ACS?

The acronym **ROMANCE** may be helpful:

- *Reassure*
- *Oxygen: High-flow oxygen via a non-re-breathing mask (if saturations are below 94%)*
- *Morphine 1-10mg IV, titrated intravenously (to avoid sedation or respiratory depression) with an anti-emetic*
- *Aspirin 300 mg*
- *Nitroglycerine (should be used cautiously in aortic stenosis, hypotension, or right ventricular infarction)*
- *Clopidogrel 300 mg*
- *Enoxaparin (or Fondaparinux)*

What are the indications for primary PCI in ACS?

- Reperfusion therapy should be achieved without delay either by percutaneous coronary intervention (PCI) or thrombolysis (thrombolysis should only be considered if PCI is not available)
- Indications for reperfusion therapy include presentation within 12 hours of onset of chest pain suggestive of MI and:
  1. ST elevation >2 mm in 2 adjacent chest leads
  2. ST elevation of >1 mm in 2 adjacent limb leads
  3. New (or presumed new-onset) left bundle branch block (LBBB)
  4. Posterior MI

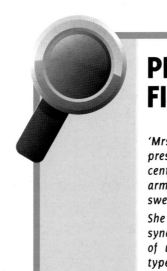

PRESENT YOUR FINDINGS...

'Mrs Jones is a 60-year-old lady who presented with a two hour history of central chest pain radiating to her left arm, with associated breathlessness and sweating.

She describes no palpitations or syncope. This is on a background history of unstable angina, hypertension and type 2 diabetes mellitus.

The most likely diagnoses I would consider at this point is an acute coronary syndrome.

I would like to admit and treat for an acute coronary syndrome, perform serial ECGs, and request a 12-hour troponin.'

Station 2:
RESPIRATORY HISTORY: PRODUCTIVE COUGH

Mr Gordon is a 60 year-old gentleman who presents with a 3 day history of a productive cough and has been finding it increasingly difficult to sleep and get around his house. He is a lifelong cigarette smoker. Please take a history from Mr Gordon and present your findings.

Chest Pain

Take a pain history; use the mnemonic 'SOCRATES' as previously described.

Chest pain due to pulmonary disease is characteristically:

- Unilateral
- Aggravated by deep inspiration, coughing and sneezing (pleuritic pain)
- Usually localised to the chest wall, although diaphragmatic pain sometimes refers to the shoulder tip or anterior abdominal wall (Nerve root C3-5 supplies diaphragm but also dermatomes as above – 'C3, 4, 5 keep the diaphragm alive!')

Cardinal Symptoms
Chest pain
Breathlessness
Stridor
Wheeze
Cough
Sputum
Haemoptysis

Right lower lobe pneumonia is an important differential diagnosis of upper abdominal pain.

Breathlessness

Current Episode of Breathlessness:

- *'When did it start?'* – Note what the patient was doing at the time and their location (e.g. important in occupational asthma)
- *'How did it start?'* Note the speed of onset:

Acute Onset (minutes/hours/days)	Intermediate Onset (days/weeks)	Chronic Onset (months/years)
Acute Asthma	Bronchial Carcinoma	COPD
Pneumonia	Pleural Effusion	Interstitial Lung Disease
Pneumothorax	Tuberculosis	
Pulmonary Embolism		

- *'How long has the breathlessness lasted?' 'Has the breathlessness gotten better or worse since it came on?' 'What makes it better?'* (e.g. rest/inhaler). *'What makes it worse?'* (e.g exercise/night time)

Previous breathing problems and baseline function

- *'How has your breathing been in the past?'*
- *'Do you get breathless on lying flat (orthopnoea)?' 'Do you ever get woken up from breathlessness during sleep (paroxysmal nocturnal dyspnoea)?' 'How many pillows do you sleep on at night?'* Check whether these have changed over time
- Establish change in exercise tolerance: *'How far can you walk without getting breathless at the moment on the flat/on an incline?' 'Were you able to walk further before?' 'If so, how long ago?'*

Stridor

- High-pitched, musical sound heard on inspiration and aggravated by coughing
- Due to obstruction of upper airways (e.g. foreign body aspiration), or sub-total obstruction of the trachea/main bronchi (that may be due to a tumour)

Wheeze

- Coarse, whistling sound usually more noticeable during expiration
- Almost invariably accompanied by dyspnoea
- Due to obstruction of small airways (e.g. asthma)
- May get *'cardiac wheeze'* due to pulmonary oedema
- Establish when the wheeze occurs. During exercise? At night? In cold?
- Monophonic? (single obstruction e.g. tumour) Polyphonic? (multiple obstructions e.g. COPD)

Cough

- Character: Harsh? Dry or productive? Paroxysmal?
- Bovine: Less explosive cough due to vocal cord paralysis (e.g tumour invasion to left recurrent laryngeal nerve)

Sputum

- Loose? Readily productive of sputum? If so, what colour, volume, frequency, consistency, and duration? Blood stained (haemoptysis)?
- Mucoid: grey, white, clear
- Purulent: yellow, green
- Mucopurulent: mixture of mucoid and purulent
- When does it occur? (e.g. night – heart failure, post-nasal drip)

Haemoptysis

- Differentiate between blood-stained sputum (blood in sputum), frothy pink sputum (pulmonary oedema), haematemesis (vomiting blood), nose bleeds
- *'How much blood did you cough up?'* It can be helpful to ask the patient to quantify this by something familiar e.g. a teaspoon of blood. *'How often have you coughed up blood?'*

Past Medical History

- Childhood asthma/wheeze/bronchiolitis
- Malignancy
- Infections (TB, pneumonia)
- Chest trauma or operations (including problems with intubation)
- Asthma/COPD
- Thromboembolic disease (DVT/PE)

It is helpful to check whether the patient has had any previous respiratory investigations (e.g. lung function tests, CT scans, or allergen testing).

Social History

- Recent travel: (could indicate atypical infections and long-haul travel is associated with DVT/PE)
- Occupational history: all jobs, NOT just the most recent one (e.g. asbestos exposure, coal mining, paint spraying, farming, baking)
- Pets
- Hobbies (e.g. pigeon racing)
- Alcohol consumption
- Illicit drugs: whether inhaled or smoked?
- Sexual history: HIV/AIDS and respiratory implications

Smoking History

- Calculate the pack year history (see section 1.1)

Family History

- Atopic illness, cancer, DVT/PE or infectious diseases such as TB
- Current health of close contacts (infections)

Drug History

- Use of inhalers (assess compliance and inhaler technique)
- Use of steroids (dose, route, number of courses in last year)
- Other drugs relevant in respiratory disease in terms of side effects (e.g. ACE inhibitors and cough; aspirin and NSAIDs inducing wheeze in some patients with asthma)

Allergies

- Not only to drugs but also food, inhaled allergens and pets

Systematic Enquiry

- Loss of appetite
- Malaise
- Weight loss
- Night sweats
- Fever/rigors
- Upper respiratory tract symptoms (e.g. nasal obstruction, bleeding or discharge?)
- Urinary symptoms: stress incontinence secondary to cough
- Cardiovascular symptoms: angina or ankle swelling (cardiac disease often causes respiratory symptoms, and chest pain can be cardiac in origin)
- Rheumatoid arthritis/other connective tissue diseases
- Neuromuscular diseases

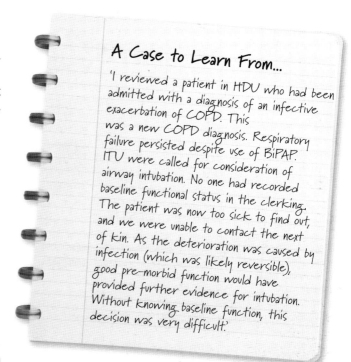

A Case to Learn From...

'I reviewed a patient in HDU who had been admitted with a diagnosis of an infective exacerbation of COPD. This was a new COPD diagnosis. Respiratory failure persisted despite use of BiPAP. ITU were called for consideration of airway intubation. No one had recorded baseline functional status in the clerking. The patient was now too sick to find out, and we were unable to contact the next of kin. As the deterioration was caused by infection (which was likely reversible), good pre-morbid function would have provided further evidence for intubation. Without knowing baseline function, this decision was very difficult.'

What further investigations might you consider in this patient?

- Blood tests: Full blood count, urea and electrolytes, calcium, liver function tests, and CRP
- ECG
- Peak flow
- Arterial blood gas
- Chest imaging: Chest X-ray (first line), CT chest (assessment of lung malignancy) and ultrasound scans (especially useful when clinically a pleural effusion is suspected)
- Sputum culture, microscopy, and sensitivities (especially useful in chronic infectious processes such as bronchiectasis, COPD and CF)
- Spirometry: diagnosis and monitoring of asthma, COPD, and interstitial lung disease (useful before considering lung volume reduction surgery)
- Bronchoscopy and mediastinoscopy: may be used for lung cancer staging

How can you grade the severity of Community Acquired Pneumonia?

Using the CURB 65 Score, 1 point is given for each of the following:

- Confusion (Abbreviated Mental Test (AMT) a score less than 8/10, of new onset)
- Urea (greater than 7mmol/l)
- Respiratory rate (greater than 30 per minute)
- Blood pressure (less than 90 mmHg systolic or 60 mmHg diastolic)
- Age (65 or older)

A higher score equates with a greater mortality.

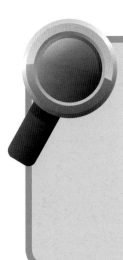

PRESENT YOUR FINDINGS...

'Mr Gordon is a 60-year-old gentleman who presents with a three day history of a gradually worsening cough productive of mucopurulent sputum. He reports breathlessness at rest, wheeze, pleuritic chest pain and a decreased exercise tolerance. There is no haemopytsis. He has lost 3kg in the last two months, and is increasingly reliant on his wife for activities of daily living. He has a 50 pack year smoking history. He has had COPD for five years, for which he takes a regular long-acting muscarinic antagonist (tiotropium), and a short acting beta agonist (salbutamol) as required. Mr Gordon has no previous hospital admissions and is normally fully independent. My differential diagnosis includes community acquired pneumonia, acute exacerbation of chronic obstructive pulmonary disease and neoplastic disease.'

Station 3: GI HISTORY: ABDOMINAL PAIN

Mrs Smith is a 25 year-old patient complaining of abdominal pain and vomiting. Please take a history from Mrs Smith and present your findings.

Pain History

- **Site:** *'Where is the pain?'* Ask the patient if they can point to a specific site. Localising the pain to a quadrant (e.g. right upper quadrant) helps narrow the differential diagnosis
- **Onset:** What was the patient doing when the pain came on? Large fatty meal (e.g. gall stones)? Exercise? Alcohol binge? *'Did the pain come on gradually* (e.g. endometriosis) *or suddenly* (e.g. renal colic)?*'*
- **Character:** *'What does the pain feel like?'* Sharp (e.g. ectopic pregnancy)? Tight band? Dull? Electric shock? *'Is the pain at a constant level* (e.g. bowel perforation), *or does it increase and decrease* (in a colicky pattern e.g. small bowel obstruction, biliary colic)?*'*
- **Radiation:** *'Does the pain spread anywhere?'* (e.g. from the epigastrium through to the back (pancreatitis)). *'Has the pain shifted from one site to another?'* (e.g. periumbilical pain localising to the right iliac fossa (appendicitis))
- **Associated Symptoms** (as outlined in table on page 19)
- **Timing:** *'How long does the pain last?'* *'How frequently does it occur?'* *'Is it constant?'*
- **Exacerbating and relieving factors:** *'What worsens the pain?'* *'What eases the pain?'* (e.g. paracetamol, movement, position, food). Peritonitic pain is worsened by movement
- **Severity:** *'How severe is the pain on a scale of 1 to 10 (with 10 being the worst)? 'Is it getting better or worse?'*

Has the patient ever had this pain before? Was the cause identified at that time?

Past Medical and Surgical History

- *'Any previous bowel problems?'* Has the patient ever been investigated for bowel problems? (E.g. endoscopy, CT scan, colonoscopy)
- *'Any previous surgery?'* (adhesions from previous surgery are an important cause of bowel obstruction)
- Previous radiotherapy treatment

Drug History

- Document all drugs currently being taken, and allergies. Ask about recent use of NSAIDs (including aspirin) and blood thinning agents (warfarin, clopidogrel) if concerned about GI bleeding. Steroids are also associated with gastric upset

Cardinal Symptoms

Weight Loss

Anorexia

Abdominal Pain

Dysphagia

Nausea and Vomiting

Haematemesis

Reflux/Dyspepsia

Altered Bowel Habit

Rectal Bleeding

Jaundice

Nausea, Vomiting and Abdominal Distension

- How much has been vomited?
- How often?
- What colour? Is there any haematemesis (fresh blood/ coffee-ground vomiting)? Was it in the first vomit, or only after several vomiting episodes?
- What is the relationship with food?
- Is vomiting associated with nausea?
- Has the patient noticed their abdomen being more swollen than normal? (bowel obstruction, ascites)

Change in Bowel Habits

- If diarrhoea, ask about the exact meaning: increased frequency or loose consistency or both?
- How many times have they opened their bowels? How much do they pass each time? Is there any blood or mucus?
- Does the patient feel that they don't completely empty their bowel on straining? (tenesmus)
- With constipation, when was the last bowel movement? When did they last pass wind?

Anorexia and Weight Loss

- If present, how much? Was it deliberate?
- Over what time period?

Dyspepsia

- Any problems with indigestion?
- Use of over the counter antacids?

Dysphagia

- Solids or liquids? If difficulty swallowing liquids comes first, the problem may be neurological rather than obstructive (liquids provide less sensory stimulation to the swallow reflex)
- Sudden onset or gradual onset?
- Intermittent or progressive?

Blood or Mucus Per Rectum

- If so, how much?
- Is it mixed in with the stool/coating stool/on the toilet paper?
- Is it fresh blood (lower GI) or is it melaena (upper GI)?

Urological Symptoms

- Frequency, dysuria, haematuria
- Look for obstructive symptoms (especially when considering prostatic obstruction) such as hesitancy and terminal dribbling

Gynaecological Symptoms

- Discharge, bleeding, dyspareunia
- **Do NOT forget to ask about the last menstrual period in females of child-bearing age (pregnancy)**

Social History

- Smoking (increased risk of GI malignancy)
- Alcohol consumption: important cause of pancreatitis
- Possible contact with infectious sources: Ill close contacts? Dietary changes? Recent travel?

Family History

- Ask about diseases that run in the family, particularly inflammatory bowel disease, coeliac disease, peptic ulcer disease (*Helicobacter pylori* infection)

Management

- Resuscitate the patient following an ABCDE approach
- Pain relief
- Full abdominal examination. If clinically indicated, perform a rectal and external genital examination
- Place nil by mouth and prescribe IV fluids if considering surgery, or in the case of obstructive symptoms such as bilious vomiting, abdominal distension, abdominal pain and constipation
- NG tube (in case of suspected bowel obstruction)
- Catheterise if urinary retention, or if urine output monitoring is required (for example in shock or in acute pancreatitis)

'You should always consider pregnancy as a cause for symptoms in a woman of reproductive age'

Colin Duncan
Consultant Obstetrician and Gynaecologist
Royal Infirmary of Edinburgh

Laboratory Tests

- **Urinalysis and pregnancy test**
- **Bloods:** Full blood count, urea and electrolytes, CRP, liver function, LDH, glucose, amylase, group and save +/– cross match. Blood cultures if pyrexial
- **CLO (Campylobacter-like organisms):** Testing (done at endoscopy) if Helicobacter pylori is suspected
- **Vaginal swabs:** If pelvic inflammatory disease is suspected
- **ABG:** If particularly unwell or if pancreatitis is suspected

Diagnostic Imaging

- **Abdominal ultrasound:** Useful for diagnosing gallstones, abdominal collections, abdominal aortic aneurysm
- **Pelvic ultrasound:** Useful for looking at ovarian/gynaecological pathology, and also appendicitis
- **Abdominal X-ray:** Looking for intestinal obstruction
- **Erect Chest X-ray:** If perforation is suspected (air under the diaphragm), but may also pick up lower lobe pneumonia, or subphrenic collection
- **CT scan:** To look for masses, and to help guide surgery in intestinal obstruction. CT KUB (kidneys, ureter and bladder) to look for renal tract stones
- **Barium meal** (hiatus hernias, oesophageal spasm, and achalasia) /**enema** (bowel tumours, polyps or diverticular disease) **follow-through** (small bowel strictures)
- **Water soluble contrast swallow:** More suitable than barium if perforation suspected
- **Endoscopy:** In the case of upper GI bleed, suspected peptic ulceration or duodenal biopsies for coeliac disease
- **Meckel scan:** Looking for the presence of gastric mucosa in the small intestine, as obscure GI bleed is often associated with a Meckel's diverticulum

What is the differential diagnosis for umbilical pain?

- *Early Appendicitis*
- *Intestinal Obstruction*
- *Acute Gastritis*
- *Peptic Ulcer Disease*
- *Acute Pancreatitis*
- *Ruptured Abdominal Aortic Aneurysm*
- *Mesenteric Adenitis*
- *Gastroenteritis*
- *Irritable Bowel Syndrome*
- *Inflammatory Bowel Disease*
- *Constipation*
- *Perforated Viscus*

What is the differential diagnosis for right iliac fossa pain?

Gastrointestinal

- Appendicitis
- Diverticulitis
- Inflammatory bowel disease (Crohn's-related terminal ileitis)
- Intestinal obstruction
- Meckel's diverticulitis
- Perforated viscera
- Obstructed or incarcerated inguinal or femoral hernia

Gynaecological

- Ruptured ovarian cyst
- Torsion of ovarian cyst
- Pelvic inflammatory disease
- Ectopic pregnancy

Urinary

- Urinary tract infection
- Renal calculi

Other

- Testicular torsion
- Musculoskeletal

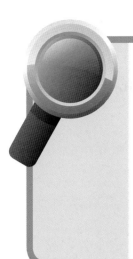

PRESENT YOUR FINDINGS...

'Mrs Smith is a 25 year-old lady who presents with abdominal pain. She is normally fit and well, apart from recurrent infections with Chlamydia trachomatis.

She has a 2-day history of sudden onset right iliac fossa pain, which is constant, sharp and does not radiate. This is associated with vomiting. She has had no changes in her bowel habits, and does not have urinary symptoms. Her last menstrual period was 7 weeks previously.

The most important diagnosis to consider is an ectopic pregnancy.

I would like to secure IV access and resuscitate if necessary, perform a urine dipstick, including beta-hCG, and organise a pelvic ultrasound.'

Station 4: GI HISTORY: DIARRHOEA

Mrs Sanderson is a 60 year-old lady who has been experiencing severe abdominal pain and diarrhoea for the last 4 days. She was recently discharged from hospital following an appendicectomy. Please take a history from Mrs Sanderson and present your findings.

Start with an open question, to find out more about the nature of the problem. For example, *'What do you mean by diarrhoea?'*

Description of Stool

- *'How much diarrhoea is being produced each time you go to the toilet?'*
- *'What is its consistency?'* *'Is it very watery?'*
- *'What colour is it?'*
- *'Does it contain any blood or mucus? Is it 'tarry'?'*
- *'Is it difficult to flush the stool away?'* *'Does the stool float?'*

Timing of the Diarrhoea

- *'How frequent are the motions?'* Compare them with the patient's normal frequency
- *'Any particular time of day?'* Nocturnal diarrhoea usually indicates organic pathology (e.g. diabetes, exacerbation of inflammatory bowel disease)
- *'Do you feel a sense of urgency to pass stool?'*
- *'How long has this change in bowel habit persisted for?'*
- *'What was your previous bowel habit like?'*
- Exacerbating and relieving factors: *'Is the diarrhoea associated with specific foods?'* *'Is the diarrhoea associated with any new medications?'*
- Take a full gastrointestinal history as detailed in section 1.3

Enquire about Specific Causes

- **Medication:** Laxatives, purgatives, antibiotics (Clostridium difficile)?
- **Recent travel (foreign and otherwise)?:** Ask about appropriate vaccinations, and about holiday diet/activities
- **Contact:** With animals? Recent contact with other individuals suffering from diarrhoea?
- **Diet:** Meats (cooked and uncooked), eggs, seafood, dairy foods, wheat, unusual foods
- **Past Medical History:** Diabetes mellitus, inflammatory bowel disease, abdominal surgery, HIV, organ transplant, malignancy, chemotherapy, radiotherapy, constipation
- **Occupation:** As a potential cause (e.g. veterinary surgeon) and implications for return to work (e.g. NHS staff have to be 48 hours free of symptoms prior to returning to work)
- **Family history:** Of bowel problems? Inflammatory bowel disease, coeliac disease

What are the principal causes of diarrhoea?

Acute Diarrhoea	Chronic Diarrhoea
DRUGS: antibiotics, cytotoxic drugs, NSAIDs, proton pump inhibitors	**SMALL INTESTINE:** (often large volume, watery stool) – inflammatory bowel disease (small bowel Crohn's), malignancy, infection, ischemia, irritable bowel syndrome
INFECTION: bacteria, viruses, parasites	**LARGE INTESTINE:** (often with blood or mucus in stool) – drugs (NSAIDs, aminosalicylates, SSRIs, laxatives), inflammatory bowel disease (UC or Crohn's colitis), infection, constipation
	MALABSORPTION: (steatorrhoea with undigested food in stool) – coeliac disease, chronic pancreatitis, diabetes, pancreatic cancer, lymphoma, tropical sprue
	INFECTION: HIV enteropathy, chronic intestinal schistosomiasis, Ileocaecal tuberculosis

Causes of chronic diarrhoea can present acutely. The causes of acute diarrhoea can be further sub divided into diarrhoea with blood, and diarrhoea without blood:

Diarrhoea without Blood	Bloody Diarrhoea (dysentery)
• *Enterotoxigenic E. coli* (commonly causing traveler's diarrhoea) • Malaria, especially *P. falciparum* • Almost any infection in a child or neonate (e.g. rotavirus) • Enterotoxin producing strains of Staphylococcus aureus • Giardiasis • Cholera • Food toxins • Drugs (e.g. proton pump inhibitors, NSAIDS)	• *Enterohaemorrhagic E. coli* (0157) • Shigella, Salmonella, Campylobacter • Clostridium difficile • Schistosomiasis *(e.g. S. mansoni, S. japonicum)* • Drugs e.g. NSAIDs (N.B. only if severe ulceration)

Note: causes of bloody diarrhoea can present with non-bloody diarrhoea, particularly if in a milder form.

What are the extra-intestinal manifestations of inflammatory bowel disease?

Site	Manifestation
EYE CHANGES	Iritis, uveitis, episcleritis
MUSCULOSKELETAL	Seronegative arthritis, osteoporosis
DERMATOLOGICAL	Erythema nodosum, pyoderma gangrenosum, aphthous mouth ulcers
OTHER	Autoimmune haemolytic anaemia, finger clubbing, growth failure, primary sclerosing cholangitis, interstitial lung disease (rare)

Arthritis is the most common extra-intestinal manifestation of inflammatory bowel disease. Extra-intestinal manifestations occur in roughly similar frequency with Crohn's and ulcerative colitis. Note that primary sclerosing cholangitis is more common with ulcerative colitis, and arthritis is more common with Crohn's disease.

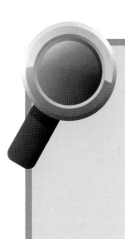

PRESENT YOUR FINDINGS...

'Mrs Sanderson is a 60 year-old lady who presents with a 4-day history of severe lower abdominal pain.

This is associated with the passage of foul-smelling watery stools approximately 8 times daily. She has been feeling nauseous and feverish, and was recently discharged from hospital after having completed a seven day course of clindamycin. There is no blood or mucus per rectum. She is otherwise well.

This is consistent with a diagnosis of infective diarrhoea, possibly Clostridium difficile given the recent antibiotic course.

I would re-admit Mrs Sanderson to hospital for IV fluids, stool analysis and, if indicated, antibiotic therapy.'

Station 5: NEUROLOGICAL HISTORY: HEADACHE

You are the junior doctor on call and have been asked to review Mrs Heart, a 25 year-old patient who has presented to Accident and Emergency with a new and severe headache. Please take a focused history and formulate a management plan.

If the patient is shielding their eyes or is in obvious discomfort because of the light in the room, offer to dim the lights or draw the curtains, and offer analgesia

It is important to differentiate between i) a new acute headache and ii) a headache that is part of a chronic or recurrent headache history. For a new acute headache, the first and essential questions should be directed towards the immediate identification or exclusion of either intracranial haemorrhage (including subarachnoid haemorrhage) or intracranial infection (meningitis/encephalitis):

Cardinal Symptoms

Headache
Syncope
Seizures
Falls
Dizziness/Vertigo
Visual disturbances
Altered sensation
Aura

Subdural Haemorrhage

- Recent head injury
- Gradual onset headache, either constant or fluctuating
- Fluctuating levels of consciousness: may have loss of consciousness at time of injury, followed by 'lucid interval', but subsequent deterioration (as haematoma forms)
- More common in elderly and alcoholics

Extradural Haemorrhage

- Recent head injury
- Gradual onset headache, either constant or fluctuating
- Fluctuating levels of consciousness: may have loss of consciousness at time of injury, followed by 'lucid interval', but subsequent deterioration (as haematoma forms)
- More common in young (dura mater less fixed to skull) and alcoholics

Intracerebral Haemorrhage

- Sudden onset, severe headache
- Symptoms of raised intracranial pressure (e.g. waking up with a headache, vomiting without nausea)
- Focal neurology (corresponding to area of brain that is damaged)

Subarachnoid Haemorrhage

- Sudden onset, severe headache
- Meningism (neck stiffness, photophobia, headache)
- Drowsiness/ loss of consciousness
- Focal neurology

Meningitis/ Encephalitis

- Fever
- Rash (non blanching rash associated with meningococcal septicaemia)
- Meningism (neck stiffness/ photophobia/ headache)
- Infective symptoms: flu-like, sweating, malaise, joint pain, diarrhoea
- Nausea and vomiting
- Drowsiness/ loss of consciousness

Pain History

Site

- Where in the head do they feel the pain?
  - Generalized, occipital, or temporal? Is it bilateral or unilateral?
  - Migraines tend to be unilateral, while subarachnoid haemorrhages tend to be occipital, although these are not absolute rules: for example, a migraine can be occipital
- 'Does the pain spread anywhere else?'

Severity

- 'How severe is the headache on a scale of 1 to 10?'
- 'How does this headache compare in severity to previous headaches?'

Onset

- What were they doing when the headache occurred?
- Recent head trauma or drug intake?
- 'Was it sudden in onset or did it occur gradually?'
- 'How long did the headache take to reach its peak intensity?'

Aggravating and Relieving Factors

- What has the patient done to relieve their headache? e.g. lying in the dark
- Has simple analgesia (if taken) helped?
- Triggers for migraines include cheese, chocolate and red wine (though this has very limited diagnostic value)

Associated Symptoms and Systemic Enquiry

- Neurological history: Loss of (or altered) consciousness, motor or sensory deficit, gait, disturbances in vision, speech, hearing, incontinence
- Enquire about symptoms of meningism (neck stiffness, photophobia, headache)
- Fever
- Rashes
- Scalp tenderness when brushing their hair or pain on chewing (these symptoms might indicate temporal arteritis)
- Nausea or vomiting
- Infective symptoms: Increasing the possibility of meningitis or encephalitis (e.g. fever, diarrhoea, malaise)
- Visual disturbance or 'aura' before onset of headache?
- Watering of the eyes or nasal congestion (associated with cluster headaches)?
- Use of glasses and last visual acuity test

'In relation to subarachnoid haemorrhage, the truly sudden onset of the headache is critical: how long it took from the very first moment of the headache to its peak intensity. This is a vital indicator of whether a subarachnoid haemorrhage has to be considered.'

Richard Knight
Professor of Neurology
University of Edinburgh

Past Medical History

- Enquire about the patient's general past health
- Hypertension
- Kidney disease in the past (damaged kidneys could lead to hypertension and polycystic kidney disease is associated with berry aneurysms and subsequent subarachnoid haemorrhages)
- TIAs or strokes
- Migraines or tension headaches
- If the patient has previously experienced a similar episode, enquire about the investigations and treatments that were previously performed

Drug History

- Enquire about regular medications (as well as any medications they have taken acutely to relieve the headache)
- Is the patient on anticoagulants?
- Is the patient on the oral contraceptive pill?
- Over-the-counter medications
- Allergies

Family History

- Any history of headaches (particularly migraines), kidney disease or hypertension?

Social History

- Smoking and alcohol history
- Occupation is important (is the headache likely to be aggravated by/ interfere with their job?)
- Any recent stresses which could be contributing to the symptoms? Any contact with confirmed cases of meningitis or encephalitis?

Management

Immediate Treatment

- Resuscitate using an ABCDE approach. Is the patient stable? Establish IV access (if necessary)
- Offer to give analgesia and anti-emetics
- If meningitis is suspected, administer antibiotics as soon as blood cultures and lumbar puncture have been taken – do not wait for a CT scan (unless there is a important reason for requiring one – see below)

Investigations

a) Suspected Intracranial Bleed

- A CT scan is helpful in identifying a subarachnoid haemorrhage (SAH), a subdural haematoma, an extradural haematoma, or a space occupying legion
- A negative CT scan does not completely rule out SAH
- You might then want to consider a lumbar puncture at 12 hours to look for:
  A. Xanthochromia (yellow colour after CSF is centrifuged, indicative of haemoglobin breakdown products)
  B. Request spectrophotometry to detect bilirubin (another breakdown of haemoglobin; greater sensitivity than xanthochromia)
- Referral to neurosurgeons if intervention may be required e.g. for extra dural haematoma

b) Suspected Intracranial Infection

- FBC, urea and electrolytes, glucose, coagulation screen, blood cultures and CRP
- If history suggests meningitis, perform lumbar puncture and blood cultures: a CT scan should only be done if indicated. Raised intra cranial pressure (causing a pressure gradient between the supratentorial and infratentorial compartments of the brain, increasing the risk of transtentorial herniation) is the major concern. This may be suspected, for example, by the presence of focal neurological signs
- A CT scan (if necessary) must NOT delay antibiotic treatment in serious illness such as potential meningococcal meningitis
- Skull X-rays: for example, to support a diagnosis of paranasal sinus infection

What is your differential diagnosis in this patient?

1. Subarachnoid haemorrhage (SAH) or intracerebral haemorrhage
2. Meningitis or encephalitis
3. Migraine or tension headache
4. Cluster headache
5. Space-occupying lesion
6. Temporal arteritis

'Given the gradual onset, generalized nature of headache, meningeal signs and the local outbreak of meningococcal infection, meningitis is my working diagnosis. However, I would also like to exclude a sub-arachnoid haemorrhage. Other causes of headache include space occupying legions, migraines and tension headache.'

What characteristics from lumbar puncture help to differentiate likely cause of meningitis?

	NORMAL	VIRAL	BACTERIAL	TUBERCULOUS
Appearance	Clear	Clear/Turbid	Turbid/Purulent	Turbid/Viscous
Predominant cell type	Lymphocytes	Lymphocytes	Polymorphs	Polymorphs/ lymphocytes (mixed)
White cell count	0-4 x 10^6/L	10-2000 x 10^6/L	1000-5000 x 10^6/L	50-5000 x 10^6/L
Protein	0.2-0.4 g/L	0.4-0.8 g/L	0.5-2 g/L	0.5-3 g/L
Glucose	2/3-1/2 blood glucose	>1/2 blood glucose	<1/2 blood glucose	<1/2 blood glucose

Meningitis Prophylaxis

- Notify public health authorities of meningococcal infection
- Seek advice about immunization and prophylaxis of contacts (normally rifampicin for 'kissing contacts')

Features of Other Specific Causes of Headache

Space Occupying Legion

- Absence of other clear diagnosis for the headache
- Older age at onset
- Focal neurological symptoms and signs
- Headache on waking (though this is more commonly caused by migraine)
- Vomiting without nausea

Temporal Arteritis

- Usually in patients over 60 years old
- Frontal or occipital
- Jaw pain (whilst eating or talking), scalp tenderness, visual disturbances
- Malaise and proximal muscle weakness

Cluster Headache

- Localised around one eye and associated with autonomic features such as lacrimation and nasal congestion
- Occurs for 15 minutes to 2 hours daily for 6-8 weeks, then subsiding for months

Cervical Spondylosis

- Headache associated with neck pain
- Worsens with neck movements

Migraine

- Chronic or recurrent headache
- May have a prodrome or aura (though only around 10% of those with migraines will have neurological aura)
- Trigger, (e.g. cheese, chocolate, stress) though none are very specific
- May be related to oral contraceptive pills
- Photophobia or other visual disturbances such as zigzag lines
- Nausea and vomiting
- Family history

Tension Headache

- Band-like dull headache, sometimes with sharp exacerbations
- In the scalp rather than the cranium
- Can last throughout the day, worsening in the evenings
- May get tired or dizzy

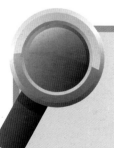

PRESENT YOUR FINDINGS...

'Mrs Heart has presented with a six hour history of a generalised headache that was gradual in onset, aching in character, and 9/10 in severity. There is no radiation, but the pain is associated with fever, general malaise, photophobia and neck stiffness. Bright lights intensely aggravate the pain, and nothing seems to make it better. She has never had this before. There are no associated rashes.

She has no significant past medical history, and is on no regular medication. There are no sick close contacts of note, but there has been a recent outbreak of meningococcal meningitis in the community.

This is consistent with a possible diagnosis of meningitis'.

Station 6: INTERMITTENT CLAUDICATION

Mr Brown is a 63 year-old gentleman who presents with worsening leg pain on exertion. He is a long-term cigarette smoker and has type II diabetes, with a recent HbA1c of 9%. Please take a history from Mr Brown and present your findings.

Pain History

- **Site:** *'Where is the pain?'* The site is suggestive of the ischaemic territory, and therefore if the pain is vascular, the culprit artery can be predicted
- **Onset:** *'Did the pain come on gradually or suddenly?'* Sudden onset pain is suggestive of an embolic rather than a thrombotic event. What was the patient doing when the pain came on? Does the patient get any rest pain? What triggers the pain? Is it related to exercise? If so, how far can the patient walk before getting pain? Does it come on at a fixed distance?
- **Character:** Cramping? Dull ache? Stabbing? Sharp?
- **Radiation:** *'Does the pain radiate anywhere?'* If so, ask the patient to delineate the area. If this is in a dermatomal distribution, consider nerve compression
- **Associated symptoms:** See below
- **Timing:** *'How long does the pain last?'*
- **Exacerbating/relieving factors:** *'Is the pain worse with bending/twisting?'* more suggestive of musculoskeletal pain/spinal stenosis) *'Is the pain worse at night?'* Patients with peripheral vascular disease often hang their legs off the side of the bed to reduce pain. This improves circulation because of assistance from gravity. *'Is the pain relieved with simple analgesia or rest?'*
- **Severity:** *'How severe is the pain on a scale of one to ten?'*

Associated Symptoms

Ask about factors relating to peripheral vascular disease:

- Does the patient have any foot ulcers?
- Do the patient's feet ever feel numb or cold? If collateral vessels have developed, the feet may be warm
- Is the patient impotent? (Need to phrase carefully to avoid offending the patient)
- Any muscle weakness?

Systemic Enquiry

- Those with peripheral vascular disease are more generally at risk of vascular disease. Ask specifically about symptoms of angina. Palpitations may be present in the context of atrial fibrillation. Malignancy is associated with an increased risk of thrombotic disease. Ask the patient as well about cardiovascular risk factors, as detailed in Station 1.1
- Take a drug history
- Ask about the effect of the disease process on the patient's day-to-day life

Pattern of Pain and Site of Stenosis

- Buttock/thigh pain: aorto-iliac disease
- Calf pain: femoro-popliteal disease

Symptoms Suggestive of Acute Embolism

- Sudden onset of symptoms
- Known embolic source (e.g. atrial fibrillation, mural thrombus post myocardial infarction)
- Absence of previous symptoms of intermittent claudication
- Cold leg (no time for collateral blood supply to develop)
- Normal vascular exam in the other leg

What investigations might be done in a patient with intermittent claudication?

- Resting Doppler pressure indexes
- Urinalysis (glycosuria), blood pressure and ECG
- Bloods: Full blood count (anaemia, polycythemia), urea and electrolytes (renovascular disease), lipid profile, fasting glucose
- Exercise testing: Foot pressure normally rises with exercise but is reduced in the presence of occlusive arterial disease
- Non invasive imaging: Doppler ultrasonography, magnetic resonance angiography (MRA) and computed tomography angiography (CTA)
- Echocardiography: Detect cardiac disease, if concerned about cardiac emboli

What management options are there for a claudication?

Best Medical Therapy	Revascularisation
• Risk factor management (stop smoking, lose weight and manage hyperlipidaemia with modified diet) • Exercise (to open and develop the collateral circulation) • Take care not to injure the leg (since healing is generally poor) • Aspirin, statins, ACE inhibitors • Treat risk factors: Hypertension and diabetes	• Percutaneous balloon angioplasty and stent insertion • Bypass surgery: for example aorto-iliac bypass or femoral-popliteal bypass • Amputation

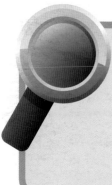

PRESENT YOUR FINDINGS...

'Mr Brown is a 63 year-old gentleman with poorly controlled type 2 diabetes mellitus. He presents with gradual onset, cramping left calf pain on exertion. This comes on predictably after walking 30 metres. It is relieved on resting for 5 minutes and by simple analgesia. He does not have any rest pain. He has a 20 pack year smoking history and is otherwise fit and well. He is on metformin, but no other regular medications.

This is consistent with a diagnosis of intermittent claudication.'

Station 7: BACK PAIN HISTORY

Mrs Fletcher is a 60 year-old lady who is suffering from back pain. She has also become incontinent and is feeling unsteady on her feet. Please take a history from this patient.

Pain History

- **Site:** *'Where is the pain?'* Can the patient point to a specific point? Ask about bone pain
- **Onset:** *'When did the pain come on (acute or chronic)?'* What was the patient doing at the time the pain came on this time?
- **Character:** *'What does the back pain feel like e.g. a tight band, dull, sharp, electric shock?'*
- **Radiation:** *'Does the pain radiate?'* E.g. down the buttock and thigh? Or does it radiate all the way down to foot?
- **Timing:** *'How long does the pain last for, how frequently does it occur?'* *'When does it occur?'* E.g. first thing in the morning or after exercise
- **Exacerbating/alleviating factors:** *'What worsens the pain?'* E.g. exercise, rest, movement. *'What helps the pain?'* E.g. exercise, rest, movement, simple analgesia
- **Severity:** Ask the patient to rate their pain on a scale of 1 to 10. This is very subjective, but it can be useful in monitoring that particular patient's pain over time

> 'It is crucial that you ask whether the pain radiates as far as the foot. This helps differentiates referred and sciatic pain'
>
> **Mark Rodrigues**
> *Orthopaedics FY2 (2010)*
> *Edinburgh Royal Infirmary*

Associated Symptoms

- *'Are there any other changes that you have noticed?'*
- If there is a history of cancer, what type? Has the patient received any treatment?
- *'Have you had any problems walking?'*
- *'Have you experienced any incontinence of urine or faeces or difficulty passing urine?'*
- Ask about other bowel and bladder symptoms
- Numbness, tingling, leg weakness? Peri-anal numbness ('saddle anaesthesia')

Ensure that past medical history, drug history (including allergies), family history and social history are all covered

Sinister Back Pain: Red Flags

Onset age >55 or <20 years	Constant or progressive pain
Nocturnal pain	Morning stiffness
History of carcinoma	Constitutional symptoms (fevers, unexplained weight loss, night sweats)
Progressive neurological deficit	Current or recent infection
Disturbed gait, saddle anaesthesia	Bladder or bowel dysfunction
Leg claudication	Immunosuppression

Causes of Back Pain by Age

15-30 years	Trauma, fracture, prolapsed disc, ankylosing spondylitis
30-50 years	Degenerative disease, prolapsed disc, malignancy (metastases e.g. breast, lung, prostate, kidney and thyroid cancer)
>50 years	Degenerative disease, osteoporosis (wedge fracture), malignancy, myeloma

Management

- Examination
- Pain relief
- Lumbar X-ray or MRI scan
- Bone scan/skeletal survey
- Specialist input dependant on aetiology e.g. clinical oncologists for spinal cord compression secondary to metastatic deposits or neurosurgeons for cauda equina syndrome secondary to a herniated intervertebral disc

	Aetiology	Clinical Presentation
Mechanical Back Pain	1. Low back pain arising from an anatomical structure such as a muscle, ligament, or intervertebral disc due to trauma, deformity, or degenerative change 2. Osteoporotic fracture	• Sudden onset • Eased by rest • Unilateral symptoms • Increased by coughing/ sneezing • Previous episodes, clear mechanical precipitant e.g. heavy lifting
Inflammatory Back Pain	1. Inflammatory spondylitis 2. Infection (epidural abscess) 3. Malignancy 4. Paget's disease	• Predominant stiffness (greater than 30 minutes in the morning) • Gradual onset and progressive • Increased pain with rest • Disturbs sleep • Stiff/rigid spine on examination, symmetrical restriction +/- sacroiliac joint tenderness

Other Important Aetiologies

Cauda Equina Syndrome

- This is caused by compression of the cauda equina; it can be caused for example by posterior disc herniation or metastatic deposits
- Persistent and progressive, bilateral leg pain, normal leg pulses, pain eased by leaning forward, stiff spine on examination, bladder/bowel dysfunction
- Requires urgent assessment and management: including an MRI and consideration for surgery/ radiotherapy

Sciatica

- Pain that radiates from the buttock down the back of the leg and into the foot, often accompanied by paraesthesia with the same distribution; it usually occurs due to compression of a lumbosacral nerve root by a protruding disc
- This is usually managed conservatively, with analgesia, physiotherapy, and monitoring of the pain. Chronic sciatica may require input from the chronic pain team. Surgery may be of benefit for some patients with sciatica

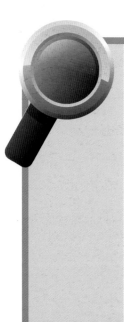

PRESENT YOUR FINDINGS...

'Mrs Fletcher is a 60 year old lady who presents with back pain. She has recently been diagnosed with breast cancer.

She has been experiencing new onset, gradually progressive lower back pain over the last 2 days. It radiates down both legs, and is associated with urinary and faecal incontinence. Her legs feel weak, and she is unsteady on her feet.

This is consistent with a diagnosis of cauda equina syndrome secondary to lumbar spine metastases. This is a medical emergency, requiring an urgent MRI, steroid therapy, and consideration for further neurosurgical/oncological intervention'

How would you manage probable mechanical back pain?

- If <55 years of age or previous episodes, trial of analgesia, e.g. NSAIDs, and review after three months
- Ten percent of patients are still symptomatic at 3 months; in these cases, address any contributing factors and consider further investigation for systemic illness
- If the patient is >55 years or <20 years of age, investigate for systemic illness

If a non mechanical cause is suspected:

- Investigations: CRP/ESR, full blood count, calcium, phosphate, ALP, protein electrophoresis (multiple myeloma), blood cultures if appropriate, imaging (X-ray/CT/MRI); rheumatoid factor and anti-CCP antibodies to test for rheumatoid arthritis
- Treatment depends on the cause: NSAIDs may be useful in the short term, but steroids and anti-inflammatory drugs such as methotrexate may be necessary in the long term
- Facet joint injections/local anaesthetic injections around nerve roots may be useful in some cases

Station 8: HAEMATOLOGY HISTORY

Mrs Bee is a 44 year-old lady who reports feeling increasingly tired over the last few weeks. She has lost a considerable amount of weight and also reports increased sweating. Her partner notes that she appears more pale than usual. Please take a history from Mrs Bee and present your findings.

Presenting Complaint

Symptoms of Anaemia

- Tiredness
- Light-headedness
- Breathlessness
- Palpitations
- Worsening of pre-existing ischaemic conditions (e.g. angina, claudication)

Weight loss

- Quantify either exact weight loss (e.g. 5kg in 3 months) or subjective weight loss (e.g. now requires a belt for trousers, which, was not needed 3 months previously)
- Ask whether there has been a conscious effort to lose weight

Sweating

- Duration: when did it start?
- Quantity: needing to change clothes/bed sheets?

Other Symptoms

Bleeding

- Haemoptysis
- Gum bleeding
- Haematuria
- Epistaxis
- Blood blisters
- Prolonged menstrual bleeding, bleeding post surgery/ trauma

Bruising

- Site(s)
- Amount
- Petechiae, purpura, ecchymoses
- Precipitating causes (e.g. new medications, infection)

Noticeable lumps (enlarged lymph nodes)

- Where?
- When were they noticed? How quickly are they enlarging?
- Tenderness (though this does not differentiate infective and malignant causes of lymphadenopathy)

It is also important to enquire about fever, itching, bone pain and jaundice

Past Medical History

- Is this the first time the patient is presenting with these symptoms?
- Any known malignancy, or family history of malignancy?
- Chemotherapy: what treatment, and when was the last treatment?
    - Patients undergoing chemotherapy or bone marrow transplantation may be neutropenic and require early, aggressive, specific combination antimicrobial therapy
- Recurrent infections: patients with haematological disease may be immunocompromised and susceptible not only to common pathogens, but also to opportunistic organisms
    - Myeloma and chronic lymphocytic leukaemia: may be hypogammaglobulinaemic so can have bacterial infections that require aggressive antimicrobial therapy. Patients are potentially susceptible to other infections of any type (e.g. viral infections such as herpes zoster)
    - Asplenic patients are susceptible to infections from encapsulated organisms – prior to elective splenectomy, patients should have received:
        - **Haemophilus influenzae type B vaccination**
        - **Pneumococcal polysaccharide vaccination**
        - **Vaccination against meningococcus**
- Recent illnesses/ infections
- Antimicrobial/ antiviral treatments
- Vaccinations

Drug History

- Any drugs that could affect bleeding:
    - Warfarin; consider drugs that may affect warfarin metabolism
    - Antiplatelet agents: aspirin, clopidogrel, dipyridamole

Social History

- Alcohol intake
- Smoking
- Occupational history: carcinogen exposure (e.g. pesticides (containing aromatic hydrocarbons) used by farmers)
- Recent travel, and infective contacts
- Ask additional questions to further assess risk of HIV and other blood borne viruses (BBVs):
    - Sexual history
    - Intravenous drug use
    - Tattoos/piercings – where and when?
    - Blood transfusions – where and when?

Haematological Investigations

Blood Tests

- Full blood count
    - WBC (include differential of white blood cells)
    - Platelets
    - Haemoglobin and mean cell volume
    - Blood film (size, shape, structure and colour of blood cells)
- Liver function tests: unconjugated bilirubin may be elevated if there is increased haemolysis
- Renal function
- Coagulation screen
- Lactate dehydrogenase (raised in lymphoma, though is non-specific)
- Iron studies, vitamin B12, folate
- Protein electrophoresis
- Immunoglobulins
- Calcium
- HIV test

Imaging

- Ultrasound: for hepatomegaly, splenomegaly
- CT thorax, abdomen and pelvis (with contrast): for organomegaly and lymphadenopathy

Biopsies

- Bone marrow examination (for staging of haematological malignancy)
- Lymph node biopsy and spleen biopsy

Histories

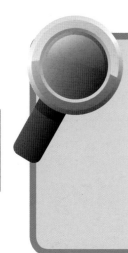

PRESENT YOUR FINDINGS...

'Mrs Bee presents with general malaise, fever, drenching night sweats and unintentional weight loss of around 8kg over the last 3 months. She has noticed painless swellings in her neck and axillae. She was previously fit and well.

This is consistent with a possible diagnosis of lymphoma.

Following examination of the lymphoreticular system, I would like to check blood for full blood count, urea and electrolytes, coagulation, LDH, a blood film, and arrange a chest X-ray and a lymph node biopsy. I would also like to request a HIV test after informed consent and counselling has been provided.'

Station 9: BREAST HISTORY

Mrs Patterson is a 45 year-old lady who has noticed a lump in her left breast. Please take a history and consider her risk factors for breast cancer.

Features of a Breast Lump

- Site
  - 'Where have you felt a lump?'
  - 'Have you noticed any other lumps – in particular, in the other breast, your neck, or in your armpits?'
- 'When did you first notice the lump?'
- Change in size or consistency
- Painful or painless
- Preceding trauma
- Breast or nipple changes
- Nipple discharge
  - 'Have you noticed any discharge from your nipples?'
  - If so, ask them to describe the discharge – is it bloody?
- Changes throughout the menstrual cycle
- 'Have you had a similar lump/any other breast problem in the past?'
- Parity? Last menstrual period? (LMP)
- Breast feeding? Duration?

Associated Symptoms

- Shortness of breath
- Skin changes elsewhere
- Weight loss
- Swelling (especially arm on the affected side)
- Malaise
- Backache

Drug History

- Oral contraceptive pill
- Hormone replacement therapy

Breast Cancer Risk Factors

- Previous breast cancer
- Smoking
- Early menarche
- Late menopause
- Nulliparity
- Family history of breast/ovarian cancer; age of affected relative at the time of diagnosis; relation (1st or 2nd degree)
- Note: breast-feeding is protective

Further Investigation

Referral to the one-stop breast clinic for 'Triple Assessment'

Triple Assessment

History and Examination: in particular breast and lymph node examination

Imaging: X-ray mammography or USS

Sampling: Fine needle aspiration or core biopsy

What are the management options for breast cancer?

Medical
- CMF (cyclophosphamide, methotrexate, fluorouracil 5FU) chemotherapy regime
- Herceptin
- Tamoxifen
- Aromatase inhibitors (e.g. letrozole, anastrozole, exemestane)

Surgical
- Wide local excision of the breast lump (ensuring clear margin and taking sentinel lymph node biopsy)
- Simple mastectomy (plus or minus sentinel node biopsy)

Axillary node clearance is additionally done:
- If pre-operative ultrasound of the axilla and fine needle aspiration cytology (FNA)/core biopsy of the axillary node is positive for metastasis OR
- If sentinel node biopsy is positive for metastasis
- Note: morbidity is significant with axillary node clearance (e.g. lymphodema/bruising, shoulder stiffness, and reduced movement)

Cosmetic
- Secondary reconstruction should always be discussed: nipple tattoo, latissimus dorsi flap/abdominal sheath flap

Typical Age Ranges For Breast Lump Differentials

Condition	Age
Fibroadenoma	20 – 35
Fibrocystic change	20 – 40
Abscess	20 – 30 (Child bearing age)
Cyst	40-50 (Peri-menopausal)
Malignancy	40-70

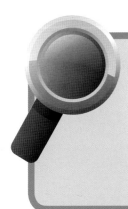

PRESENT YOUR FINDINGS...

'Mrs Patterson is a 45 year-old peri-menopausal female with a 3 month history of a painless left breast lump which is increasing in size. She has noted a blood-stained discharge from her left nipple. She is a smoker of 40 pack years, experienced menarche at 15 and is nulliparous. She is on no regular medications, and is otherwise well. Her sister had breast cancer at the age of 50.

Mrs Patterson is at high risk of breast cancer and further investigation in the form of Triple Assessment at the one-stop breast clinic is required.'

Station 10:
SEXUAL HISTORY

Margaret Ford is a 23 year-old woman who has developed vaginal discharge for the last few days. Take a full sexual history from her, and state a management plan.

Remind patients again that these are standard questions asked of everyone before asking about areas which are likely to be particularly sensitive: i.e. paying for sex, same-sex relationships, injecting recreational drugs, terminations, miscarriages and abortions

Good GUM histories depend on showing that you can be sensitive in asking the following questions: *'I need to ask you some personal questions today. Please don't be embarrassed – we ask everybody the same questions.'*

History

GUM Symptoms: Discharge (urethral or vaginal; colour, odour), lumps or bumps, rashes or ulcers, dyspareunia (pain on sexual intercourse – superficial or deep), lower abdominal pain (in women)

Systemic: Jaundice, eye problems, joint problems, rashes, mouth ulcers, fever, lethargy, reduced appetite, menstrual irregularity urinary symptoms, bowel symptoms

'Has your partner had any symptoms?' 'Does your partner have any STIs that you know of?'

Sexual Relations

- *'When did you last have sex?'*
- *'Was your partner a man or a woman?'*
- *'Have you had sex with them before?'*
  - If a regular partner, ask about length of the relationship
- *'What type of sex did you have – oral/vaginal/anal?'*
- *'Did you use a condom?'*
  - Ask about condom usage with each type of sex, as above
  - *'Have you noticed if any condoms have ever broken?'*
- *'Do you use any other forms of contraception?'*
- *'Have you had sex with anyone else in the last three months?'*
  - If not, ask about sexual partners prior to this. You must establish at least the last two partners
  - Ask the same questions about oral/vaginal/anal intercourse, and whether protected/unprotected intercourse, for each partner. For male-male anal sex, ask whether penetrative or receptive
- *'Have you travelled abroad recently?'*
  - If yes, *'did you have sex with anyone whilst abroad?' 'Where were they from?'* Then ask the same questions as above, for each partner
  - *'Have you had any partners born outside of the UK?'*
- *'Have you ever paid for sex?'*
- *'Have you ever had a same-sex relationship?'*
- *'Are you aware of your partner ever having a same-sex relationship?'*

Previous Tests

- *'Have you ever been tested for STIs in the past?' 'What was the result?'*
- *'Have you ever had an HIV test?' 'What was the result?' 'Why were you tested?'*
- *'Have you ever been tested for, or vaccinated against Hepatitis B?'*

HIV Risk Factors

- *'Have you ever received a blood transfusion?'*
  - Where? When?
- *'Do you have any tattoos?'*
- *'Have you ever injected recreational drugs?'*

Past Medical History

- Specifically ask about diabetes (increased risk of infections)

Drug History

- *'Any antibiotics in the last month?'*
- *'Are you allergic to anything?' 'What happens when you're exposed to it?'*

Obstetric and Gynaecological History

- *'How regular are your periods?' 'How long is there, usually, between the first day of one month's period, and the first day of the next month's period?'*
- *'How many days does your bleeding last?'*
- *'When was your last period?' 'Was it a normal period?' 'Is there any chance you could be pregnant?'*
- *'Do you use tampons or pads?'*
  - Tampons can, very rarely, be retained, potentially leading to toxic shock syndrome
- *'Have you ever been pregnant?'*
  - Ask about all pregnancies, whether delivered/miscarried/terminated

Social History

- Smoking and alcohol
- *'What do you do for a living?'*
- *'Do you live with anyone at the moment?'*

How would you manage this patient?

Follow the 6-point plan:

1. Accurate diagnosis
2. Treat symptomatic disease and prevent complications
3. Bring back to test for cure
4. Contact tracing
5. Screen for other STIs (2 weeks after a sexual encounter)
6. Education: counsel appropriately

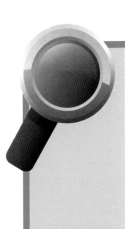

PRESENT YOUR FINDINGS...

'Margaret Ford is a 23 year-old lady who presents with vaginal discharge. She is normally fit and well. She has a 3 day history of white thick vaginal discharge. This is odourless, and associated with a severe itch. There is no associated dyspareunia, swelling, rashes or lumps.

She has had 10 sexual partners in the last 3 months, and did not use any contraception with any of these partners. All sexual encounters have been in the UK; however, one sexual partner was visiting from south-east asia. She has previously had multiple partners who were bi-sexual and she has two tattoos.

This is consistent with a diagnosis of candida albicans infection.

I would like to follow the six point management plan: confirm the diagnosis, treat the infection (and bring back to test for cure), encourage contact tracing, screen for STIs, and counsel about safe sex.'

Station 11: VAGINAL DISCHARGE

Mrs Peters is a 26 year-old lady who has developed vaginal discharge over the previous week. Please try and establish a cause for the discharge by taking a history. Tell the examiner what investigations you might request to help with your diagnosis.

Take a GUM history as detailed in section 1.10.

Causes of Vaginal Discharge

Pathological

Vulval	candidiasis, trichomoniasis, herpes, trauma
Urethral	gonorrhoea, chlamydia, non-specific genital infection (NSGI), trichomoniasis
Vaginal	candidiasis, bacterial vaginosis, trichomoniasis, senile discharge, foreign body
Cervix	gonorrhoea, chlamydia, herpes, erosion, polyp secondary to supra-cervical lesions

Always consider cervical infection in women presenting with discharge. Many of the cervical causes of vaginal discharge are serious and if not diagnosed and managed effectively, can result in serious morbidity: pelvic inflammatory disease, infertility, ectopic pregnancy, or disseminated infection

Investigation of Possible Cervicitis

Speculum insertion and examination. Obtain cervical cell samples for:

- *Neisseria gonorrhoea*
- *Chlamydia*
- *Herpes* virus

Above infections are screened for using nucleic acid amplification tests e.g. PCR rather than culture

What are the physiological causes of vaginal discharge?

- *Menstrual cyclical variation*
- *Pregnancy*
- *Smegma*
- *Sexual stimulation*

Vaginal Discharge

- Look for evidence of vulval irritation, excoriation, colour of discharge at the vulva, odour
- With the aid of a speculum, observe for consistency, location, and colour of discharge

Tests that can be done with sample from vagina:
- pH
- Mix discharge into saline and use microscopy to look for clue cells, neutrophils, *trichomoniasis, fungi*
- Mix discharge with 10% potassium hydroxide: sniff for release of amines
- Gram-stained specimen of discharge
- Vaginal culture

Common Pathogens

Candidiasis	gram stain reveals hyphae spores and neutrophils, pH normal, sniff test negative
Trichomoniasis	offensive frothy discharge, purulent, involvement of cervix, pH raised, sniff test positive, microscopy reveals presence of flagellate protozoans, neutrophils observed on Gram staining
Bacterial Vaginosis	grey discharge, fishy odour, clue cells, pH over 4.5, sniff test positive, vaginal culture yields *Gardnerella*

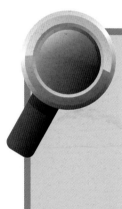

PRESENT YOUR FINDINGS...

'Mrs Peters is a 26 year-old lady who presents with vaginal discharge. She is normally fit and well. She has a 5 day history of grey vaginal discharge which has a 'fishy' odour. She reports no pain, itch or bleeding. She has had at least 20 sexual partners (heterosexual males) in the last 3 months and has, in the last 2 weeks, not been using any contraception. The odour is more pronounced after intercourse.

This is consistent with a diagnosis of bacterial vaginosis. I would like to follow the six point management plan: confirm the diagnosis, treat the infection (and bring back to test for cure), encourage contact tracing, screen for STIs, and counsel about safe sex.'

2 Examination

Time to get hands on! The best way to practice is to examine people, whether this is a patient or a friend. Some universities close the main hospital off to students for a while before the OSCEs, so you may not be able to practice there. You can, however, go to GP practices or other hospitals where you may have had attachments at and practice there. If you are well organised, you can contact someone in advance and arrange some bedside teaching or – more usefully, someone can grill you and point out your weaknesses. This will make you work harder and is therefore better than having someone be very nice and telling you to relax because you are already really good. So choose a contact that you were always a little bit scared of and ask them – the more intimidating, the better in the long run.

Remember to ask permission to perform any examination, and to ask whether the patient has any pain before starting. It is helpful to check whether the examiner prefers a running commentary during the OSCE, or whether they would prefer you to present the case at the end. Also, if you are in any doubt, ask the patient if they would like a chaperone to be present.

Study Action Plan

- Start by familiarising with the routine for examination: practising on friends is a good way of doing this
- Then try to identify real patients with real clinical signs to examine
- You don't necessarily need to exclusively examine patients to learn clinical signs, for example CDs are available for listening to heart murmur recordings
- Always try to practice presenting your findings at the conclusion of an examination routine

This chapter contains notes on the following systems:

Station 1: CARDIOVASCULAR EXAM

You are the junior doctor on-call, and have been asked to review a 60-year-old patient who has presented to the Emergency Department with shortness of breath and a new murmur. Please examine them. You may assume there is no hepatomegaly, peripheral oedema, or basal lung crackles.

- The patient has a heart murmur so you will need to prioritise auscultating the chest
- Think about the signs related to a heart murmur and do your cardiovascular examination with these at the back of your mind
- Ensure the patient is comfortable at 45 degrees, with neck muscles relaxed

General Observations

'The patient is comfortable at rest. She is on 2 litres of oxygen, in a monitored bed. She is not breathless, pale or cyanosed.'

- Assess the hands
- Both hands can be felt for temperature at the same time
- Do a capillary refill. Push down on the finger pulp for five seconds to ensure an accurate reading
- Look for signs of infective endocarditis. Look for clubbing and splinter haemorrhages. Turn the hand around and feel for Osler's nodes in the pulps of the fingers, and look for Janeway lesions on the palms

'The patient's hands are warm and well perfused. There are no peripheral stigmata of infective endocarditis.'

- Feel both radial pulses at the same time. Comment on whether they are regular/ irregular, and whether there is a radio-radio delay
- Feel for a collapsing pulse. Ask the patient if they have any shoulder pain before lifting the arm (with the forearm above the head)
- Feel the brachial or carotid pulse for the volume and character of the pulse. You will be thinking about whether the pulse is slow-rising (aortic stenosis) or collapsing (aortic regurgitation)

Say that you would want to check blood pressure (relevant to a valvular pathology: aortic stenosis is associated with a narrow pulse pressure, and aortic regurgitation is associated with a wide pulse pressure). Look at the face.

'There is no xanthelasma or corneal arcus. The patient is not centrally cyanosed and has no malar flush.'

Look in the eyes for pallor, and say that you would perform fundoscopy to look for Roth spots.

Then move on to the chest.

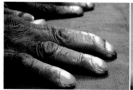
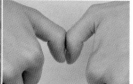

Fig 2.1: Capillary refill: note the loss of colour in pulp of thumb

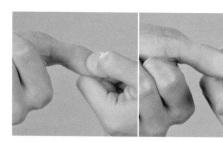
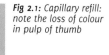

Fig 2.2: Clubbed fingers, with increased convexity of nail fold, and loss of angle between nail bed/ fold, (left), assessing for clubbing: look for a diamond formed between thumbnails (right)

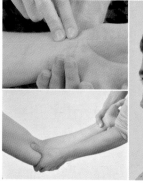
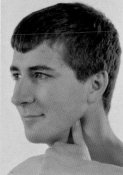

Fig 2.3: Feeling for pulses: radial (between radial styloid, and tendon of flexor carpi radialis) (top left), brachial (medial to bicep tendon) (bottom left), carotid (between sternocleidomastoid and angle of jaw) (right)

Causes of Atrial Fibrillation

Cardiac	Non Cardiac
Heart Failure	Infection
Myocardial Infarction / Ischemic Heart Disease	Thyrotoxicosis
Atrial Dilatation (secondary to mitral stenosis or regurgitation)	Alcohol
Cardiac Surgery	Pulmonary Embolism
Hypertension	

Inspection

- Look for a pacemaker/ICD, for scars (median sternotomy, lateral thoracotomy, pacemaker, mitral valvotomy, chest drains), chest wall deformities, and visible pulsations. Also look at legs/wrists for blood vessel grafts

Jugular Venous Pressure

- Look for pulsation behind the sternocleidomastoid. Positioning is very important. Sit the patient at 45 degrees if possible. Ask them to relax. Ask them to turn their head slightly away from the side of the neck that you are inspecting. Look for the JVP
- If the JVP is not seen assess hepatojugular reflux: place the hand inferior to the liver edge and press gently to accentuate the JVP. Ask about abdominal pain first!

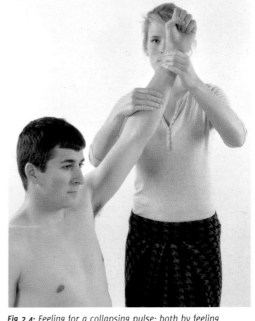

Fig 2.4: Feeling for a collapsing pulse: both by feeling character of the pulse with one hand, and with the other hand feeling for pulsations in the anterior forearm muscles

How does JVP differ from the carotid pulse?

Use the acronym 'MOPHAIR'

Multi-waveform: for each cardiac cycle, there are two JVP 'waves' ('a' wave and 'v' wave), compared to one carotid wave

Occludable: lightly pressing on the internal jugular vein occludes the JVP

Positional variation: falls on sitting up

Hepatojugular reflux: the JVP rises with light pressure on the liver

Fills from Above: after being occluded *(since this is the direction of blood flow)*

Impalpable: a pulse cannot be felt in the JVP

Respiratory changes: the JVP falls on inspiration

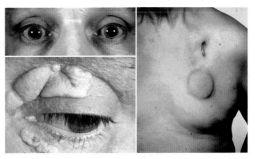

Fig 2.5: Corneal arcus (top left) xanthelasma (bottom left) Pacemaker/ ICD (right)

Palpation

- Palpate for the apex beat. If you feel it, count down the ribs to see if it is displaced. If you do not, state, *'I cannot palpate the apex beat'*
- Feel for a parasternal heave and thrills

Auscultation

- Auscultate all four areas of the precordium. Check for radiation to both the carotids and axillae
- Think about the heart sounds (including presence of S3 and S4) as well as any murmurs

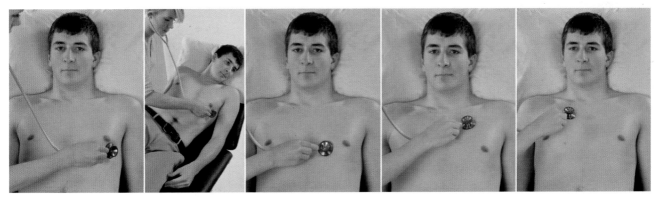

Fig 2.6: Auscultation: from (left to right), start at the apex (which you have just identified). Listen in mitral area. Listen in mitral area again with bell, and in mitral area with patient rolled onto left (for mitral stenosis). Listen in tricuspid, listen in pulmonary, and listen in aortic areas
ALWAYS FEEL A CENTRAL PULSE e.g. CAROTID TO TIME HEART SOUNDS/MURMURS

Grade of Murmur	Audibility	Thrill
1	Barely audible	No
2	Audible after a few seconds of auscultation	No
3	Immediately audible. Moderate intensity	No
4	Loud intensity	Yes
5	Very loud (may be heard with stethoscope slightly off thoracic wall)	Yes
6	Loudest (may be heard with stethoscope entirely off thoracic wall)	Yes

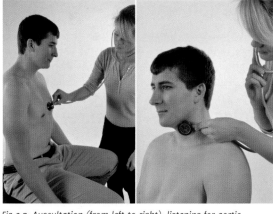

Fig 2.7: Auscultation (from left to right): listening for aortic murmur, and for radiation into the neck

- Roll patient onto their left side. Auscultate the mitral area to listen for mitral stenosis
- Ask the patient to sit up, breathe in, breathe out and then hold their breath. Listen at lower left sternal edge for aortic regurgitation

Because of the specific details of this particular cardiovascular scenario, it is not necessary to listen to the lung bases or feel for peripheral oedema. You had already been told no peripheral oedema/hepatomegaly. However, this should be done as part of the routine examination.

'When introduced to a patient with a murmur, most students will only listen to the murmur on one occasion. I found that, providing the patient was happy, going back and listening to the murmur a second or third time really helped consolidate my pattern recognition skills'

Zeshan Qureshi
Paediatric Trainee, London Deanery

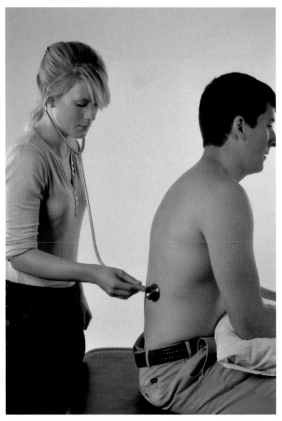

Fig 2.8: Auscultation of the lung base

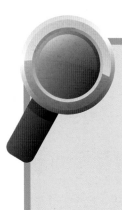

PRESENT YOUR FINDINGS...

'This is Mrs Smith, who has presented with shortness of breath and a heart murmur.

She is comfortable at rest, on 2 litres of oxygen. There are no stigmata of infective endocarditis. Her pulse is regular at a rate of 60BPM. It is slow rising and normal volume. Pulse pressure is normal. On auscultation, she has an ejection systolic murmur in the aortic area, radiating to both her carotids. S1 is normal with a quiet S2. There are no additional heart sounds. There is no evidence of heart failure.

This is consistent with a diagnosis of aortic stenosis.

I would like to confirm this with an echocardiogram, perform a chest X-ray, and an ECG.'

Systolic Murmurs: Comparison of Aortic Stenosis and Mitral Regurgitation

	Aortic Stenosis	Mitral Regurgitation
Aetiology	**Valvular (most common)** • Congenital (bicuspid valve most common cause in 40-60) • Senile calcification (over 60s) • Inflammatory valvulitis e.g. rheumatic fever **Subvalvular** • Fibromuscular ring • Hypertrophic cardiomyopathy **Supravalvular** • William's Syndrome	**Annulus** • Senile calcification **Mitral Valve Leaflets** • Mitral valve prolapse syndrome • Connective tissue disorders • Infective endocarditis **Chordae Tendinae** • Connective tissue disorders • Infective endocarditis **Papillary Muscles** • Post myocardial infarction
Symptoms	**Asymptomatic** **Breathlessness:** left ventricular failure **Angina:** due to increased myocardial work **Dizziness and syncope:** on exertion **Systemic Emboli:** retinal or cerebral **Sudden Death**	**Acute (not compensated)** • Pulmonary oedema – severe dyspnoea **Chronic (partially compensated)** • Fatigue • Dyspnoea (on exertion)
Pulse	• Low volume • Slow rising • Faint • Pulsus alternans (severe cases)	May have: • Atrial fibrillation • Atrial flutter
BP	• Low BP • Narrowed pulse pressure	Not typically effected unless heart failure
Precordium	• Systolic thrill in aortic area (leaning forward/ expiration) • Heaving (rarely displaced) apex	• Systolic thrill in mitral region • Laterally and downwardly displaced thrusting apex (dilated LV) • JVP raised • Pulmonary hypertension
Heart Sounds	• Ejection systolic murmur (left sternal edge, expiration, leaning forward, cresecendo, decrescendo, radiating to carotid) • Ejection click (if valve mobile and bicuspid) • Soft A2, may be inaudible if valve calcified • S4	• Pansystolic murmur (apex, expiration, blowing, patient leaning back at 45 degrees, radiating to back/axilla) • Soft S1 • S3 • Loud P2 if pulmonary hypertension develops • Midsystolic click (if mitral prolapse)
ECG	• Left ventricular hypertrophy • Left axis deviation • First degree heart block (extension of calcification across AV node)	• Left ventricular hypertrophy • Atrial fibrillation may be present • P mitrale (if significant atrial dilatation)
CXR	• Calcified valve	• Calcified valve • Left ventricular dilatation • Left atrial dilatation
Echo	• Unicuspid or bicuspid valve • Calcified valve • Increased blood flow velocity across aortic valve (on Doppler)	• Left atrial dilatation • Left ventricular dilatation • Mitral valve prolapse • Infective vegetation • Pulmonary hypertension
Complications	• Arrhythmias • Myocardial infarction • Heart failure • Infective endocarditis • Emboli (from endocarditis or calcification)	• Arrhythmias • Heart failure • Pulmonary hypertension • Infective endocarditis

Diastolic Murmurs: Comparison of Aortic Regurgitation and Mitral Stenosis

Examination

	Aortic Regurgitation	Mitral Stenosis
Aetiology	**Valve disease** • Infective endocarditis • Connective tissue disorders **Aortic Root disease** • Aortic dissection • Connective tissue disorders • Syphillis **Mixed stenosis/regurgitation** • Rheumatic fever • Rheumatoid arthritis	• Rheumatic heart disease (almost all) • Congenital
Symptoms	Similar presentation to aortic stenosis • Angina and syncope less common • Breathlessness • Generally well tolerated unless acute	• Breathlessness (pulmonary hypertension) • Fatigue • Haemopytsis • Systemic emboli • Chronic bronchitis (due to oedematous bronchial mucosa) • Chest pain • Palpitations • Enlarged atria (and subsequent compression of recurrent laryngeal nerve/ oesophagus/ left main bronchus)
Pulse	• Collapsing ('water-hammer') pulse • Throbbing peripheral pulses	• Small volume • Atrial arrhythmia (atrial fibrillation is more common than with mitral regurgitation)
BP	• Wide pulse pressure	• Not typically effected unless heart failure
Precordium	• Diastolic thrill in aortic area • Diffuse, displaced, forceful apex	• Diastolic thrill in mitral region • Tapping apex • Raised JVP if right heart failure • Parasternal heave due to right ventricular hypertrophy
Heart Sounds	• Early diastolic murmur (left lower sternal edge, high pitched, expiration, leaning forward) • May be an ejection systolic 'flow' murmur (volume overload) • Soft A2	• Mid diastolic murmur (apex, rumbling, expiration, radiating to axilla) • Opening snap • Loud P2 • Split S2
ECG	• Left ventricular dilatation (due to volume overload) • P mitrale (if significant atrial dilatation)	• Right ventricular hypertrophy • Atrial fibrillation
CXR	• Possible widened medistinum (aortic dissection) • Left ventricular dilatation	• Left atrial dilatation +/- right heart dilatation • Pulmonary hypertension and pulmonary oedema
Echo	• Dilated aortic root • Dilated left ventricle with vigorous contractions	• Mitral valve calcification • Left atrial dilatation • Pulmonary hypertension • Right ventricular hypertrophy, dilatation and failure
Complications	• Arrhythmias • Heart failure • Infective endocarditis	• Arrhythmias • Pulmonary hypertension • Right heart failure • Infective endocarditis

Station 2: RESPIRATORY EXAM

Please examine this lady's respiratory system, and present your findings.

General Inspection

- Environmental clues: O_2 mask or nasal cannula. Inhalers/ nebulisers/ spacers/ peak flow meter/ sputum pot
- Evidence of weight loss
- Is the patient breathless at rest? (tachypnoea >15 breaths per minute)
- Scars from surgery or drain insertion. Also look in both axillae

Nature of Breathing

- Hyperventilation: multiple causes including anxiety, metabolic acidosis (Kussmaul respirations), toxins, and head injury
- Hypoventilation: indicating ventilatory failure
- Use of accessory muscles (sternocleidomastoid, pectoralis, and platysma) is characteristic of patients with respiratory distress
- Any cough, wheeze or stridor?

Hands

- Clubbing
- Peripheral cyanosis
- **Tremor:** there may be a fine tremor caused by excessive use of beta-agonists or theophylline bronchodilators
- Tar staining
- **Pulse:** check the rate, rhythm and volume of the pulse at the wrist. In chronic CO_2 retainers, these patients will have warm peripheries and large volume pulses due to the actions of CO_2 as a vasodilator
- **CO_2 retention flap/flapping tremor:** test by asking patient to lift arms in front of them and cock their wrists back. State that you would assess this for thirty seconds

Axilla

- Palpate for enlarged axillary lymph nodes (whilst taking the weight of the arm with your non-palpating hand)

Face

- Anaemia (conjunctival pallor)
- Horner's syndrome (interruption in sympathetic chain in the neck or brainstem – commonly due to a lung cancer at apex of the lung invading the sympathetic chain)
- Check at the lips and tongue for central cyanosis
- Check mouth for oral thrush (e.g. secondary to steroids)

Neck – Elevated JVP

- Assess as described in Station 2.1
- Causes include, Cor Pulmonale, elevated intrathoracic pressures (acute severe asthma or tension pneumothorax), and SVC obstruction

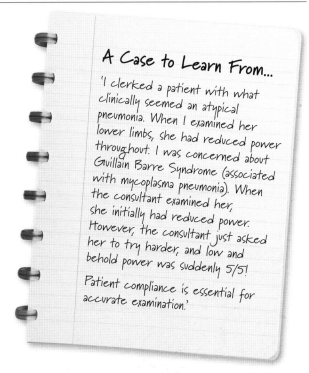

A Case to Learn From...

'I clerked a patient with what clinically seemed an atypical pneumonia. When I examined her lower limbs, she had reduced power throughout. I was concerned about Guillain Barre Syndrome (associated with mycoplasma pneumonia). When the consultant examined her, she initially had reduced power. However, the consultant just asked her to try harder, and low and behold power was suddenly 5/5!

Patient compliance is essential for accurate examination.'

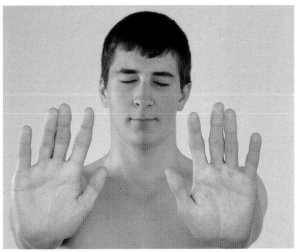

Fig 2.9: Assessing for CO_2 retention flap

Causes of Clubbing

- *Carcinoma of bronchus*
- *Chronic suppurative lung disease e.g. cystic fibrosis, empyema, bronchiectasis, lung abscess*
- *Fibrosing alveolitis*
- *Cyanotic heart disease*
- *Infective endocarditis*
- *Liver cirrhosis*
- *Inflammatory bowel disease*
- *Idiopathic*
- *Familial*

Lymph Nodes

- Palpate the lymph nodes of the neck from standing behind the patient. If a node is palpable, then describe its nature: Is it rubbery (as in Hodgkin's disease), tender (tonsillitis), or matted together (TB and metastatic disease)?

Inspection of Chest

- Fully expose the evenly illuminated chest, with the patient sitting (though minor asymmetry of the chest is best seen with the patient lying supine)
- Ask permission to inspect BOTH axillae, followed by the patient's back. Note: when inspecting the back the patient's arms should be folded across the chest (to ensure scapulae are opened up)
- Look for lesions in the chest wall (possible metastatic tumour nodules, and neurofibromas)
- Scars from thoracic surgery (lateral thoracotomy, chest drain)
- Dilated superficial veins (SVC obstruction – elevation of JVP does not vary with breathing (unlike with heart failure) since there is a fixed obstruction)

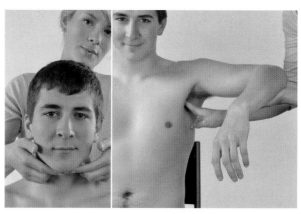

Fig 2.10: Feeling for lymph nodes in the neck (left) and in the axilla (right)

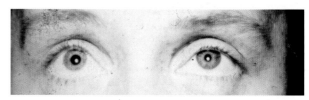

Fig 2.11: Horner's syndrome: note ptosis and pupil constriction on left; associated with apical lung tumours

Chest Wall Shape

Barrel Chest	Pectus Excavatum	Thoracic Kyphoscoliosis	Pectus Carinatum
Increased AP diameter compared to lateral diameter, typically associated with lung hyperinflation or kyphoscoliosis	Depressed sternum (usually benign). May be associated with pulmonary hypertension	Excessive AP and lateral curvature of the spine. May be idiopathic or secondary to childhood poliomyelitis or spinal TB. Causes decreased ventilatory capacity and increased work of breathing	Prominent sternum (pigeon chest) which may be an indicator of chronic respiratory disease in childhood

Chest Wall Movements

- Generalised indrawing of intercostal muscles (implying that the patient cannot achieve adequate ventilation by normal inspiratory efforts). This is seen in patients with gross hyperinflation secondary to emphysema or asthma
- Local indrawing of a portion of the chest wall ('flail chest' usually seen in trauma patients who have sustained double fractures of a series of ribs or sternum)
- Purse-lipped exhalation (this prevents bronchial wall collapse and minimises work done in breathing). This is seen in patients with severe airway narrowing

Palpation

- Palpate any local abnormalities seen on inspection
- Assess tracheal position. Insert the tip of your finger into the suprasternal notch and press gently into the trachea. Check that your fingertip fits easily into both sides, and that the trachea is central. Warn patients that this might feel uncomfortable
- Palpate for an apex beat. If it is impalpable, consider diagnosis such as emphysema, obesity, dextrocardia and a large pleural effusion
- Chest Expansion: assess upper, middle and lower zones. Any change is difficult to detect if it is bilateral. Unilateral causes of reduced expansion included pneumothorax, pleural effusion, pneumonia and collapse

'I don't think it is easy to assess hypoventilation clinically. Many COPD patients with hypercapnia can look like they are hyperventilating even when they have alveolar hypoventilation'

Simon Watkin
Consultant Respiratory Physician
Borders General Hospital

Trachea Deviated Towards Pathology	Trachea Deviated Away From Pathology
Lobar Collapse Pneumonectomy	Large Pleural Effusion Tension Pneumothorax

Percussion

- All movement should come from your wrist joint, and your middle finger should remain partially flexed. Compare the note at equivalent positions on both sides
- Start at the supra-clavicular fossae and work down. Map out any area of altered resonance by going from the normal to the abnormal area

Percussion Notes

Resonant	Hyper Resonant
Normal	Large air filled space e.g. markedly emphysematous lung, pneumothorax

Dull	Stony Dull
Lung separated from the chest wall e.g. pleural fluid/thickening or pulmonary consolidation/collapse	Characteristic of a large pleural effusion

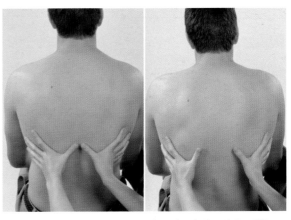

Fig 2.12: Assessing chest expansion. Place thumbs loosely in midline, and fingers on peripheral chest. After taking a deep breath out (left), ask the patient to take a deep breath in (right)

Auscultation

- Listen with the patient relaxed and breathing normally through an open mouth
- Auscultate the anterior chest wall, alternating between each side of the chest wall (to compare like with like), starting above the clavicle and finishing below the 11th rib (do not forget the lateral chest wall prior to auscultating the posterior chest wall)
- In each area, assess the quality and amplitude of breath sounds whilst noting any added sounds

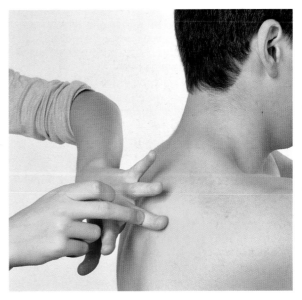

Fig 2.13: Percussion: striking the middle phalanx of the middle finger (left hand) with the distal phalanx of the middle finger (right hand). The other fingers are not touching the chest

Types of Breath Sounds

	Normal Vesicular Breathing	Diminished Vesicular Breathing	Bronchial Breathing
Causes	Normal	Occurs if there is a thick chest wall e.g. pleural thickening or if there is a reason for conduction of sound to the chest wall to be reduced e.g. emphysema or simply shallow breathing	Associated with pneumonic consolidation, which produces a uniform conducting medium. Also present at the border between lung and a pleural effusion (due to an underlying compressed lung)
Character	Said to have a rustling quality: the sound should increase steadily during inspiration, and then quickly fade during the first third of expiration	Similar in character to normal vesicular breathing, but quieter	Breath sounds are loud and blowing. Similar pitch and length of inspiration and expiration. Unlike normal vesicular breath sounds, there is an audible gap between inspiration and expiration

Crackles

- Non-musical sounds with a crackling quality, due to a loss of stability of peripheral airways, which collapse on expiration
- The high pressures of inspiration cause the abrupt re-opening of alveoli and small bronchi, which produces the characteristic crackling noise

Pleural Rub

- Creaking sound, produced by the movement of the visceral over the parietal pleura, when both sides have been roughened by fibrinous exudates or acute inflammation
- Sounds like crunching snow, or the creaking of leather
- Typically not audible on shallow breathing, but becomes clear on deep breathing
- Causes include pneumonia, and pulmonary embolism

Wheeze

- Musical quality sound caused by continuous oscillation of opposing airway walls implying narrowing of the small airways
- Typically present at the end of expiration as airways normally narrow on expiration
- If present on inspiration (when the airways are normally dilated) it implies severe airway narrowing, although in extremely severe airway obstruction wheeze may be absent due to severely reduced airflow
- Monophonic wheeze may be caused by an obstructing lesion, classically a tumour. Polyphonic wheeze is associated with more diffuse airway disease e.g. asthma

Whispering Pectoriloquy

- This is performed by asking the patient to whisper '99' whilst auscultating the chest
- Usually sounds of this volume are not heard, but in the setting of consolidation an increased transmission of sound occurs, and thus louder 'whispering pectoriloquy' in the affected area
- This is a useful way of differentiating pleural effusion (where there is reduced transmission of sound) from consolidation
- Tactile vocal fremitus in principle assesses the same thing, but transmission of sound is felt rather than auscultated

What are the causes of Inspiratory crackles?

Where they occur during inspiration may offer a clue to their cause:
- *Early inspiration* – small airway disease such as bronchiolitis
- *Mid-inspiration* – pulmonary oedema
- *Late inspiration* – interstitial lung disease, COPD, pneumonia
- *Throughout inspiration and expiration* – bronchiectasis

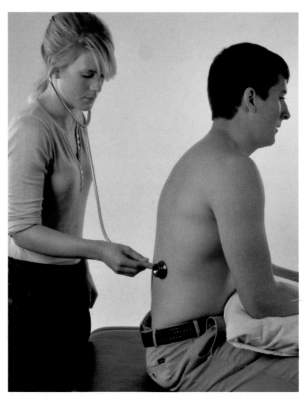

Fig 2.14: Auscultation of lower zones, whilst asking the patient to say '99'

PRESENT YOUR FINDINGS...

'This patient has reduced breath sounds, dull percussion note and reduced whispering pectoriloquy at the left base.

This is consistent with a left pleural effusion, but may also be lobar collapse.

I would want to order a chest x-ray to narrow my differential.'

Causes of Interstitial Lung Disease

Idiopathic (cryptogenic)
Extrinsic allergic alveolitis
- Pigeon fancier's lung
- Farmer's lung

Sarcoidosis
Autoimmune
- Rheumatoid arthritis, systemic sclerosis, ankylosing spondylitis

Occupational
- Asbestosis, pneumoconiosis, silicosis

Drugs
- Methotrexate, amiodarone, nitrofurantoin

Familial

Station 3: CRANIAL NERVE EXAM

Mr Wade is a 48 year-old smoker with progressive left-sided neck and arm pain. Please examine this man's cranial nerves and then present your findings.

General Inspection

- Ptosis (III)
- Eye position (III, IV, VI)
- Pupil symmetry (II, III)
- Facial symmetry (VII)
- Sternocleidomastoid/trapezius bulk (XI)
- Speech (V, VII, IX, X, XII)

Appearance of the Eye

- **Ptosis** – drooping of upper eyelid; due to Horner's syndrome, 3rd nerve palsy, congenital abnormality, senile ptosis, Myasthenia Gravis
- **Exophthalmos** – anterior bulging of the eyeball; secondary to Grave's disease or retro-orbital mass
- **Enophthalmos** – eyeball recession within the orbit; congenital, traumatic causes or secondary to Horner's syndrome

CN I: Olfactory

- *'Have you noticed any changes in how food tastes or in your sense of smell?'*
- Could be tested formally by covering each nostril and testing with a battery of standardised smells, e.g. peppermint

CN II: Optic

- *'Do you wear glasses?'*
- Test one eye at a time with a Snellen chart or, as a simple bedside screen, get the patient to read something
- **Visual Fields:** sit opposite the patient and ask them to look straight ahead. Test 4 quadrants of both eyes separately (*'which finger am I moving?'*), then see if there is evidence of neglect by testing both eyes simultaneously
- Blind spot: test using a red hat pin
- Offer to perform fundoscopy

CN III, IV, VI: Oculomotor, Trochlear, Abducens

- Eye movements: *'keeping your head still, follow the movements of the end of my pen with your eyes'* (pursuit movements). Test slow pursuit movements to 8 areas as follows; ask about double vision and look for nystagmus

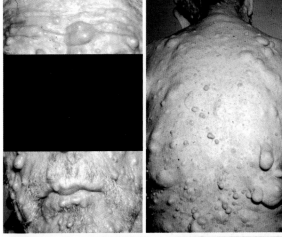
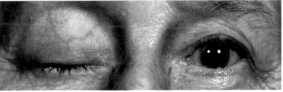

Fig 2.15: Skin lesions of neurofibromatosis (above) ptosis (below)

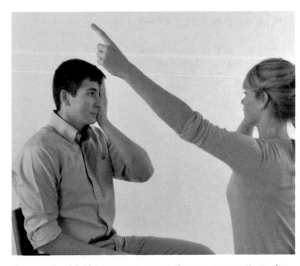

Fig 2.16: Visual field assessment: ensure that you cover your eye that is directly OPPOSITE the one that isn't being tested (i.e. cover your right eye if testing the patient's right eye)

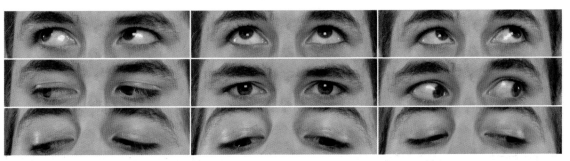

Fig 2.17: Assessing ocular movements (III, IV, VI), look in eight directions as above

- Accommodation reflex: ask patient to look to at distant point e.g. a curtain, then at something closer e.g. your pen torch
- Pupillary light reflexes: direct and consensual; look for a relative afferent pupillary defect
- For both reflexes above, the sensory limb is dependent on CN II and the motor limb on CN III

CN V: Trigeminal

- *'Clench your jaw'* – feel contraction of masseter and temporalis under your fingers
- *'Open your jaw against my hand'*
- Sensation of face: demonstrate centrally (e.g. sternum), then test light touch to corresponding areas for ophthalmic, maxillary, mandibular branches on both sides whilst patients eyes are closed
- Offer to assess pain and temperature sensation in the same areas
- Offer to assess corneal reflex and jaw jerk

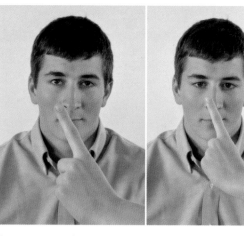

Fig 2.18: Accommodation: ask the patient to focus on an object in the distance (left) and then to focus on your finger (right). Look for a) convergence of the eyes and b) constriction of the pupils

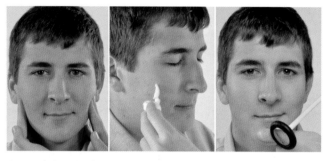

Fig 2.19: (Left to right) Masseter palpation whilst teeth being clenched, sensation in the maxillary division of trigeminal nerve. Note the patient's eyes are shut to prevent cheating! Jaw jerk reflex

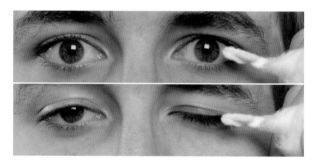

Fig 2.20: Corneal reflex: blink in response to stimulation of the cornea with a cotton wool wisp

CN VII: Facial

- **Test in order of branches:** *'raise your eyebrows'* (temporal) *'scrunch up your eyes'* (zygomatic) *'blow out your cheeks'* (buccal) *'show me your teeth'* and *'whistle'* (mandibular) *'stick forward your chin as if shaving'* (cervical). Ask patient to relax between tests

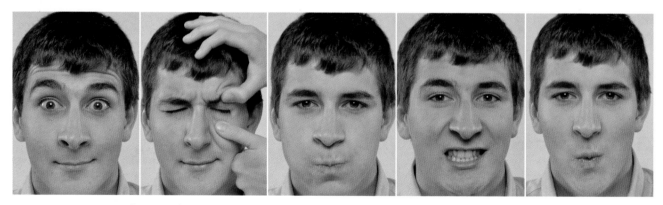

Fig 2.21: Facial nerve testing: (Left to right) Raising eyebrows (temporal), scrunching up eye (with examiner trying to open them) (zygomatic), blowing out cheeks (buccal), bearing teeth, whistling (mandibular)

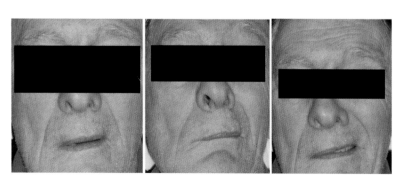

Fig 2.22: Facial nerve palsy: (Left to right) Baseline, raising eyebrows (temporal), smiling (mandibular). This is consistent with a lower motor neuron legion since there is no forehead sparing

CN VIII: Vestibulocochlear

- Sit to the side of your patient (remember to start with the good side first)
- With one hand, obscure the entrance to the contralateral ear canal and rub gently (do this by pushing the tragus in to the canal). This will muffle this ear and ensure that you are only testing one ear at a time. With the other hand, cover the patient's eyes (so they cannot lip read)
- Ensure that you are at full arm's length
- Whisper a combination of a number and a letter e.g. 'N4' and ask the patient to repeat what you are saying. Get increasingly louder until they can hear you
- Perform Rinne's and Weber's tests (see 2.24 Ear Examination)
- Offer to assess balance

CN IX/X: Glossopharyngeal and Vagus

- *'Please can you cough'*
- *'Please swallow this cup of water'*
- Ask the patient to open their mouth and say 'ahh' – look for uvula deviation
- Offer to test the gag reflex

CN XI: Accessory (spinal root)

- Ask the patient to shrug their shoulders against resistance
- Ask the patient to put their chin onto their left shoulder and then onto their right shoulder; ask the patient to do both of these against resistance

CN XII: Hypoglossal

- *'Please open your mouth'* – inspect the patient's mouth; any tongue fasciculations?
- Ask the patient to stick out their tongue: inspect for wasting and deviation
- Ask the patient to push their tongue into their cheek (resist the movement by pushing on the outside of the cheek)

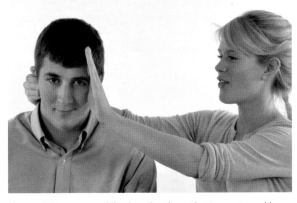

Fig 2.23: Whisper test, while obscuring the patient's eyes to avoid any lip reading

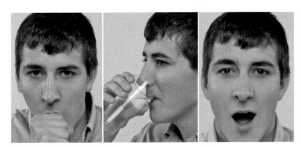

Fig 2.24: (Left to right) Ask patient to cough, assessing swallow, and asking the patient to say 'ahh' so you can look in the mouth

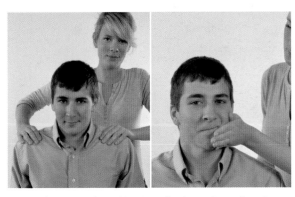

Fig 2.25: (Left to right) Shoulder shrug, (against resistance) putting chin onto left shoulder (against resistance)

> 'It is actually much more reliable to look for fasciculations when the tongue is resting in the mouth, rather than when it is protruded.'
>
> **Richard Knight**
> *Professor of Neurology*
> *University of Edinburgh*

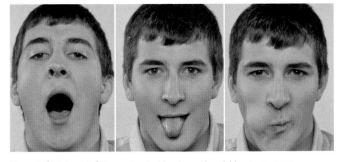

Fig 2.26: (Left to right) Inspecting inside of mouth, sticking tongue out, and sticking tongue into cheek

How would you differentiate an upper motor neuron VII lesion from a lower motor neuron VII lesion?

The muscles of the forehead have bilateral cortical representation. Therefore, in an upper motor neurone lesion, e.g. a cerebral infarct, there is sparing of the forehead. The patient would still be able to raise their eyebrows equally on both sides.

What are the causes of a facial nerve palsy?

Lower Motor Neuron	Upper Motor Neuron
Bell's Palsy	Cerebrovascular Disease
Ramsay Hunt Syndrome	Tumour
Trauma	
Parotid Tumour	
Sarcoidosis	

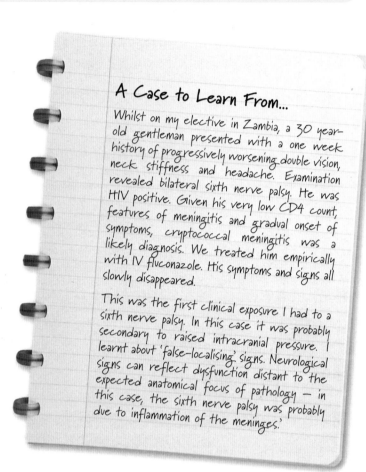

A Case to Learn From...

Whilst on my elective in Zambia, a 30 year-old gentleman presented with a one week history of progressively worsening double vision, neck stiffness and headache. Examination revealed bilateral sixth nerve palsy. He was HIV positive. Given his very low CD4 count, features of meningitis and gradual onset of symptoms, cryptococcal meningitis was a likely diagnosis. We treated him empirically with IV fluconazole. His symptoms and signs all slowly disappeared.

This was the first clinical exposure I had to a sixth nerve palsy. In this case it was probably secondary to raised intracranial pressure. I learnt about 'false-localising' signs. Neurological signs can reflect dysfunction distant to the expected anatomical focus of pathology — in this case, the sixth nerve palsy was probably due to inflammation of the meninges.'

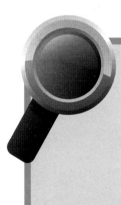

PRESENT YOUR FINDINGS...

'Mr Wade has a left-sided miosis, enophthalmos and a partial ptosis. There was a slow direct pupillary response to light on the left side compared with the right. There were no other significant abnormalities.

The findings are most consistent with Horner's Syndrome. Given the history of tobacco use, I would be concerned about a Pancoast tumour.

To complete my examination, I would like to assess sweating on both sides of the face and perform examinations of the peripheral neurological and respiratory systems'

Station 4: PERIPHERAL NERVE EXAM (UPPER LIMB)

Mr Reilly recently had a fall and fractured his humerus. He is now struggling to perform everyday tasks with his right hand. Please perform a neurological examination of this patient's upper limbs.

Communication is very important in neurological examination. Particularly when you are assessing power, ensure that you give clear instructions to the patient. Demonstrate movements that you want the patient to do, if necessary.

Inspection

- Look around for walking aids or wheelchairs
- Wasting, hypertrophy, asymmetry, abnormal movements, posture, fasciculations (best spotted in the triceps)
- Ask the patient to hold their arms out in supination (palms facing the ceiling) and close his eyes – if you see pronator drift (palm(s) turning involuntarily to face the floor), think upper motor neuron lesion

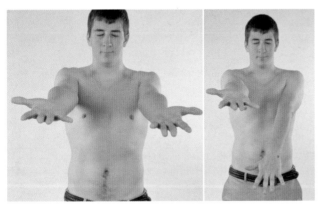

Fig 2.27: Pronator drift

Tone

- Ensure that the patient is relaxed: hold the patient's hand in a handshake position, then use your other hand to support their elbow, taking the weight of their arm
- Ask if the patient has any pain
- Explain to the patient *'I'm going to move your arm for you, so just relax and don't resist my movements'*
- Test tone: i) flexing elbow, ii) supinating (slow then feel for supinator 'catch') iii) wrist circumduction (feel for cogwheeling)

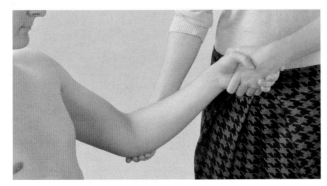

Fig 2.28: Taking the weight off the arm for tone assessment

Power

- Power is most easily tested by giving the patient specific instructions. Always make sure that you localise the joint appropriately by careful positioning of the patient and stabilising the patient's limb above the joint you are testing.

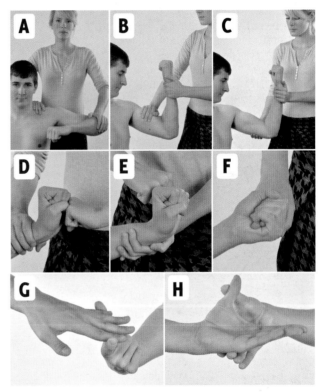

Fig 2.29: A: shoulder abduction, B: elbow flexion, C: elbow extension, D: wrist flexion, E: wrist extension, F: grip strength, G: finger abduction, H: thumb abduction. Note that, in each assessment, the joint being tested is isolated using the other hand if necessary (ensuring the test is specific for the joint in question)

A. *'Put your arms out (like a chicken) and don't let me push them up or down'*

B. *'Put your arms up in front of you and bend your elbows (like a boxer)';* hold their arms and ask them to pull you towards them;

C. Ask them to push their forearm away from them (from same position as 'B')

D. *'Put your arms out straight and cock your wrists back';* with your fists clenched; push down on their fist from above, (using your fist to compare like with like)

E. Then push up from below (from same position as 'D')

F. *'Now open your hands and squeeze my fingers as hard as you can with your palms'*

G. *'Spread your fingers and do not let me close them'*

H. *'Face your palms upwards and bring your thumb to the ceiling; do not let me push it down'*

MRC Scale of Muscle Power

When scoring power at each joint, the following standardised scale is used by clinicians.

0 – No movement
1 – Flicker of movement
2 – Isogravitational movements only
3 – Able to move against gravity
4 – Able to move against resistance but not fully
5 – Full power

One of the problems with this scale is that 4 encompasses such a wide range of power that its utility can be limited. Also, testing movements specifically against and with gravity is difficult to do properly.

Reflexes

- Biceps (musculocutaneous nerve/C5)
- Brachioradialis (radial nerve/C6)
- Triceps (radial nerve/C7)
- Reinforce as necessary (clench teeth)

Reflexes are best obtained when the patient is relaxed. Biceps and brachioradialis are best elicited when the arms are positioned in the lap. Triceps is best elicited when the elbow is bent at 90 degrees; with one hand supporting the wrist, strike the triceps tendon just above the olecranon.

Co-ordination

See cerebellar exam (section 2.6) for detail.

- Cerebellar rebound
- Finger-nose testing
- Dysdiadochokinesia

Sensation

A number of factors limit reliable testing of sensation. These include the challenge of getting the patient to keep their eyes shut, the difficulty in applying the same amount of pressure each time you touch the patient, and the presence of calloused skin. Different modalities test different tracts; normally light touch, proprioception and pain suffice, but vibration and temperature can also be tested. Do all of these with the patient's eyes shut.

- **Light Touch:** reference stimulus by touching the sternum first. Then test by dabbing (rather than stroking) in each dermatome (see box). Ask the patient to say if both sides are the 'same' or 'different' and if 'different' to clarify further
- **Proprioception:** start with small amplitude movements in most distal joint (i.e. distal interphalangeal joints)
- **Pain:** use a neurotip

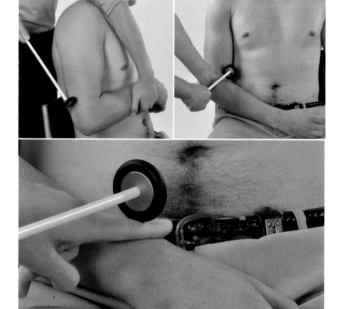

Fig 2.30: Tricep (left top) bicep (right top) brachioradialis (bottom) reflexes

Dermatomes

Some dermatomes are tested twice to ensure all major nerves are tested:

- 'Regimental patch': upper, lateral aspect of the arm (axillary nerve/C5)
- Outer forearm (lateral cutaneous nerve of forearm/C6)
- Middle finger (median nerve/C7)
- First dorsal web space (radial nerve/C7)
- Little finger (ulnar nerve/C8)
- Medical aspect of antecubital fossa (medial cutaneous nerve of forearm/T1)

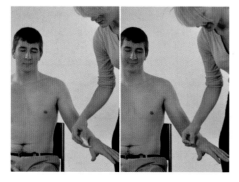

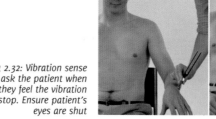

Fig 2.31: Assessing light touch and pain. Ensure patient's eyes are shut

Fig 2.32: Vibration sense – ask the patient when they feel the vibration stop. Ensure patient's eyes are shut

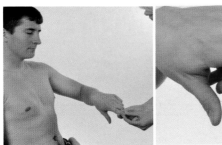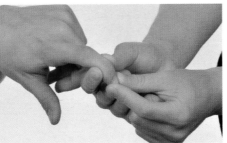

Fig 2.33: Proprioception: ensure you hold the finger from the sides to avoid excessive sensory stimulation. Ensure patient's eyes are shut

How would you differentiate between an upper and a lower motor neuron lesion?

	Upper Motor Neuron	Lower Motor Neuron
Inspection	Pronator Drift	Muscle Wasting and Fasciculation
Tone	Increased (may be reduced in severe acute upper motor neurone lesions in the initial stages)	Decreased or normal
Power	Not often useful in differentiation between Upper and Lower Motor Neuron lesions	Not often useful in differentiation between Upper and Lower Motor Neuron lesions
Tendon Reflexes	Increased (may be reduced in severe acute upper motor neurone lesions in the initial stages) Presence of clonus	Decreased or absent
Plantar Reflexes	Upgoing	Downgoing

What muscles in the hand are supplied by the median nerve?

LOAF muscles: First and second Lumbricals   Thenar Eminence (Opponens pollicis, Abductor pollicis brevis, Flexor pollicis brevis)

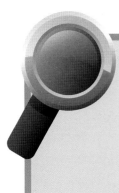

PRESENT YOUR FINDINGS...

'Mr Reilly has 0/5 power of wrist and finger extension on the right side. Furthermore, there is reduced sensation in the first dorsal web space on the right hand. There is loss of the brachioradialis reflex on the right side, despite reinforcement. There are no other abnormalities.

Given the sparing of triceps power and reflex, this would be most consistent with a right radial nerve palsy due to damage to the nerve secondary to humeral fracture.

To complete my assessment, I would like to examine the cranial nerves and lower limbs, perform a vascular assessment of the upper limb and examine for fractures elsewhere.'

Station 5: PERIPHERAL NERVE EXAM (LOWER LIMB)

Mr Romberg has long-standing diabetes mellitus. He is concerned that he is continually injuring his feet without realising it. Please perform a neurological examination of this patient's lower limbs.

Inspection

- Walking aids, wheelchairs, shoes (especially tailor made orthoses)
- Wasting (particularly evident in hip girdle and quadriceps)
- Posture
- Abnormal movements (e.g. pill-rolling tremor in Parkinson's disease)
- Fasciculation (most easily identified in quadriceps and peroneal muscles)

Walk (can be done at the beginning or the end of examination)

- If possible, get the patient up and see how they can manage to walk from one end of the room to the other. Look for gaits such as festinant (Parkinson's disease), antalgic (e.g. due to osteoarthritis of hip), scissoring (cerebral palsy), ataxic (cerebellar dysfunction), marche-à-petit-pas (diffuse cerebrovascular disease) or foot-slapping (sensory polyneuropathy)
- Consider additional examinations whilst the patient is standing e.g. tandem walk and Romberg's test as appropriate: see cerebellar examination (section 2.6)

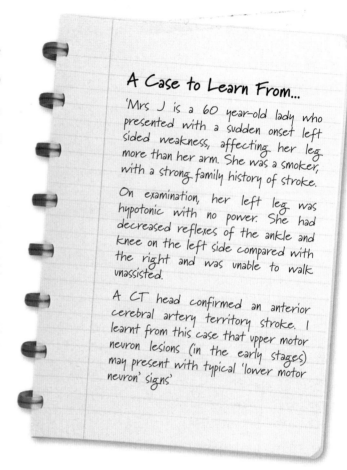

A Case to Learn From...

'Mrs J is a 60 year-old lady who presented with a sudden onset left sided weakness, affecting her leg more than her arm. She was a smoker, with a strong family history of stroke.

On examination, her left leg was hypotonic with no power. She had decreased reflexes of the ankle and knee on the left side compared with the right and was unable to walk unassisted.

A CT head confirmed an anterior cerebral artery territory stroke. I learnt from this case that upper motor neuron lesions (in the early stages) may present with typical 'lower motor neuron' signs'

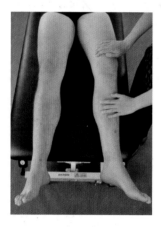

Tone

- Ask the patient to lie flat on their back
- Ensure that the patient is relaxed and the limbs are floppy
- Roll the patient's legs from side to side, looking at feet for resistance
- Abruptly lift the knee and note the movement of lower leg – in hypertonia, the ankle will come off the examination couch, even if the patient is relaxed
- Passively flex and extend the knee joint

Fig 2.34: Assessing tone by gently rolling the leg from side to side

Power

Movement	Muscle (s)	Nerve	Root
Hip Flexion	Iliopsoas	Lumbar sacral plexus	L1, L2
Hip Extension	Gluteus maximus	Inferior gluteal	L5, S1
Knee Flexion	Hamstrings	Sciatic	L5, S1
Knee Extension	Quadriceps	Femoral	L3,4
Ankle Plantar Flexion	Gastrocnemius	Posterior tibial	S1
Ankle Dorsiflexion	Tibialis anterior	Deep peroneal	L4, L5
Hallux Extension	Extensor hallucis longus	Deep peroneal	L5

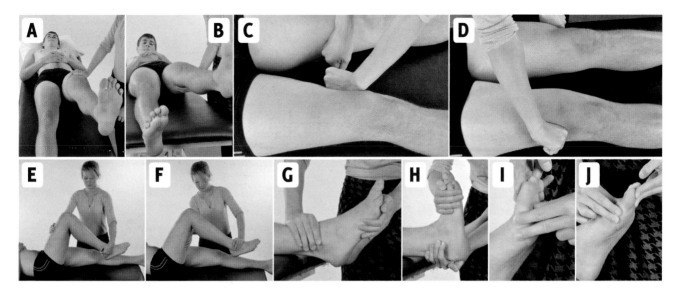

Fig 2.35: (Top: left to right) A: hip flexion, B: extension, C: adduction, D: abduction (Bottom: left to right) E: knee flexion, F: knee extension, G: ankle plantar flexion, H: ankle dorsiflexion, I: toe extension, J: toe flexion. Note isolation of knee and ankle joints.

A. 'Lift your leg up off the bed without bending your knee. Do not let me push you down'

B. 'Now push your thigh down towards the bed'

C. 'Push your knees together'

D. 'Push your knees apart'

E. 'Bend your knees and pull your heel into your body'

F. 'Now straighten your leg as though you're kicking a football'

G. 'Push your foot down like you're pushing down on an accelerator'

H. 'Now bend your foot up towards your head'

I. 'Push your big toe up'

J. 'Push your big toe down'

Reflexes

- Reinforce if reflexes absent (Jendrassik manoeuvre)
- Knee tendon reflex (L3/4)
- Ankle tendon reflex (S1/2)

When eliciting a knee reflex, look for contraction of quadriceps muscle. Obtaining ankle reflexes can be difficult: the foot should be pulled up with one hand into dorsiflexion, before striking the Achilles with the tendon hammer. Another method is to get the patient to kneel on a chair, with ankles dangling off the side.

- Plantar reflex: use the blunt end of an object, e.g. reverse end of a pen to run up the lateral aspect of the sole of an unsocked foot
- Ankle clonus (more than 3 beats is abnormal)

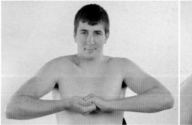

Fig 2.36: Reinforcement with the Jendrassik manoeuvre (left); knee reflex (right)

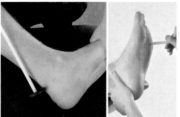

Fig 2.37: Ankle reflex (left) plantar reflex (right)

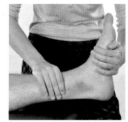

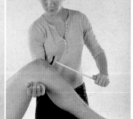

Fig 2.38: Ankle clonus testing

Co-ordination

- In the supine position, ask the patient to 'run your left heel from the right knee down along the shin of your right leg'
- Ask them then to make an arc in the air with their heel and repeat the above
- This should then be repeated with opposite legs

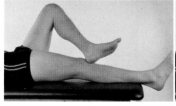

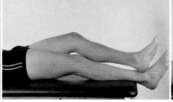

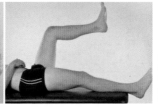

Fig 2.39: Coordination testing: the ankle should be placed on the knee, (left) rolled down the shin, (middle) lifted back up to the knee in an arc (right), and the cycle repeated

Sensation

Provide a reference stimulus by touching the sternum first. Then test by dabbing (rather than stroking) in each dermatome whilst the patient's eyes are closed. Regularly ask if one side is any different from the other. To ensure that you're covering all dermatomes and the major nerves, test the following areas:

- Upper outer thigh (lateral cutaneous nerve of thigh L2)
- Inner aspect of thigh (femoral nerve L3)
- Medial lower leg (saphenous nerve L4)
- Upper outer aspect of lower leg (common peroneal nerve L5)
- Dorsal surface, medial aspect of big toe (superficial peroneal nerve L5)
- Heel of foot (tibial nerve S1)
- Posterior aspect of knee (sciatic nerve S2)

Repeat for pain (using a neurotip), then test proprioception (start with small amplitude movements in the most distal joint). If spinal cord pathology is suspected, e.g. demyelinating lesion from Multiple Sclerosis, then it's important to assess the sensory level at which sensation changes (decreases, increases or alters) when moving in a caudal to cranial direction.

If abnormalities are present, consider vibration and temperature testing, and cerebellar function testing e.g. Romberg's test

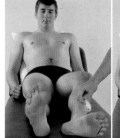
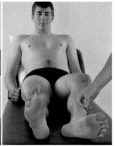

Fig 2.40: Assessing light touch (left) and pain (right). Ensure that the patient's eyes are shut

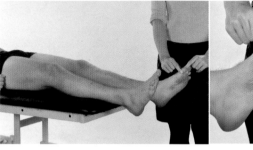

Fig 2.41: Proprioception: ensure you hold the toe from the sides to avoid excessive sensory stimulation. Ensure that the patient's eyes are shut

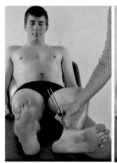
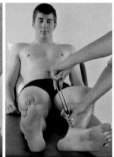

Fig 2.42: Vibration sense – ask the patient when they feel the vibration stop. Ensure that the patient's eyes are shut

What is the Brown-Sequard syndrome? Describe the pattern of sensory loss.

The Brown-Sequard syndrome is the clinical presentation that results from lateral disruption to only one side of the spinal cord.

This leads to ipsilateral loss of light touch, proprioception and vibration, and contralateral loss of pain and temperature. This is because the fibres of the spinothalamic tract cross early on entry to the spinal cord, whereas the dorsal columns do not decussate until they ascend to the medulla.

Causes of Brown-Sequard syndrome include trauma, pressure effects of vertebral metastases, cervical spondylosis, transverse myelitis and multiple sclerosis.

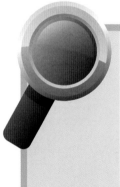

PRESENT YOUR FINDINGS...

'Mr Romberg is an overweight gentleman who walks with the aid of one stick. He has a foot-slapping gait and a positive Romberg's test.

He has decreased sensation to light touch and pain up to the ankle, in a stocking distribution. Motor examination is unremarkable.

Mr Romberg has a bilateral symmetrical sensory neuropathy. Given the stocking distribution of sensory loss, the findings are consistent with diabetic polyneuropathy.

In order to complete my assessment, I would like to examine the upper limbs and cranial nerves, check the fundi, dip the urine and check the other organ systems for complications of diabetes.'

Station 6: CEREBELLAR EXAM

Mr Gordon presents to you because of persistent falling whilst walking. He also finds that when reaching for objects, he keeps missing them. Examine his cerebellar function and then present your findings.

General Inspection

- Walking aids
- Dishevelled appearance (may suggest alcohol excess)
- Signs of chronic liver disease (e.g. palmar erythema, spider naevi)

Gait

- Ask the patient to walk up and down the room: look for a broad-based gait and irregular stride rhythm and length
- If you fail to detect any abnormality, then also ask the patient to tandem walk – *'please walk placing one foot in front of the other as if on a tightrope'* – this may bring out an ataxic gait

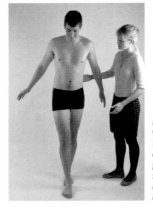

Fig 2.43: Tandem walking – ensure that you remain close to the patient, to support them in case they become unstable

Eye Signs

Slow pursuit movements: *'please follow the movements of my pen, while keeping your head still'*. Test in all directions (as for ocular muscle examination), holding gaze at lateral and vertical positions to try and elicit nystagmus. To test rapid eye movements, make a fist with one hand, and an open palm with other. Rapidly shout 'fist' and 'palm', while asking the patient to look at the respective hand in response.

- Look for square-wave jerks (SWJ) and saccadic intrusions (SI)
- A saccade is a fast eye movement. SWJ are inappropriate saccades that take the eye away from its focus. There is then a subsequent pause, followed by a corrective saccade back to the original target
- Saccadic intrusions are similar, but not necessarily followed by a return movement. They may be associated with cerebellar disease

Fig 2.44: Rapid eye movement testing: the patient alternates between looking at the fist and palm on the examiner's command

Speech

- Say: *'British constitution'*; now say: *'West Register Street'*; now say: *'Baby hippopotamus'*; listen for slurring of the speech
- Longer speech: ask them *'how do you make a cup of tea?'*; listen for staccato

Upper Limb Examination

- **Cerebellar rebound:** with the patient's arms held out in front of them, say to them that you're going to press their arms downward and let go and that they should try to restore their arms to the original position; look for overshoot
- **Finger-nose test:** *'bring your index finger out to touch my finger, now touch your nose, repeat that as quickly and accurately as you can'*; hold index finger out at arm's length; look for intention tremor and dysmetria
- **Dysdiadochokinesis:** *'slap your hand with the palm of the other hand, now slap it using the other side, back to the palm, keep repeating that as fast as you can'*

> 'The evaluation of cerebellar signs is rather dependent on a prior motor and sensory examination. Some features of cerebellar disease such as incoordination can indeed be an expression of proprioceptive loss or weakness'
>
> **Richard Knight**
> *Professor of Neurology, University of Edinburgh*

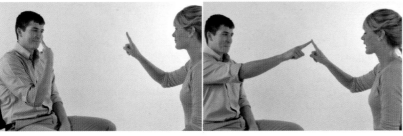

Fig 2.45: Finger nose testing: ensure that the patient is at full arm's length when touching your finger

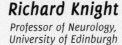

Examination

What is nystagmus?

Nystagmus describes a rhythmical, involuntary, oscillatory movement of the eye that can be elicited when the eyes look horizontally or vertically. This can be a normal variant at extremes of horizontal gaze. However, if nystagmus is pathological, then it should occur less than 30 degrees from the midline.

Causes of a Cerebellar Syndrome

- *Alcohol*
- *Drugs e.g. phenytoin*
- *Multiple sclerosis*
- *Hereditary ataxias e.g. Friedreich's ataxia*
- *Tumours of the posterior fossa*
- *Metastatic disease e.g. lung/ breast primary*
- *Infection e.g. varicella zoster and legionella*

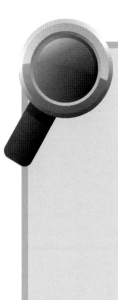

PRESENT YOUR FINDINGS...

'Mr Gordon has an ataxic gait. On testing ocular pursuit movements, nystagmus was elicited at mid-lateral gaze and he demonstrated ocular dysmetria on testing fast saccadic eye movements. He has slurred speech, intention tremor and past-pointing. I also note that he has stigmata of chronic liver disease.

This is consistent with cerebellar dysfunction, perhaps secondary to ethanol excess.

In order to complete my assessment, I would like to do a full neurological examination, take an alcohol history and complete an abdominal examination.'

Station 7: PARKINSON'S EXAM

Mr Smith has been referred to your neurology clinic. His GP is concerned that Mr Smith has signs of Parkinsonism. Please examine the patient for this and present your findings.

General Inspection

- Start, if possible, with the patient sitting in a chair, hands on their lap
- Look around for walking aids
- Look and listen for hypomimia (reduced degree of facial expression), hypophonia (soft speech), drooling, resting tremor of hands and/or feet

Tremor

- Ask the patient to close their eyes and slowly count backwards from twenty (this should elicit/accentuate any tremor)
- See if any other tremor is evident: *'hold out your arms straight with the palms facing the floor'* (postural); finger-nose test (intention tremor due to cerebellar disease)
- Note that the finger-nose test should dampen a Parkinson's disease (PD) tremor, but accentuate a benign essential tremor
- A PD tremor is normally markedly asymmetrical. Remember that up to a third of patients with idiopathic Parkinson's disease will not have a tremor

Bradykinesia

- Using one hand first, ask the patient to *'move your fingers towards your thumb as though closing a duck's beak, then open it up, close it; repeat as fast and accurately as you can'*
- *'Using both hands, imagine you are playing the piano in mid-air/on this table; lift your fingers as high as you can; and play as fast as you can'*
- Look for bradykinetic fade in both of the above
- Micrographia (abnormally small writing): *'write the sentence "Little red riding hood" on this paper'; 'repeat it below'; 'and again'* – stop after about five sentences

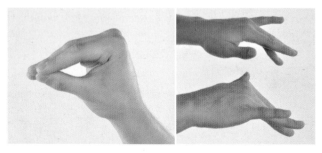

Fig 2.46: Testing for bradykinesia: duck beak movements (left) piano playing movements (right)

Rigidity

- Passively circumduct a wrist and then flex/extend at the elbow; repeat on the other side: feel for lead-pipe rigidity and cogwheeling

Gait and Postural Instability

- Ask the patient to walk normally from one side of the room to the other, and then to turn around and come back; look for gait ignition failure, festinance, reduced arm swing, stooped posture and en bloc turning
- Pull test: with the patient still standing warn them that you need to test their tendency to fall backwards (retropulsion) and will need to pull them back, but you will be behind to support them; then, with both hands on each of the patient's shoulders, pull them back sharply
- In idiopathic Parkinson's disease, postural instability is a late sign to develop; therefore, if this was present early/at onset, an alternative diagnosis should be sought

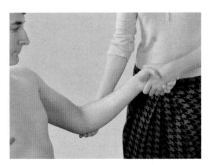

Fig 2.47: Taking the weight off arm for tone assessment

Parkinson-Plus Syndromes

The Parkinson-plus syndromes are all neurodegenerative disorders, in which Parkinsonian features occur alongside other symptoms and signs.

- Eye movements: look for vertical downward ophthalmoplegia (Progressive Supranuclear Palsy)
- Assess speech (any nasal or staccato quality?); feel temperature of the hands and measure capillary refill time; consider erect and supine blood pressure (Multiple System Atrophy)

Progressive Supranuclear Palsy: vertical gaze dysfunction; frequent falling
Multiple System Atrophy: urogenital problems (i.e. incontinence and/or erectile dysfunction), and/or orthostatic hypotension. Cerebellar, as opposed to Parkinsonian, features may occur

Fig 2.48: 'Pull test' – patient sharply pulled back from shoulders

Glossary of Terms

- **Bradykinetic fading:** performed movements get progressively slower
- **Cogwheeling:** intermittent, regular elicitation of resistance on passive movement of a limb, due to co-occurrence of tremor and rigidity
- **Festinant gait:** involuntary acceleration of rate of steps
- **Gait-ignition failure:** difficulty initiating walking
- **Lead-pipe rigidity:** increased tone throughout range of passive movement
- **Micrographia:** small, spidery handwriting
- **Retropulsion:** the tendency to step backwards involuntarily if pulled from behind

What are the differential diagnoses of idiopathic Parkinson's disease?

- Vascular Parkinson's disease
- Dementia with Lewy Bodies
- Anti-dopaminergic drugs (e.g. phenothiazines, metoclopramide)
- Parkinson-plus syndromes
- Wilson's disease
- Dementia Pugilistica

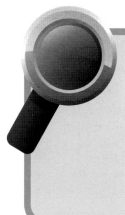

PRESENT YOUR FINDINGS...

'Mr Smith has a unilateral, pill-rolling, rest tremor of his right hand, dampened by movement. He has bradykinesia of his right side and has marked micrographia. He has bilateral rigidity with noticeable cogwheel rigidity at the right wrist. He walks with the aid of one stick and has a stooped, festinant gait. There is no evidence of Parkinson-plus syndromes.

Given the clinical features and asymmetrical nature of his tremor and bradykinesia, the most likely diagnosis is idiopathic Parkinson's disease.'

Station 8: GASTROINTESTINAL EXAM

Mr McClintock has been feeling increasingly tired and confused. His wife feels that Mr McClintock doesn't look like himself anymore. He has been bruising more easily, and has a long history of excessive alcohol consumption. Please perform a gastrointestinal examination on this gentleman.

General Inspection

- Expose patient from nipple to knee ideally, but maintain their dignity
- Ensure that the patient is lying flat
- Inspect for wasting, distension, scars
- Look generally for spider naevi, gynaecomastia, bruising, tattoos, and peripheral oedema

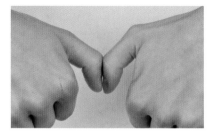

Fig 2.49: Assessing for clubbing: look for a diamond formed between thumbnails

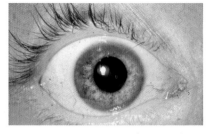

Fig 2.50: Kayser-Fleischer rings (yellow brown ring at corneo-scleral junction) – associated with Wilson's syndrome

Hands

- Clubbing, palmar erythema, Dupuytren's contractures, leukonychia, koilonychia
- Liver flap: a sign of hepatic encephalopathy
- Pulse and blood pressure: particularly important if a gastrointestinal bleed is suspected

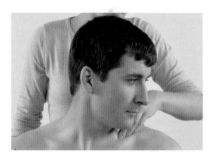

Fig 2.51: Palpating for Virchow's node: this is more easily palpable with the head turned to the left

Face

- Eyes: jaundice, anaemia, Kayser-Fleischer rings
- Mouth: gingivitis, ulcers, hydration, peri-oral pigmentation, hepatic fetor

Causes of Hepatomegaly

- *Primary hepatocellular carcinoma*
- *Metastatic liver disease*
- *Cirrhosis*
- *Nonalcoholic fatty liver disease*
- *Hepatitis*
- *Leukaemia*
- *Lymphoma*

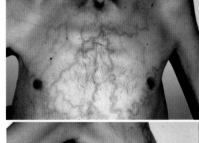

Fig 2.52: Grey-turner's sign: retroperitoneal bleeding associated with pancreatitis, and ruptured abdominal aortic aneurysm

Neck

- Supraclavicular nodes: a palpable Virchow's node in the left supraclavicular fossa is known as 'Troisier's sign'. It is suggestive of gastric carcinoma

Abdominal Inspection

- *'Please put your hands by your side and breathe normally'*
- Ensure the patient is lying flat and ask if there is any pain
- Look for scars anteriorly, posteriorly, and in the flanks
- Look for distension, dilated veins, and areas of fullness (masses, organomegaly, and ascites)
- Ask patient to blow out there tummy and/or ask them to cough. If either action elicits abdominal pain, it may be a sign of peritonism

Causes of Splenomegaly

- *MASSIVE: Chronic Myeloid Leukaemia, Myelofibrosis, Kala-azar*

- *MODERATE: Lymphoma, Chronic Lymphocytic Leukaemia, Malaria*

- *MILD: Epstein-Barr virus, Hepatitis, Portal Hypertension, Rheumatoid Arthritis (Felty's Syndrome)*

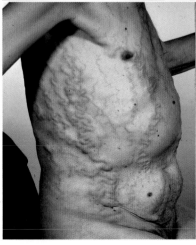

Fig 2.53: Dilated abdominal wall veins (due to portal hypertension) from front (top) and side (bottom) profile

Surgical Scars (example of corresponding operations in brackets)

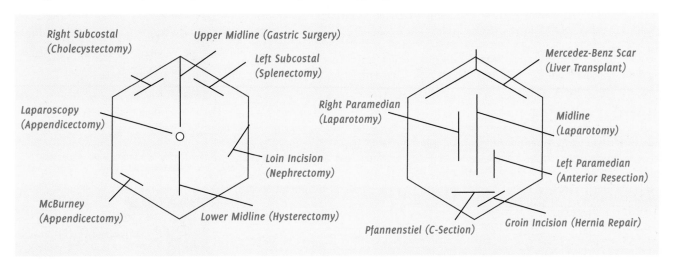

Right Subcostal (Cholecystectomy)

Upper Midline (Gastric Surgery)

Left Subcostal (Splenectomy)

Laparoscopy (Appendicectomy)

Loin Incision (Nephrectomy)

McBurney (Appendicectomy)

Lower Midline (Hysterectomy)

Right Paramedian (Laparotomy)

Mercedez-Benz Scar (Liver Transplant)

Midline (Laparotomy)

Left Paramedian (Anterior Resection)

Pfannenstiel (C-Section)

Groin Incision (Hernia Repair)

Palpation

- Palpate whilst at the level of the patient. Look at the patient's face whilst palpating for evidence of pain
- Light followed by deep palpation
- Palpate liver, spleen, and kidneys
  - Hepatomegaly: edge, consistency, and size measured in finger-breadths
- Palpate for abdominal aortic aneurysm (pulsatile and expansile)

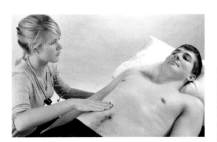

Fig 2.54: Palpating the abdomen: looking at the face for signs of pain, and positioned at the level of the patient

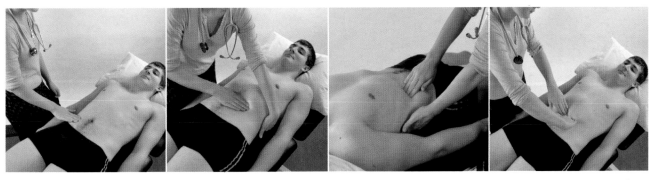

Fig 2.55: (Left to right) liver (starting in right iliac fossa), left kidney, right kidney, palpating for an aortic aneurysm

Percussion

- Percuss all four quadrants of the abdomen
- Percuss the liver (from the right iliac fossa and from the chest), and percuss spleen
- Percussion tenderness

Shifting dullness/fluid thrill to look for ascites

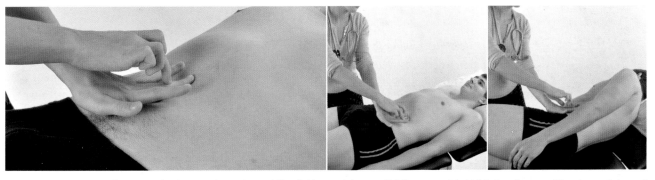

Fig 2.56: Shifting dullness: (left to right) percuss abdomen from midline (left) to periphery until dullness noted (middle). Keep finger at this point, and then roll patient toward you. Percuss again after 30 seconds, and note if now the note is resonant (positive test)

Auscultation

- Listen for bowel sounds over the ileo-cecal valve (for 30 seconds)
- Bruits: listen over aorta and renal arteries (use bell)
- If you find hepatomegaly, you may listen for bruit over the liver (suggestive of a hepatoma, acute alcoholic hepatitis or Transjugular Intrahepatic Portosystemic Stent Shunt (TIPSS))

Hernial Orifices

- Mark out midway between the anterior superior iliac spine and pubic symphysis. Place your hand over this point and ask the patient to cough

To complete the examination, say you would like to do a rectal examination and examine the external genitalia.

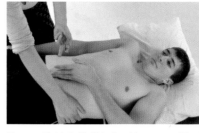

Fig 2.57: Fluid thrill: flick the skin on one side of the abdomen and feel for a 'thrill' on the other side with your hand. Place the patients hand in the midline to stop transmission through the skin (since you only want to measure transmission through fluid)

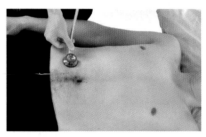

Fig 2.58: Auscultation over the ileo-cecal valve

Causes of Ascites

- *HYPOALBUMINAEMIA: Cirrhosis (commonest), Protein malnutrition or malabsorption, Nephrotic syndrome*
- *PORTAL HYPERTENSION: Chronic liver disease*
- *INFLAMMATION: Metastatic carcinoma, Pelvic carcinoma (ovary), Infection, e.g. peritoneal tuberculosis*

'Don't forget that loud cardiac murmurs may be heard (and mistaken) as bruits over the liver'

John Plevris
Consultant Gastroenterologist
University of Edinburgh

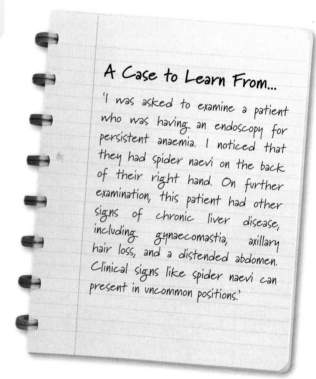

A Case to Learn From...

'I was asked to examine a patient who was having an endoscopy for persistent anaemia. I noticed that they had spider naevi on the back of their right hand. On further examination, this patient had other signs of chronic liver disease, including gynaecomastia, axillary hair loss, and a distended abdomen. Clinical signs like spider naevi can present in uncommon positions.'

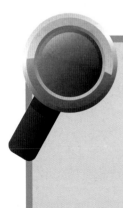

PRESENT YOUR FINDINGS...

'This is Mr. McClintock who presented with worsening bruising on a background of alcohol excess.

On examination, he looks well. He has bilateral palmar erythema and dupuytren's contractures, bruising and scratch marks on both arms and 8 spider naevi on his upper chest wall. Mr McClintock is also jaundiced, with axillary hair loss, and gynaecomastia. His abdomen is soft and non-tender. It is distended, with shifting dullness. There is no organomegaly. Bowel sounds are normal. Examination is otherwise unremarkable.

This is consistent with a diagnosis of chronic liver disease. To complete my examination, I would review his observation chart, inspect external genitalia, examine hernial orifices, perform a PR exam and request an abdominal USS.'

Station 9: HERNIA EXAMINATION

Mr Jarral is a 91 year-old gentleman who has presented with abdominal pain and distension. He has also been vomiting and has noticed a lump in the groin. Please examine this gentleman's groin and present your findings.

General Inspection

- Expose from the umbilicus down to knees and ask the patient to stand, as this will make swellings more obvious
- Look for any scars, visible masses or redness of the skin: pay particular attention to the inguinal, femoral and scrotal regions
- Next, ask the patient to cough to accentuate any hernia

Palpation

- Gently feel the hernia, assessing for tenderness and observing their face for discomfort
- Ask for a cough, feeling over the mass for a palpable cough impulse
- Define the local anatomy, highlighting each bony prominence in turn with a finger placement: this will help you appreciate the course of the inguinal ligament:

  - **Pubic tubercle**: hernias **above and medial** to your finger are likely to be inguinal, whereas those **below and lateral** are more likely femoral
  - **Anterior superior iliac spine**: thus allowing you to find the midpoint between the **anterior superior iliac spine and the public tubercle**: midpoint of the inguinal ligament (the site of the deep inguinal ring)
  - Note: the 'mid-inguinal point' is different: this is halfway between the **anterior superior iliac spine and the pubic symphisis**

- Ask the patient if their hernia ever 'goes back in'. First ask the patient to reduce it on their own, and if they cannot, attempt to do it yourself. The patient ideally should be supine in the Trendelenberg position (with the feet higher than the head) when trying to reduce an inguinal hernia. Standing up will make it pop out
- Once reduced, keep fingers held over the site of reduction
- Then apply firm pressure with two fingers over midpoint of the inguinal ligament, which you have just located (whilst still pressing on the site of reduction)
- Release the patient's fingers (or your fingers) from the site of reduction (whilst keeping other fingers on the midpoint of the inguinal ligament)
- Ask the patient to cough once more. For an inguinal hernia, this will allow you to differentiate direct from indirect hernia:

  - **If the hernia is controlled (it does not reappear)** ➤ Indirect hernia
  - **If the hernia is uncontrolled (it reappears)** ➤ Direct hernia
  - The only *definitive* way to differentiate between the two is intra-operatively

Auscultate

- Listen over the hernia for bowel sounds, particularly in large hernias

To Complete your Examination

- If time allows, examine the contralateral side for herniae, perform an abdominal examination, and examine the scrotum (see station 2.10). Thank the patient and cover them up

> 'Key points: Examine the patient both standing and lying. Start with whichever is convenient. Expose the scrotum in a male (other lumps may be there, to trick you!) Check the other side while you're there'
>
> **Bruce Tulloh**
> Consultant General Surgeon
> University of Edinburgh

Groin Lump Differentials

- *Hernia*
- *Lymph node*
- *Saphena varix*
- *Femoral aneurysm*
- *Abscess*
- *Undescended testis*
- *Lipoma*

Indirect Inguinal Hernia (80%)	Direct Inguinal Hernia (20%)
Viscus passes through the deep ring into the inguinal canal (therefore it is controlled by pressure over deep ring)	Viscus passes through a defect in the abdominal wall, sometimes bulging into the inguinal canal

What is the definition of a hernia?

A **Hernia** is a protrusion of a viscus (or part of a viscus) through a defect in the wall of its containing cavity and into an anatomically abnormal position.

'Auscultation maybe useful for a large hernia, but I don't think it is necessary. Contents are either bowel or omentum (rarely other small things; e.g. appendix or ovary, bladder)'

Bruce Tulloh

Consultant General Surgeon, University of Edinburgh

Common Hernia

Inguinal Hernia	A protrusion of a viscus (commonly bowel) through the inguinal canal
Femoral Hernia	A protrusion of a viscus (commonly bowel) through the femoral canal
Incisional Hernia	A protrusion of a viscus (commonly bowel) through an acquired defect, which is iatrogenic (previous surgery) or from injury (knife wounds)

Complications of Hernia

Irreducible Hernia	Cannot be reduced, but not necessarily causing bowel obstruction or vascular compromise
Obstructed Hernia	Intestine within the hernia sac is obstructed
Strangulated Hernia	Irreducible hernia which results in vascular compromise, and infarction of the obstructed bowel

Rare Hernia

Richter's hernia	A hernia involving only one side of the bowel wall (also known as partial enterocele)
Amyand's hernia	Inguinal hernias where the hernia contains the appendix
Spigelian hernia	A hernia protruding through the spigelian fascia (aponeurosis of transversus abdominis muscle, which fills the space between the edge of the rectus and the muscle belly of the transversus). The fascia is widest (and therefore weakest) just below the level of the umbilicus, but Spigelian hernia can occur anywhere along this line
Littre's hernia	A hernia involving Meckel's diverticulum

Anatomy

The Inguinal Canal

The communicating passage running obliquely from the deep ring to the superficial ring. The four walls can be remembered as follows:

- **Posterior**
  Transversalis fascia and conjoint tendon (medially)
- **Anterior**
  External oblique
- **Inferior**
  Inguinal ligament
- **Superior**
  Conjoint tendon (of the internal oblique and the transversus muscles)

Midpoint of the Inguinal Ligament

- The site of the deep inguinal ring, found halfway along the inguinal ligament – demarcated by the imaginary dashed line from the **anterior superior iliac spine** (ASIS) to the **pubic tubercle** (PT) (see diagram)

Mid Inguinal Point

- The site of the femoral artery, found halfway along the imaginary dashed line (see diagram) drawn from the **anterior superior iliac spine** (ASIS) to the **pubic symphysis** (PS) (see diagram)

In men, the inguinal canal conveys the spermatic cord and in women the round ligament; it also contains the ilioinguinal nerve, the genital branch of the genitofemoral nerve and lymphatics.

Hesselbach's Triangle

- The defined anatomical region within which hernias are direct. The borders are:

  - **Inferiorly:** Inguinal ligament
  - **Superiorly:** Inferior epigastric blood vessels
  - **Medially:** Rectus abdominis

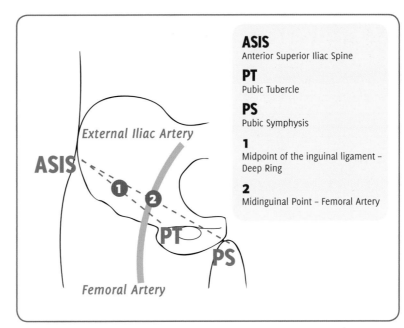

ASIS
Anterior Superior Iliac Spine

PT
Pubic Tubercle

PS
Pubic Symphysis

1
Midpoint of the inguinal ligament – Deep Ring

2
Midinguinal Point – Femoral Artery

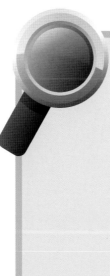

PRESENT YOUR FINDINGS...

'Mr Jarral is comfortable at rest. He has a distended abdomen, with a visible lump over the right inguinal region. There are no associated skin changes. The lump is tender, reducible and controlled with pressure over the deep ring. Bowel sounds are present over the lump.

This is consistent with a diagnosis of a right sided indirect inguinal hernia (although the question of being direct or indirect can only be confirmed during surgery).

To complete my examination, I would like perform a full abdominal examination, examine the external genitalia and perform a rectal examination'

Station 10: TESTICULAR EXAMINATION

Mr Smith is a 20 year-old gentleman who has noticed swelling of his right testicle. Please perform the appropriate examination and present your findings.

Introduction

- Introduce yourself to the patient
- Wash your hands and put on gloves
- Ask for a chaperone
- Whilst allowing the patient privacy, ask them to remove all of their clothing from the waist down and provide a modesty sheet

The remainder of the examination involves INSPECTION and PALPATION.

Inspection

General Inspection

- Is the patient visibly in pain?
- Note any gynaecomastia (exposing the patient above the waist)
- Look for secondary sexual characteristics (hormone secreting tumours)

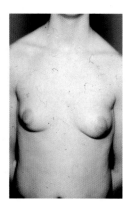

Fig 2.59: Gynaecomastia

Inspection of the Scrotum

- Assess the size and shape of the scrotum: comment on any obvious swelling, asymmetry, or lumps
- Note that the left testicle often is lower than the right in normal people
- Look for ulcers, swelling, rashes and scrotal oedema
- Assess the distribution of pubic hair
- Look for scars (previous hernia surgery, previous exploration of scrotum)
- Ensure that both the front and back of the scrotum are inspected

Inspect the Penis

- Examine for ulceration and discharge
- Assess the position of urethral meatus

Palpation

General Principles

- Ask the patient if they are in any pain
- Warm your hands
- Ask the patient to stand up
- Examine the normal side first

Testes

1. Are they present?
- Causes of impalpable testis: undescended testis, retracted testis (due to cold hands, for example), previous orchidectomy

2. What size are they?
- Are they symmetrical or asymmetrical?
- If one is larger, is the whole testis larger or is there a discrete mass?
  - Small: hypogonadism, cold temperature (muscles contracted)
  - Large: hydrocele, varicocele, tumour

3. If there is a lump – can you get above the lump?
- If not, consider an inguinal hernia as the cause of the lump. For a suspected hernia, elicit a cough impulse at this point and perform hernia examination (see station 2.9)
- If you can get above it, the lump is scrotal in origin – consider the following four questions to help with your diagnosis:
  1. Is it separate from, or part of, the testis?
  2. Is it cystic or solid?
  3. Is it tender or non-tender?
  4. Does it transilluminate? (hydrocele)

Consistency	Testicular	Separate from Testes
Solid	**Tender** orchitis testicular torsion **Non-Tender** tumour granuloma	**Tender** epididymitis
Cystic	**Non Tender** hydrocele	**Non-Tender** epididymal cyst hydrocele of spermatic cord varicocele spermatocele

- **Orchitis and epididymitis:** have different aetiologies depending on age group. In young adults/adolescents, consider sexually transmitted infections, tuberculosis and mumps. In the elderly, consider E. coli infection
- **Spermatocele:** smooth, soft, well circumscribed. Typically arises from the head of the epididymis (superior aspect of testicle). Fluid usually contains sperm
- **Cyst of the epididymis:** similar to spermatocele, smooth, soft, well circumscribed, but well above the testis and separate from it. Contains clear straw-coloured fluid. Transilluminates and if multilocular gives a "Chinese lantern" appearance
- **Hydrocele:** fluid collection, covering the anterior and lateral aspects of the testis. Presents as soft, non-tender fullness, which transilluminates

- **Varicocele:** dilated venous plexus along spermatic cord, like a 'bag of worms'. More common in the left than the right (due to anatomical factors e.g. the lack of antireflux valves at the juncture of the left testicular vein and the left renal vein)
- **Haematocele:** haemorrhage into tunica vaginalis usually secondary to trauma. Presents with pain; tenderness and rapid refilling of the sac on examination, poor or absent transillumination because it is generally solid clot
- **Torsed epididymal appendix:** exquisite tenderness localized to the upper pole of the testis. Appears as a black dot on transillumination

Completing Your Examination

- Feel the epididymis head, body and tail
- Feel the spermatic cord using two fingers, tracing it from the testes to the inguinal region
- Feel **inguinal lymph nodes** for scrotal pathology – *NB testicular infection/malignancy tends to spread to the para-aortic nodes, not the inguinal nodes*
- Ask the patient if they'd like to learn how to do a self examination, so they can pick up problems on their own
- Cover the patient up again when you finish

What investigations would you do next and how would you manage this patient?

Investigations:
- Consider secondary causes of a hydrocele e.g. fluid retention, infection
- Ultrasound scan to differentiate spermatocele from hydrocele
- Ultrasound is also useful for assessing the likelihood of malignancy

Management:
- May only require conservative management
- Fluid may be aspirated, but to ensure no further recurrence, surgery is required

How would you explain to this patient how to self-examine his testicles in the future?

- Examine whilst in the bath or shower (as heat softens the skin making it easier to feel the testicles)
- Feel for lumps on the skin
- Feel for swellings inside the scrotum
- Examine each testicle separately and then compare both testicles (noting that it can be normal to have one that is larger and lower)
  - Use both hands and roll the testicle between the thumb and forefinger
- If there are any abnormalities or any concerns, seek medical advice

Common Testicular Malignancies

	Teratoma	Seminoma	Lymphoma
Definition	A germ cell tumour, with tissue components not normally found at that site	Germ cell tumour. Histological diagnosis of 'pure seminomatous elements' (large round cells with vascular nuclei) and normal alpha-fetoprotein blood levels	A solid tumour of the lymphoid cells
Age	Mainly affects 20-30 year olds	Mainly affects 30-40 year olds	Mainly affects the elderly
Relative Incidence	40-50%	40-50%	0-10%
Management	Chemotherapy, Surgery	Radiotherapy, Chemotherapy, Surgery	Surgery, Chemotherapy, Radiotherapy
Prognosis	Intermediate Prognosis	Highly curable if detected early	Poorest Prognosis: around 50% have systemic disease at presentation

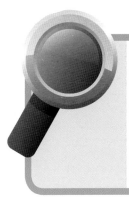

PRESENT YOUR FINDINGS...

'Mr Smith has a smooth, well circumscribed lump measuring 4cm by 6cm on the anterior aspect of his right testicle. It is soft, non-tender and transilluminates. It is not separate from the testes. Examination of the external genitalia is otherwise unremarkable.

These findings are consistent with a right hydrocele.'

Station 11: STOMA EXAMINATION

Mr Pouch has attended a general surgery outpatient clinic. Please examine the stoma bag, and present your findings.

Definition

- A stoma is an artificial (deliberate) connection between a hollow viscus and the skin surface

General Inspection

- Expose the patient as you would for an abdominal examination and continue to take stance at the foot of the bed
- Inspect the area around stoma for signs of infection, fistula or skin excoriation
- Describing a stoma is best done in a systematic manner. Paying attention to the following attributes in turn will allow you to deduce the stoma type:

SITE

- Describe in relation to quadrants of the abdomen

BAG

- Contents may be nothing, solid stool, liquid stool or urine

SURFACE

- Either flush with the skin (minimally raised/less protuberant) or with a protruding spout
- In terms of openings, may have a single lumen (end) or double lumen (loop)
- Note the health of the mucosa (colour) and surrounding skin

ABDOMEN

- Describe as you would in an abdominal examination, especially scars that can give vital clues as to the operative history

Palpation

- This would normally not be expected, however, if you are asked to palpate remember to be gentle, enquiring about pain and observing their face for signs of pain
- Be cautious about removing a bag as you would not want to cause leakage
- Put on a pair of gloves and squeeze some lubricant onto your index finger, then gently insert your finger into the opening:

STENOSIS

- Feel for narrowing of the opening conduit

END TYPE

- Confirm the number of openings as they are not always easy to visualise

To Complete Your Examination

- Asking the patient to cough shows that you appreciate some of the potential complications that can arise from stoma surgery, namely parastomal and incisional herniae
- Place a new ostomy appliance at the site (or the patient may prefer to do this for themselves)
- Thank the patient, cover them, wash your hands and turn to the examiner
- Mention that you would like to examine the rest of the abdomen including the perineum. Does the patient have an anus? This is important for assessing colostomy bags

What type of stoma do you think this is?

	Ileostomy	Colostomy	Urostomy
SURGICAL PROCEDURE (INDICATION)	Panproctocolectomy (e.g. ulcerative colitis) END ileostomy Anterior Resection (e.g. colorectal cancer) – usually a temporary LOOP ileostomy	Abdominoperoneal Resection – i.e. with no anus (e.g. colorectal cancer) Hartmann's procedure – i.e. with anus present (e.g. colorectal cancer)	Total Cystectomy (e.g. bladder cancer)
SITE	Right lower quadrant	Left lower quadrant	Usually right sided but can vary
BAG CONTENTS	Liquid stool	Semi-formed stool	Urine
SURFACE OPENING	Raised from the skin in a spout	Flush with the skin/ minimally raised	Usually as a spout like an ileostomy

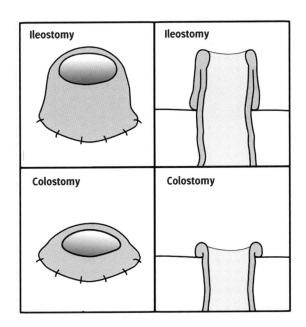

| Ileostomy | Ileostomy |
| Colostomy | Colostomy |

Complications of Stoma Bags

Immediate
- Haemorrhage

Early
- Ischaemia
- Adhesions
- Diarrhoea

Late
- Skin excoriation
- Parastomal hernia
- Stenosis
- Fistulas
- Psychosexual complications
- Nutritional deficiency
- Prolapse

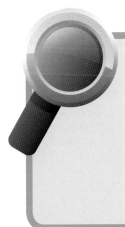

PRESENT YOUR FINDINGS...

'Mr Pouch is comfortable at rest and has a stoma located in the lower right quadrant of his abdomen. The stoma appears healthy, with liquid stool bag contents and a single lumen, which is raised from the skin. There is a midline laparotomy scar and no evidence of incisional or parastomal hernias.

These findings are consistent with an end ileostomy.

To complete my examination, i would like to examine the perineum (to look for the presence of an anus)'

Station 12: RECTAL EXAMINATION

You are an FY1 seeing an elderly gentleman who has presented with a history of altered bowel habits and PR bleeding. Treat and address the model as you would a real patient and perform a digital rectal examination, stating your positive and negative findings. He has already consented to the procedure.

General

- Ask for a chaperone
- Ask the patient to undress themselves from the waist down
- Only remove underwear when necessary: just before examination
- Position the patient in left lateral position, with their knees drawn to their chest
- Wash and glove both of your hands
- It is worthwhile placing an incontinence sheet between the patient's buttocks and the bed. This ensures that no faecal staining of the bed occurs during the exam

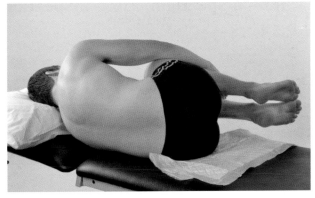

Fig 2.60: Positioning of patient for rectal examination. Note only remove underwear when necessary

Examination

Inspection

- With your left hand, gently separate the buttocks
- Inspect the anus and perianal area. Look for:
  - Fissures
  - Skin tags
  - Erythema
  - Sinuses or fistulae
  - Pilonidal sinuses
  - Haemorrhoids

What are the common causes of rectal bleeding?

- *Haemorrhoids*
- *Anal fissures*
- *Colon polyps*
- *Colorectal cancer*
- *Inflammatory bowel disease*
  - *Crohn's disease*
  - *Ulcerative colitis*
- *Intestinal infections*
- *Diverticular disease*
- *Angiodysplasia*
- *Blood loss from upper GI tract that has transited through the GI tract e.g. oesophageal varices, gastritis, gastric carcinoma*

Examination

- Lubricate your right index finger
- Separate the buttocks with your left hand and gently apply pressure with pulp of the finger to enter the anus. This will overcome sphincter tone. Insert your finger through the anus, aiming towards the umbilicus
- Palpate the anterior, right lateral, posterior and left lateral walls in turn
- Note any pain that may be elicited
- Comment on size, surface and consistency of the prostate gland (in males)
- Comment on presence of any other masses or stool in rectum
- Test anal tone: ask patient to squeeze or bear down on your finger
- Withdraw finger: inspect for faeces, blood, mucus or melaena
- Offer patient paper towel to clean themselves. The patient may require assistance if they are unable to do this independently

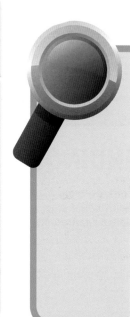

PRESENT YOUR FINDINGS...

'I performed a digital rectal examination on this gentleman in the presence of Staff Nurse Sarah Smith.

There was evidence of a fistula in the 9 o'clock position, with tenderness of the rectum on palpation. There was soft stool in the rectum, with blood and mucus mixed in.

Given the presence of the fistula, this is consistent with a diagnosis of Crohn's Disease.'

Station 13: PERIPHERAL ARTERIAL EXAMINATION

Mr Smith is a 60-year-old smoker who has developed pain in his right leg on walking. It is present at rest. Please examine the arterial system in his lower limbs and present your findings.

General Inspection

- Adequately expose: should remove trousers
- Tar stains
- Corneal arcus
- Xanthelasmata and/or xanthoma
- Previous surgical scars
- Pulse: atrial fibrillation?
- Say that you would also like to measure blood pressure and look at the fundi

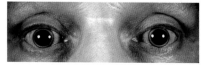

Fig 2.61: Corneal arcus

Inspection of Legs

Lay the patient on the bed and expose the legs:
- Expose and inspect both legs. Look between the toes – note any scars/ulcers/breaks in skin, examine the heels
- If a dressing is present, indicate that you would like to look underneath it
- What colour is the skin? Pale, blue, dusky red or black (ischaemic), brown
- Assess muscle bulk, particularly looking for asymmetry

Look for:
- Scars from previous surgery. Don't miss an amputation!
- Skin changes: hair loss, thickening of skin, dry skin
- Swelling
- Nail changes
- Varicose veins and signs of chronic venous disease
- Ulcers

For ulcers, describe:
- Site
  - Arterial ulcers generally appear on pressure areas such as the malleoli, 5th metatarsal base, metatarsal heads, toes and heel
  - Venous ulcers usually appear in the gaiter region of the lower leg (80% medial, 20% lateral)
- Shape, depth and edge
  - Arterial ulcers are small, regularly shaped, deep and with a "punched out" appearance and a sloughy or necrotic base
  - Venous ulcers are shallow, irregularly shaped, large with a green sloughy appearance over a pink and granulating base

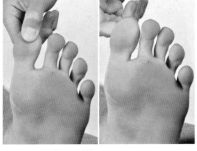
Fig 2.62: Capillary refill

Palpate

- Temperature: may be cool if the vascular supply is compromised
- Capillary refill - <2 seconds is normal after pressing the nail bed for 5 seconds
- Oedema
- Sensation
- Squeeze the calf gently – it will be tender in acute limb ischaemia
- Pulses: femoral, popliteal, dorsalis pedis, posterior tibial. If pulses are absent, use a handheld Doppler

Auscultate for femoral bruits. Palpate for AAA

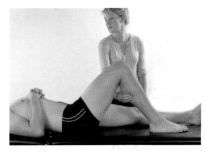
Fig 2.63: Squeezing calf

Buerger's Test

- Raise the limb slowly (up to an angle of 45°), flexing at the hip joint
- Once the limb appears pale, note the angle (Buerger's angle: smaller = more severe). If the limb does not appear pale, wait two further minutes when you reach 45°. The limb should not turn pale in a healthy individual
- After this, ask the patient to sit with their legs hanging off the side of the bed
- Normally, the legs will turn a pink colour. An abnormal result is signified by 'sunset rubor' (dusky red colour). This is reactive hyperaemia (due to arteriole dilatation to remove toxic metabolites)
- Note that this can be painful for patients, so be gentle and remember to ask if they are experiencing any pain

Tell the examiner that to complete the examination, you would like to do a full cardiovascular examination, palpate for an abdominal aneurysm, measure Ankle Brachial Pressure Index (ABPI), dip the urine for glucose (diabetes), protein, and blood (renal disease), and assess functional ability in a corridor walking test.

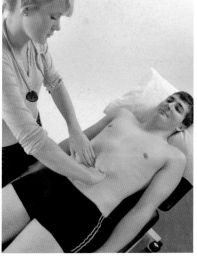
Fig 2.64: Palpating for an abdominal aortic aneurysm

Further Investigations

- Angiography/spiral CT or MRI
- Doppler/duplex assessment

Tips on Examining Pulses

Femoral

- Situated at the mid-inguinal point midway between the anterior superior iliac spine and the pubic symphysis. Remember the acronym **NAVAL**, from lateral to medial; **N**erve, **A**rtery, **V**ein **A**nd **L**ymphatics
- Press firmly down and towards the patient's head in the groin crease. Use 2 or 3 fingers

Popliteal

- This is notoriously difficult to palpate even though it is quite large and strong
- Flex the patient's knee to **30 degrees** but don't let them bend it themselves
- Place your thumbs on the patella, place your other fingers in the popliteal fossa and try to sandwich the popliteal pulse between your fingers and the back of the tibia
- If the popliteal pulse is very easy to feel, this should alert you to a possible aneurysm

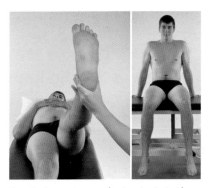
Fig 2.65: Buerger's test: a) raise the limb b) patient sitting on the edge of bed with legs hanging off the end

Posterior Tibial

- Best palpated posterior to the medial malleolus
- Place your fingers on the artery and push it up against the bony medial malleolus to feel its pulse

Dorsalis Pedis

- Draw an imaginary horizontal line between malleoli
- Drop a perpendicular line down from this to meet the first interspace (between the big toe and 2nd toe). The dorsalis pedis is palpated one third the way down this perpendicular from the malleoli

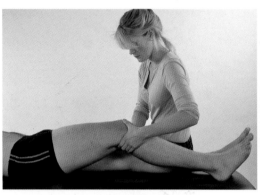
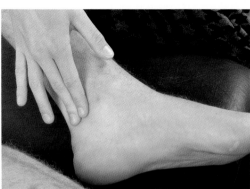

Fig 2.66: Popliteal (left), posterior tibial (right) pulses

Note: Make sure that you appreciate the difference between intermittent claudication (calf pain on walking, limb not at risk) and critical limb ischaemia (rest pain, ulceration or gangrene: limb at risk).

A Case to Learn From...

'A patient with known atrial fibrillation developed an embolic stroke. Whilst an inpatient, he then developed an acutely ischaemic left arm. This was initially missed, because the upper limb sensation loss was felt to be due to the stroke. However, a more careful examination revealed signs of acute ischemia, with loss of sensation as well as pain, pallor, reduced radial pulse and a cold limb. The patient required urgent vascular intervention.

Patients with atrial fibrillation can develop multiple emboli in close succession, and possible signs of an ischemic limb need to be thoroughly evaluated'

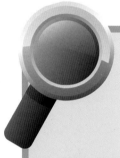

PRESENT YOUR FINDINGS...

'This is Mr Smith who presented with right leg pain at rest.

On examination, Mr Smith has tar-stained fingers and corneal arci in both eyes. His right leg is thin, pale and cool up to the knee. There is evidence of hair loss. Capillary refill is 3 seconds. The right femoral pulse is palpable, but no pulses distal to this are present. Power is normal but there is reduced sensation at the toes. There is a small, painful, necrotic looking ulcer on the tip of the big toe of his right foot. It is of regular shape, about 0.5cm deep and has the punched out appearance of an arterial ulcer. Buerger's angle is 30° with sunset rubor seen at 15 seconds. Examination of the left leg was unremarkable.

My examination findings are consistent with a diagnosis of critical limb ischemia of the right leg.'

What are the key features of an acutely ischemic limb?

Soft Signs (which tend to come first):
- *Pulseless, pallor and perishingly cold*

Hard Signs:
- ***Pain*** - *such as calf muscle tenderness, spasms or pain on squeezing the limb*
- ***Paraesthesia*** - *loss of sensory function (e.g. the patient is unable to feel a light touch over the dorsum of the hand or forefoot)*
- ***Paralysis*** - *loss of motor function (e.g. the patient can't wiggle the toes or fingers)*

Station 14: VARICOSE VEINS

Mr Wilson is known to suffer from varicose veins. Please examine his legs, and describe any changes that may be associated with venous disease.

Inspection

Adequately expose the patient. You should ask permission to remove trousers for lower limb examination. Ask for a chaperone.

Varicose veins follow the path of the two major veins:

- **Long Saphenous:** ascends in front of the medial malleolus and runs along the medial side of the leg, going behind the medial condyles and along the medial side of the thigh, passing through the fossa ovalis and ending in the femoral vein at the sapheno-femoral junction (SFJ)
- **Short Saphenous:** ascends behind the lateral malleolus and runs laterally, crossing to the middle at the lower part of the popliteal fossa, and ending in the popliteal vein, between the heads of the gastrocnemius. Also gives off a branch that joins the long saphenous vein
- **Thread Veins:** these may also be visible: thin, thready, superficial varicosities

Signs of Chronic Venous Disease

- **Lipodermatosclerosis:** indurated areas of brown/red/orange thickened skin caused by fibrosis of subcutaneous fat (need to palpate for this)
- **Saphena varix:** a dilatation at the top of the long saphenous vein due to valvular incompetence. Can reach the size of a golf ball or larger
- **Venous eczema:** caused by leakage of irritant venous contents onto skin surface
- **Venous/malleolar flare:** spider-like venous tortuosities around the malleoli
- **Skin pigmentation from haemosiderin deposition**
- **Atrophie blanche:** white scar tissue with 'dotted' capillaries
- **Oedema**
- **'Inverted champagne bottle' appearance:** narrow around ankle, due to chronic venous insufficiency leading to fibrosis
- **Venous ulcers**

Palpation

- Temperature and tenderness (heat and tenderness of superficial thrombophlebitis)
- Pitting oedema
- Lipodermatosclerosis (scarring and contraction of the subcutaneous fat) may only be appreciated by gentle palpation. Compare the consistency of the subcutaneous fat on one leg with that on the other leg

Feel for saphenofemoral junction – 4 cm below femoral veins:

- Get the patient to cough whilst feeling at the SFJ (follow the vein up along its path)
- Feel for phlebitis along the veins
- Sapheno-popliteal junction (SPJ) incompetence – check for cough impulse

Percussion

Tap Test: tap the vein above (proximally) whilst feeling below with a finger held on the more distal portion of the vein (allows assessment of valvular incompetence)

Trendelenberg's Test

To assess for SFJ incompetence:

- With the patient lying flat on a couch, lift the leg up to drain veins
- Tie the tourniquet initially at the SFJ high in the thigh
- Ask patient to stand – the aim is to see if you can stop the veins re-engorging when the leg is lowered again
- If the varicosities refill once the leg is lowered (with the tourniquet at the SFJ), then any distal perforators are incompetent
- The 'modified test' involves subsequently attaching the tourniquet distally, at varying distances along the leg, to identify the location of the incompetent perforators

Tell the examiner that, to complete the examination, you would like to examine the abdomen. Abdominal masses may be causing the lower limb venous disease.

Venous duplex ultrasound may also be of use. Reflux is demonstrated by the reversal of the direction of blood flow (normally prevented by valves). Blood flow can be elicited by squeezing the calf. If valves are incompetent, when pressure is released from the calf, blood flow will occur in the direction of gravity.

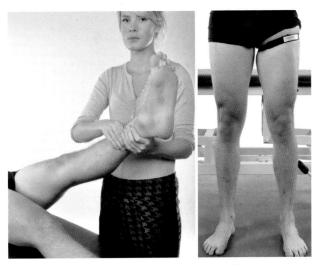

Fig 2.67: Trendelenberg's test: Lifting the leg up, and 'milking' the veins (left), and then after applying a tourniquet at the SFJ, and asking patient to stand (right)

Other sets of perforators include: ***Hunterian perforator*** (mid-thigh), ***Dodd perforator*** (approximately 1 hand-breadth above the knee), ***Boyd perforator*** (approximately 1 hand-breadth below the knee), and ***Cockett perforators*** (5, 10 and 15 cm above the ankle).

What are the management options for varicose veins?

Conservative

- Lifestyle changes (weight loss, exercise)
- Education (keep the leg elevated, skin care, prevent injury)
- Graded compression stockings - usually Class 2 (<30 mmHg) or 3 (<40 mmHg) (these cannot be used with concomitant arterial pathology or this will lead to ischaemia – therefore, it requires ABPI)
- Regular debridement and cleaning/ dressing of ulcers

Surgical

- Indications: phlebitis, ulcers, bleeding, eczema
- Venous 'stripping' and ligation
- Newer endovenous procedures such as radio frequency or laser ablation of the long or short saphenous vein

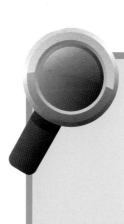

PRESENT YOUR FINDINGS...

'This is Mr Wilson who presented with varicose veins.

He has dilated superficial veins on the medial side of both legs, extending to above the knee joint. He has bilateral ulcers in the gaiter region with edges that are 'sloping' and have granulation tissue. There is also evidence of venous eczema, haemosiderosis, lipodermatosclerosis and atrophie blanche on both legs. No temperature difference, tenderness or oedema is evident. A cough impulse is palpable at both sapheno-femoral junctions. Trendelenberg's test demonstrates venous incompetence at the level of the sapheno-femoral junction.

This is consistent with a diagnosis of long saphenous varicose veins, with evidence of chronic venous disease and associated venous ulceration.

To complete my examination, I would like to palpate the abdomen for any masses.'

Station 15: ULCER EXAMINATION

Mr Smith is a 67 year-old diabetic. His wife has noticed an ulcer on Mr Smith's left foot. Please examine this gentleman's skin and present your findings.

Definition

An ulcer is a break in the normal continuity of an epithelial or endothelial surface.

General Inspection

- This is a descriptive process much like that of a lump, which can yield spot diagnoses
- Remember to look from all aspects including between the toes and soles of feet
- Take your time on the inspection and aim to comment fully before you move on to touching the patient in order to get the most marks
  - SITE   Use anatomical terms and centimetres from the nearest bony prominence
  - SIZE   Measure or estimate width
  - SHAPE   Describe the shape
  - SKIN   Surrounding skin can suggest the underlying pathology
  - SCARS   From previous ulcers (atrophie blanche), skin grafts or other surgery like stripping
  - COLOUR What colour is it?
  - BASE   Granulation tissue (red), slough (dead), pus, bone or tendon
  - EDGE   Punched out (arterial or neuropathic)
            Sloping (venous or healing)
            Undetermined – margins overhanging the ulcer (e.g. infection or pressure)
  - DEPTH   Shallow? Deep? Estimate in millimetres

Causes of Neuropathic Ulcer

Peripheral neuropathy
- Often idiopathic
- Diabetes mellitus
- Alcohol
- Vitamin deficiency

Causes of Venous Ulcer

Any cause of venous stasis:
- Varicose veins
- Deep vein thrombosis
- Immobility of the limb

Palpation

Ask the patient if they are in any pain prior to palpation:

- TENDERNESS   Look at the patient's face
- TEMPERATURE   Feel the surrounding skin with the back of your hand
- LYMPH NODES   Local drainage
- LOCAL TISSUE   Assess the neuro-vascular status of the limb for suggestive pathology

Perform a vascular examination, assessing pulses and looking for signs of chronic venous insufficiency. These include oedema, hyperpigmentation, venous dermatitis, chronic cellulitis, cutaneous infarction (atrophie blanche) and ulceration.

It is also important to measure an ankle brachial pressure index (ABPI). This may support a diagnosis of arterial ulcers, and also could be an important contraindication to compression bandages for venous ulcers.

Causes of Arterial Ulcers

Large Vessel:
- *Atherosclerosis*

Small Vessel:
- *Diabetes mellitus*
- *Vasculitides*
- *Rheumatoid arthritis*

How would you differentiate between venous, arterial and neuropathic ulcers?

	Venous	Arterial	Neuropathic
SITE	Gaiter area (around the medial malleolus and calf)	Distal extremities and pressure areas (heel and under metatarsal heads)	Pressure areas (heel and under metatarsal heads)
PAIN	Painless or Painful	Painful	Painless
EDGE and BASE	Sloping edge with red granulation base (sometimes white)	Punched out edge with no red granulation base. The base can be slough or infective	Punched out and clean edge
SKIN CHANGES	Haemosiderin deposits Venous eczema Lipodermatosclerosis	Trophic changes: hair loss and thin skin Cold	Often normal surrounding skin
OTHER	Varicose veins	Absent distal pulses	Sensory loss

Management

This will be guided by the pathology suggested from your clinical evaluation. Investigations include:

- **Punch biopsy** - to assess histological change
- **Portable 8Mhz doppler ultrasound probe**
  - Assess venous flow (reflux indicated by a second audible 'whoosh')
  - Assess arterial pulses (stenosis indicated by typical waveform)
- **Colour Duplex**
  - Define venous adequacy e.g. incompetent perforator veins
  - Visualise blood flow within arteries e.g. popliteal stenosis
- **Arteriography:** to assess branch flow within lower limb arteries

Treatment

	Conservative	Surgical
Venous Ulcer	• Four layer bandaging – heals 70% in 3 months • Keep the limb elevated and protected from injury • Regular cleaning and removal of slough to encourage granulation tissue • Once healed commence Class II compression stockings – check that ABPI is greater than or equal to 0.8	• Skin grafting • Varicose vein surgery if associated with varicosities
Arterial Ulcer	• Cardiovascular risk factor modification: lipids, hypertension, diabetes, smoking, weight loss and exercise (collaterals) • Low dose aspirin • Adequate analgesia: these can be very painful (WHO ladder) • Skin care • Foot care with the help of a chiropodist	• Endovascular - balloon angioplasty and stenting • Bypass reconstruction • Amputation • Sympathectomy (chemical or surgical)

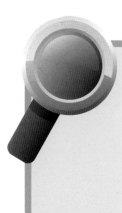

PRESENT YOUR FINDINGS...

'Mr. Smith has a 5 by 3cm round ulcer located above his left medial malleolus. There are varicose veins in the long saphenous distribution, with skin changes, namely haemosiderin deposition, eczema and lipodermatosclerosis. The base of the ulcer has red granulation tissue and is shallow, with sloping edges and an irregular margin. The skin is warm to touch, non-tender and distal pulses were present.

These findings are consistent with venous ulceration.'

Station 16: NECK LUMPS

Mr. Gardner has been complaining of a lump in his neck. Please examine him and present your findings with a differential diagnosis.

Inspection

- Introduce yourself as you would normally, but note any hoarseness in the patient's voice
- Inspect the neck looking at it from eye level. Look for masses in the front, sides or back of the neck by walking around the patient

- Describe the mass as you would any lump:
    - SITE   In relation to anatomical sites
    - SIZE   Approximate width and length in centimetres
    - SHAPE   Round, oval, irregular?
    - COLOUR   Erythematous, skin-coloured or otherwise
    - EDGE   Smooth or irregular
    - SKIN   Scars suggesting previous surgery such as thyroid or carotid incisions

- Take the time to appreciate the patient as a whole, for example noticing features suggestive of thyroid disease. The age of the patient can point towards likely pathology, for example:
    - CHILDHOOD   Congenital lesions such as branchial cysts
    - ADOLESCENTS   Lymphadenopathy from infective causes such as glandular fever
    - OLDER   Neoplastic disease

- By asking the patient to open their mouth and protrude their tongue, you may identify a thyroglossal cyst, which moves upwards with this action
- Next, ask the patient to take a mouthful of water and swallow as you are inspecting, allowing you to identify movement, which suggests a thyroid mass
- These two actions should then be repeated while gently palpating from behind, as they may be difficult to identify on inspection alone. Movement of a thyroglossal cyst, for example, is almost impossible to detect on inspection

Palpation

- Approach the patient from behind and gently place the pads of your fingers on each side of the neck. Ensure that the patient is warned, and as always observe for signs of discomfort or tenderness
- Show the examiner, in a thorough and practiced routine, the sequential palpation of the anatomical triangles of the neck including the parotid region, submandibular region and lymph nodes

'Submandibular stones are seldom palpable from the outside. One would need to palpate the floor of mouth to detect them'

David Pothier

Consultant ENT Surgeon
Toronto General Hospital

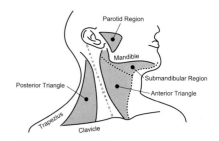

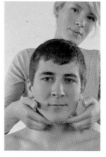

Fig 2.68: Feeling for neck lymph nodes, anatomy shown (above) and technique (below)

Example Sequence

- Palpate the submandibular area, left hand on the left, right hand on the right. Move hands progressively inward, to meet over the submental area
- Palpate down the midline to the thyroid; do the thyroid exam with swallowing, and tongue protrusion (whilst still palpating)
- Then move up both anterior borders of the sternocleidomastoid, with each hand
- At the mastoid process follow the posterior border of the sternocleidomastoid to the supraclavicular fossa
- Palpate this and finish by following the trapezius to the occiput

- Once a lump is found, identify the remaining descriptive qualities:
  - TENDERNESS   Look at the patients face (looking around from behind) and ask if pressing causes any pain
  - TEMPERATURE   Feel the surrounding skin
  - CONSISTENCY   Smooth, irregular, cystic or solid
  - MOBILITY   Mobile with the skin, or attached to deeper underlying tissue
  - PULSATILITY   Relating to vascular masses
  - BRUIT   Relating to vascular masses
  - TRANSILLUMINATION Cystic or solid

- Mention that, to complete your examination, you would want to look in the mouth as well as palpate the floor of mouth, the nose and ears. If a parotid mass is obvious, then it would be appropriate to continue to examine the face and scalp

What are you differentials for this lump?

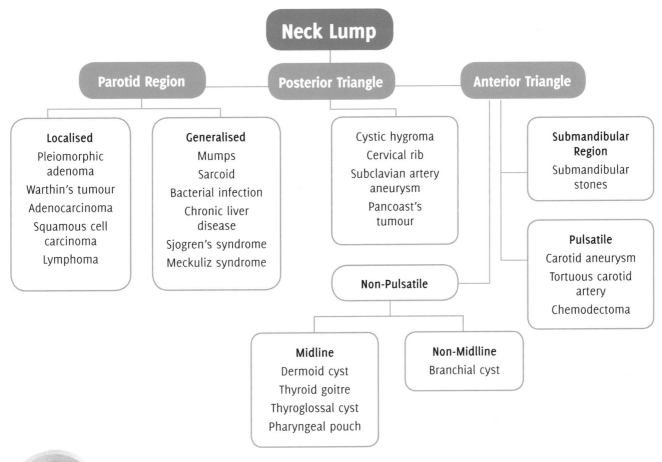

Neck Lump

Parotid Region

Localised
Pleiomorphic adenoma
Warthin's tumour
Adenocarcinoma
Squamous cell carcinoma
Lymphoma

Generalised
Mumps
Sarcoid
Bacterial infection
Chronic liver disease
Sjogren's syndrome
Meckuliz syndrome

Posterior Triangle
Cystic hygroma
Cervical rib
Subclavian artery aneurysm
Pancoast's tumour

Non-Pulsatile

Midline
Dermoid cyst
Thyroid goitre
Thyroglossal cyst
Pharyngeal pouch

Non-Midlline
Branchial cyst

Anterior Triangle

Submandibular Region
Submandibular stones

Pulsatile
Carotid aneurysm
Tortuous carotid artery
Chemodectoma

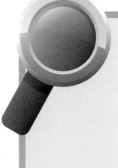

PRESENT YOUR FINDINGS...

'This is Mr Gardner who presented with an asymptomatic neck lump.

The lump is in the right anterior triangle of the neck. It measures 2 by 1 cm. It is firm, has a smooth surface, is well circumscribed, non-tender to palpation and is mobile over deep tissues. There is a central punctum. There is no pulsation or transillumination. There is no associated lymphadenopathy.

This is consistent with a diagnosis of a sebaceous cyst.'

Station 17: BREAST EXAMINATION

Mrs Dodds is a 25-year-old lady who has noticed a lump in her left breast. Perform a breast examination and present your findings.

- Ensure that you have a female chaperone present
- Ask the patient to remove her clothes down to the waist and sit on the edge of the bed
- Ask the patient on which side the problem lies
- Ask the patient if she has any pain

Examination

Inspection

- Observe for dimpling, peau d'orange, nipple retraction, scars, discharge
- Inspect in five positions
  - At rest
  - Raising both arms above head
  - Sitting and pushing body up off the bed with both hands
  - Putting hands on hips and pushing inwards
  - Asking the patient to lean forward and observe the breasts for muscle tethering of breast lumps

Palpation

- Ask the patient to lie back (45°) and relax her head on pillow while placing the arm of breast to be examined behind her head
- Start with the normal breast
- Palpate 4 quadrants in turn (with the flat of the fingers not the palm)
- Feel the area underneath nipple and areola
- Feel for the axillary breast tail tissue
- Feel the axilla: support the arm whilst doing this
- Repeat on the other breast

Ask the patient to produce discharge, if present.

- Check supraclavicular lymph nodes from behind
- Check for hepatomegaly, lymphoedema
- Palpate for bony tenderness
- Listen to the lungs

Describing Lumps

- Size
- Location
- Shape
- Colour
- Tenderness
- Temperature
- Consistency: soft/firm/hard
- Surface: smooth/irregular
- Well defined/ill defined
- Tethering, mobility
- Overlying skin changes

Causes of Benign Breast Lumps

COMMON	LESS COMMON
Fibroadenoma	Galactocele
Fibrocystic change	Lipoma
Sebaceous cyst	Fat necrosis
Acute mastitis/abscess (if in association with breast feeding/ smoking)	Gynaecomastia

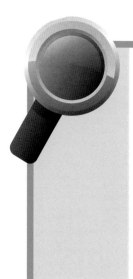

PRESENT YOUR FINDINGS...

'Mrs Dodds is a 25-year-old lady who has a 2x2cm mobile, well circumscribed lump at the six-o'clock position of her left breast. The lump is soft, non-tender and has no associated skin changes. There is no axillary or cervical lymphadenopathy.

The most likely diagnosis is a fibroadenoma.

However I would like to arrange further investigation in the form of 'Triple Assessment' at a one-stop breast clinic'

Station 18: DERMATOLOGY STATION

Mrs Barton is a 45 year-old lady who has developed a rash on her scalp and elbows. Please describe the rashes, and come up with a likely list of differentials.

Site and/or Distribution

- Psoriasis has a predilection for knees, elbows, scalp and lower back
- Eczema favours the flexures
- Acne occurs predominantly on the face and upper trunk
- Basal cell carcinomas are more common on the head and neck

Characteristics of Individual Lesions

Definitions

- **Macule:** flat, circumscribed area of skin discolouration
- **Papule:** circumscribed raised lesion less than 5mm in diameter at the widest point
- **Nodule:** circumscribed raised lesion greater than 10mm in diameter at the widest point
- **Plaque:** circumscribed, disc-shaped, elevated lesion
  - **Small:** <2 cm; **Large:** >2 cm

Note: when differentiating a nodule and plaque, there is inconsistency in describing lesions between 5-10mm

- **Vesicle:** lesion less than 5mm in diameter at the widest point, containing fluid
- **Bulla:** lesion greater than 10mm in diameter at the widest point, containing fluid

Note: when differentiating a vesicle and bulla, there is inconsistency in describing lesions between 5-10mm

- **Pustule:** lesion containing pus
- **Erosion:** loss of epidermis
- **Ulcer:** loss of epidermis and dermis
- **Weal:** circumscribed, elevated area of dermal oedema

Further Description of the Lesion

- Shape: round, oval, annular, linear, irregular
- Outline: well-demarcated vs. ill-defined
- Colour

Surface

- Smooth vs. rough
- Crust
- Scale
- Keratin horn
- Excoriation, maceration, lichenification
- Lift the scale or crust to see what is underneath
- Try to make the lesion blanch with pressure

Secondary Sites

- Look for additional features that may assist in the diagnosis, e.g. examine the nails in psoriasis, fingers and wrists in scabies, toe-webs in fungal infections and the mouth in lichen planus

Special Techniques

- Scraping a psoriatic plaque for capillary bleeding
- Nikolsky's sign in some blistering diseases e.g. toxic epidermal necrolysis or pemphigus vulgaris, rubbing of the skin results in exfoliation of the epidermis

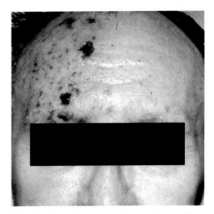

Fig 2.69: Herpes Zoster infection: note that it is confined to the ophthalmic division of the trigeminal nerve

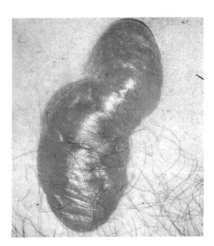

Fig 2.70: A bulla

What nail changes might you see with psoriasis?

Involved in 50% of cases
- *Pitting*
- *Ridging*
- *Discolouration*
- *Sub-ungal hyperkeratosis*
- *Onycholysis*

Psoriasis Examination

Skin

- Plaques: Salmon pink, well demarcated, silvery/white scaling, located over extensor surfaces, scalp, naval, natal clefts
- Chronic plaques, guttate, pustular, erythroderma
- Koebner phenomenon (plaque develops on a scar)
- Look behind the ears and around the scalp line (for plaques)

Joints

There are 5 different patterns of joint involvement:
- Distal interphalangeal joint swelling
- Rheumatoid arthritis pattern of symmetrical small joint swelling
- Monoarthritis
- Ankylosing spondylitis/sacroiliitis
- Arthritis mutilans

Aetiology

- A family history is present in 35% of the patients
- A child with 1 affected parent has approximately a 25% probability of being affected (approximately 60% if both parents affected)

- Risk factors (precipitating factors)
  - Koebner phenomenon: trauma, including surgical scars
  - Infection: Streptococcal sore throat may precipitate guttate psoriasis
  - Drugs: B-blockers, lithium, Non-Steroidal Anti-Inflammatory Drugs and anti-malarials can worsen or precipitate psoriasis
  - Sunlight: whilst beneficial, exposure aggravates psoriasis in 10% of cases
  - Psychological stress is said to worsen psoriasis, though there are very varied opinions on this in the dermatological community
  - Alcohol

Management

Advice

- Explain that the condition is non-infectious but long-term therapy will be needed
- Self-help group: The Psoriasis Association

Stable Plaque

- Emollients to moisturise
- Vitamin D analogue (does not smell or stain but may sometimes cause irritation)
- Dithranol stains skin, hair, linen, clothes, and bathtubs purple-brown
  - Short contact regimen – applied for 30 minutes each day and wash off in shower; avoid face and genitals
- Tar
- Corticosteroids (rebound or pustular psoriasis can possibly develop with the use of systemic corticosteroids, however topical application is used widely)
- Retinoids
- Narrowband Ultraviolet B

Severe Psoriasis

- Narrowband Ultraviolet B
- PUVA (Psoralen + Ultraviolet A light therapy)
- Methotrexate
- Cyclosporin

Observe for Complications

- Turning pustular (i.e. pustular psoriasis)
- Psoriatic arthropathy
- Erythroderma: feeling unwell, pyrexial and development of an erythematous rash that spreads to most of the body

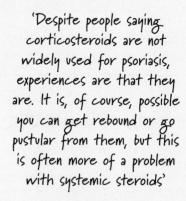

'Despite people saying corticosteroids are not widely used for psoriasis, experiences are that they are. It is, of course, possible you can get rebound or go pustular from them, but this is often more of a problem with systemic steroids'

Jonathan Rees
Professor of Dermatology
University of Edinburgh

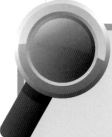

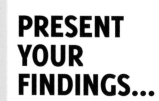

PRESENT YOUR FINDINGS...

'This is Mrs Barton, who presented with a rash on her scalp and elbows.

These are pink, well-demarcated plaques with a white-silver scaling.

She has plaques on the extensor surfaces of both elbows, her scalp, and behind her ears. There is a further plaque overlying an abdominal scar from a previous caesarean section.

Her finger nails show pitting, ridging and onycholysis.

This is consistent with a diagnosis of psoriasis.

To complete my examination, I would assess her joints for evidence of psoriatic arthropathy.'

Station 19: CUSHING'S EXAMINATION

Mrs Kain, a 30 year-old lady, presents to your GP surgery with feelings of low mood and having not had a menstrual period for three months. She has also gained weight. She is taking long term oral steroids for asthma. Please perform a relevant examination of her endocrine system.

Hand and Arms

Look for:

- Bruising: particularly on the back of the hands and forearms
- Wounds: minor injuries more likely to persist due to poor healing
- Compare the size of the limbs with that of the trunk. The centripetal adiposity associated with Cushing's Syndrome results in relatively thin arms with a large trunk ('orange on a matchstick' appearance)

Test:

- Skin fold thickness: pinch the skin, and gently lift it. Thin skin is associated with Cushing's Syndrome
- Blood pressure: may be elevated
- Muscle strength: check for proximal myopathy. Ask the patient to raise both arms out like chicken wings (demonstrate yourself). Assess for power by saying *'keep your arms up'* whilst pushing down on the arms. Check each arm individually (not both arms simultaneously)

Face

Look for:

- Facial 'mooning': look at the patient head on. With 'mooning', the cheeks may obscure the junction of the ear with the side of the face
- Acne
- Plethoric cheeks
- Hirsuitism
- Hair thinning
- Cataracts

Neck

- Inspect (and feel) supraclavicular fossae for 'fat pads'

What 3 clinical features from your examination have the best predictive value in supporting a diagnosis of Cushing's syndrome (rather than obesity or depression)?

Hypertension, myopathy, and bruising

Back

- Inspect (and feel) back for interscapular fat pads ('buffalo hump')
- Thoracic kyphosis
- Comment on stature and any clinical evidence of osteoporosis, scoliosis or loss of distance between lower ribs and top of pelvis due to crush fractures of lumbar vertebrae

Chest

- Inspect for breathlessness and auscultate for wheeze (due to respiratory illness for which long-term oral steroids may cause a Cushingoid appearance)
- In males, examine for gynaecomastia (look and feel breast tissue)

Abdomen

- Centripetal adiposity
- Scars of adrenalectomy
- Purple striae on the abdomen

Legs

- Inspect for thin legs (as for thin arms) and wasting of thigh muscles
- Proximal myopathy – *'cross your arms over your chest and please stand from sitting'*
- Thin skin
- Bruising
- Leg ulcers
- Oedema

'Remember there is a patient in front of you when you are presenting! Don't use phrases like 'buffalo hump', say 'interscapular fat pads' instead'

Zeshan Qureshi
Paediatric Trainee
London

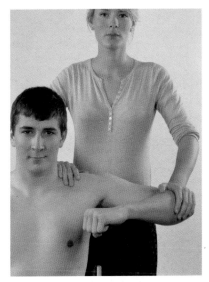

Fig 2.71: Testing for proximal myopathy

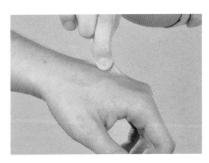

Fig 2.72: Testing for skin thinning

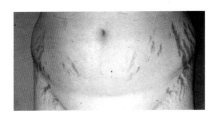

Fig 2.73: Abdominal striae

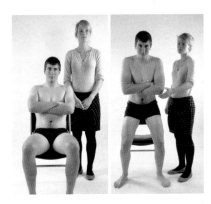

Fig 2.74: Testing for proximal myopathy. Ensure that you are close to the patient as they stand, in case they fall

Causes Of Cushing's syndrome

Exogenous Steroids

- For diseases such as rheumatoid arthritis, asthma and inflammatory bowel disease

Endogenous Steroids

- Pituitary adenoma (Cushing's **Disease**) – pituitary microadenoma producing excess ACTH, which increases cortisol production by adrenal glands
- Adrenal adenoma or carcinoma – ectopically secrete cortisol, which in turn reduced ACTH levels
- Ectopic ACTH syndrome (wasting due to carcinoma typically bronchial, small cell lung or pancreatic neuro-endocrine) – does NOT look Cushingoid, but will have pigmented skin (due to high ACTH levels) and very marked hypokalaemia

Pseudo-Cushing's Syndrome

- Excess cortisol due to another illness may result from obesity, depression and sometimes alcohol excess

> **What are the complications of transphenoidal hypophysectomy (treatment for pituitary adenoma)?**
>
> - *CSF rhinorrhoea*
> - *Diabetes insipidus*
> - *Hypopituitarism*
> - *Visual field disturbance (though only with very poor surgical technique)*
> - *Persistence of disease*
> - *Recurrence of disease*

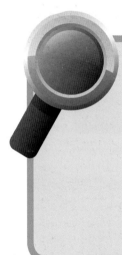

PRESENT YOUR FINDINGS...

'Mrs Kain is a 30 year-old lady on long term steroids, presenting with low mood, weight gain, and amenorrhoea.

On examination, she has centripetal obesity, dorsal fat pads, multiple bruising to the forearms, and thin skin. Her face is plethoric, and she also has acne. She has a proximal myopathy with 3/5 power for hip flexion, and 3/5 shoulder abduction.

These findings are consistent with a diagnosis of Cushing's Syndrome.

To complete my assessment of Mrs Kain, I would like to measure her blood pressure, and perform urinalysis (looking for glycosuria).'

Station 20: ACROMEGALY

Mr Black, a 34 year-old man, presents to your GP surgery after noticing his hands and feet have 'swollen up' over the last few months – his wedding ring no longer fits his finger and his shoe size has increased. He also reports increased sweating. Please perform a relevant examination of his endocrine system.

Unlike most examinations that follow the sequence of 'Inspection-Palpation-Percussion-Auscultation', endocrine examinations are often best performed in a systematic fashion, moving in a sequence from body part to body part.

Hands

Inspection

- Look at the shape and size of the hands. 'Spade like', enlarged hands are common in acromegaly. If you are unsure, compare them with your own hands

> *Before examining the hands, ask the patient if they have any pain in their hands. Arthropathy can occur in acromegaly.*

Palpation

- Ask the patient to stick their palms out in front of them. Gently feel the hands
  - The skin may feel moist and rubber-like. The palms may be boggy. This is due to increased sweating and oiliness. This is an important sign of ACTIVE disease
  - Thick skin – check skin fold thickness by gently pinching the skin on the back of the hand and comparing it with your own
- Assess for evidence of carpal tunnel syndrome. Check sensation in the median nerve distribution (lateral palm). Perform Phalen's and Tinel's test (see station 3.3)
- Feel the radial pulse. Tachycardia is associated with a high output cardiac state

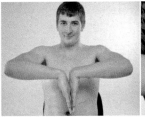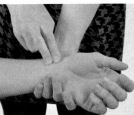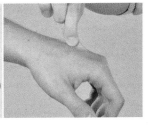

Fig 2.75: (Left to right) Phalen's test, palpating radial pulse, assessing for skin thinning

Arms

Inspection

- Check for axillary hair loss. Hypopituitarism may be associated with acromegaly

Special Tests

- Check for proximal myopathy. Ask the patient to raise both arms like chicken wings (after demonstrating the manoeuvre yourself). Check for power by saying *'don't let me push down'* whilst pushing down on the arm. Checking each arm individually, not both arms simultaneously
- Measure blood pressure. It is often increased

Face

Inspection

Look for:
- Prominent supra-orbital ridges
- Prognathism – protrusion of lower jaw/under-bite
- Large nose, ears and lips
- Coarse facial appearance

Tests

- Ask the patient to stick out their tongue. It may be large
- Ask the patient to show you their gums. Look for an increased space between the teeth (diastema)
- Ask the patient to repeat a simple phrase. They may have a husky voice
- Assess the visual fields. Optic chiasm compression may lead to a bitemporal hemianopia

Neck

- Check JVP (heart failure secondary to hypertension, cardiomyopathy or both)
- Feel for goitre (approximately 10% of patients with acromegaly have a goitre)

Chest

- Feel for apex beat (cardiomegaly)
- Auscultate the precordium (third heart sound)
- Auscultate the lung bases (left heart failure)

Abdomen

- Assess for hepatomegaly (sign of right heart failure)

Legs

- Proximal myopathy. *'Cross your arms over your chest and please stand from a sitting position'*

Ankles and Feet

Look for:
- Enlarged feet
- Increased heel pad thickness
- Oedema (heart failure)

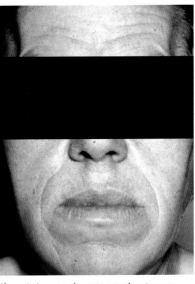

Fig 2.76: Acromegaly: note prominent supra-orbital ridges, protrusion of lower jaw, coarse facial appearance

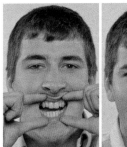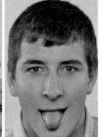

Fig 2.77: (Left to right) patient showing gums, and sticking out the tongue

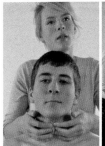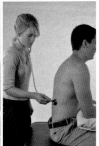

Fig 2.78: (Left to right) feeling for goitre, auscultating lung bases

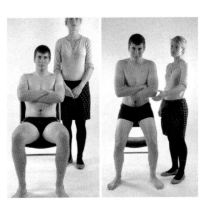

Fig 2.79: Testing for proximal myopathy. Ensure that you are close to the patient as they stand, in case they fall

How would you confirm the diagnosis of Acromegaly?

Measure growth hormone levels during an oral glucose tolerance test. In acromegaly, the growth hormone level is not suppressed after consuming the carbohydrate load. There may even be a paradoxical rise in growth hormone levels.

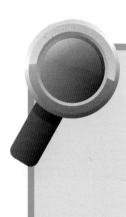

PRESENT YOUR FINDINGS...

'Mr Black is a 34 year-old gentleman who has thick, moist skin with particular 'bogginess' of both palms. He has prominent supra-orbital ridges with a relatively large nose, lips and tongue. There was evidence of reduced sensation in the distribution of the median nerve, bilaterally, with paraesthesia elicited during Tinel's test.

These findings are consistent with a diagnosis of active acromegaly, associated with carpel tunnel syndrome.

To complete my assessment of Mr Black, I would like to check his visual fields, measure his blood pressure and perform urinalysis (looking for glycosuria). A review of serial photographs of him would also help'

What treatment options are there for Mr Black?

- Surgery: trans-sphenoidal surgery to debulk the tumour
- Radiotherapy
- Medical therapies
  - Somatostatin analogues (e.g. octreotide) can cause tumour shrinkage and are often given preoperatively to increase the chances of surgical cure
  - Dopamine agonists
  - Growth hormone receptor antagonists

Station 21: THYROID EXAMINATION

Mr Pryce has recently lost weight, and has profound diarrhoea. He also has developed a lump in his neck. Please examine him and assess his thyroid status.

General Inspection

- Hair
- Skin
- Behaviour
- Build
- Clothing

Hands

- Thyroid acropachy
- Onycholysis
- Sweating
- Palmar erythema
- Fine tremor
- Pulse: Bradycardic, tachycardic, or atrial fibrillation

Eyes

- Inspect for chemosis, periorbital oedema, and erythema
- Assess for exophthalmos looking from the side and looking down on the eyes from behind the patient
- Assess for opthalmoplegia by examining cranial nerves III, IV, and VI
- Assess for lid lag. Ask the patient to follow your finger with their eyes as you sharply drop your finger from eye level downwards

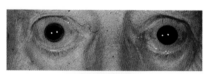

Fig 2.80: Thyrotoxicosis: note the entire white of the eye can be seen outlining the iris (due to lid retraction - above); exophthalmos (protruding eyeballs visable from side view - below)

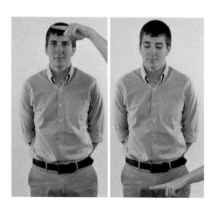

Fig 2.81: Assessing for lid lag (delay in movement of the eyelid as the eye moves downward)

Neck Inspection

- Look from front and side
- Scars, hyperaemia, swelling
- Distended neck veins
- Ask patient to sip water, hold it, and then swallow
- Ask patient to stick out their tongue

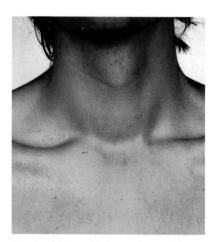

Fig 2.82: Visible neck lump consistent with a goitre

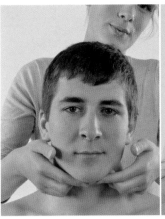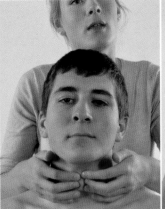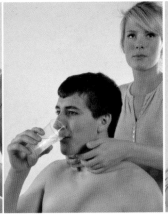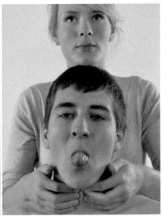

Fig 2.83: (Left to right) palpation of lymph nodes, thyroid, thyroid (whilst swallowing), thyroid (whilst sticking tongue out)

Palpation

- Palpate the neck from behind
- Temperature
- Palpate while patient is swallowing
- Palpate while the patient sticks out their tongue (a thyroglossal cyst will move with this manoeuvre)
- Swelling: site, size, shape, surface, consistency, edge, mobility, fluctuance, transillumination, relationship to skin and deep structures
- Lymph nodes: submental, submandibular, down anterior chain, supraclavicular, up posterior chain, parotid and mastoid areas, and occipital nodes
- Trachea (from front): deviated? Warn the patient that they might experience discomfort before palpating the trachea

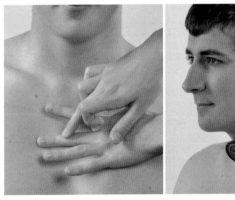

Fig 2.84: (Left to right) percussion for a retrosternal goitre; auscultation for a thyroid bruit

Finish by percussing for a retrosternal goitre and auscultating for a bruit. Ensure that any bruit is differentiated from a carotid bruit.

To complete the examination, offer to examine the legs for pre-tibial myxoedema, assess tendon reflexes and examine for proximal myopathy.

Differentials for a Thyroid Swelling

SMOOTH/DIFFUSE	SOLITARY NODULE	MULTIPLE NODULES
Hashimoto's Disease	Cyst	Multiple cyst
Graves' Disease	Colloid nodule	Multinodular goitre
Iodine Deficiency	Adenoma	
	Carcinoma	
	Dominant nodule multinodular goitre	

Treatment of Thyrotoxicosis

- Carbimazole and Beta Blockers
- Radioiodine: in a man, radioiodine would be at least second choice, but most often first choice, unless significant eye disease is present
- Surgery

Indications for Surgery

- Patient choice
- Failure of medical treatment
- Poor compliance with medication
- Intolerance of medication
- Large goitre

What are the complications of a thyroidectomy?

- *Bleeding*
- *Thyroid crisis (fast AF, pulmonary oedema)*
- *Hypoparathyroidism – hypocalcaemia*
- *Damage to the recurrent laryngeal nerve*
- *Recurrent hyperthyroidism*
- *Late hypothyroidism*

'Movement of a thyroglossal cyst on tongue protrusion is almost impossible to detect on inspection. It is essential to palpate whilst doing this manoeuvre'

David Pothier
Consultant ENT Surgeon
Toronto General Hospital

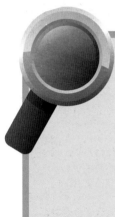

PRESENT YOUR FINDINGS...

'This is Mr Pryce, who presented with recent weight loss, diarrhoea and a neck lump.

Mr Pryce is a very thin man who appears anxious with a fine bilateral hand tremor and an irregularly irregular pulse. He has marked exophthalmos, lid lag and failure of upward gaze. He has a 2 by 2cm midline neck lump which does not move on tongue protrusion, but does elevate on swallowing. This lump is non-tender, has a well circumscribed, smooth border and is firm in consistency. There is a bruit over the lump. There is no pulsation, or retrosternal extension of the lump. He has pre-tibial myxoedema and a proximal myopathy.

This is consistent with a diagnosis of Graves' disease.

To complete my examination, I would like to look at an ECG. I would also like to look at thyroid function tests.'

Station 22: HAEMATOLOGICAL EXAMINATION

Mrs Hutchison is a 44 year-old lady who reports feeling 'under the weather' over the last few weeks. She has lost considerable weight, bruises more easily than before, and has recently been sweating profusely. Please perform a relevant examination and present your findings.

General Appearance

- Colour: pallor (anaemia); plethora (polycythaemia); unconjugated hyperbilirubinaemia in association with pallor can lead to "lemon yellow" jaundice
- Bleeding: purpura or bruising (thrombocytopaenia, reduced clotting factors)
- Breathlessness (anaemia)

Hands

- Perfusion: capillary refill time, temperature
- Skin crease pallor (anaemia)
- Telangiectasia (hepatic dysfunction)
- Koilonychia (iron deficiency anaemia)

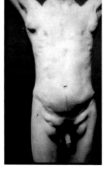
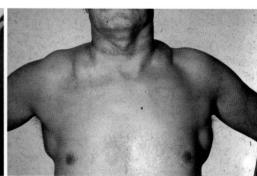

Fig 2.85: Lymphadenopathy visible on inspection, axillary and groin (left), axillary and neck (right)

Pulse

- Rate, rhythm, volume (may have sinus tachycardia with anaemia)

Mouth

- Lips: angular stomatitis, telangiectasia
- Gum hypertrophy (associated with leukaemia) or bleeding
- Tongue: colour, smoothness (atrophic glossitis and/or a fissured appearance is associated with vitamin B12 deficiency)
- Buccal mucosa: petechiae
- Tonsils: enlarged tonsils could imply infection or a palatal/pharyngeal lymphoma
- Conjunctivae: pallor, jaundice

Fundi

- Haemorrhage
- Signs of hyperviscosity (due for example to polycythaemia)
  - Engorged veins
  - Papilloedema

Neck and Axilla

Examination of lymph nodes:

- Neck: submental, submandibular, deep cervical, preauricular, postauricular, occipital, supraclavicular, infraclavicular
- Other: epitrochlear, axillary, inguinal, femoral. Assess size, consistency, and tenderness

Consistency can be divided into:
- Hard: like pressing your forehead: malignancy (lymphoma less likely)
- Rubbery: like pressing the end of your nose: malignancy (especially lymphoma)
- Soft: like pressing your lips: most likely associated with infection

Abdomen

Examine the abdomen as detailed in Station 2.3. Assess for hepatomegaly and splenomegaly. Palpate the inguinal lymph nodes.

Hepatosplenomegaly suggests lymphoproliferative or myeloproliferative disease.

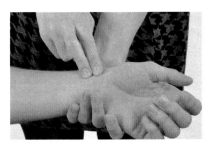

Fig 2.86: Assessing pulse

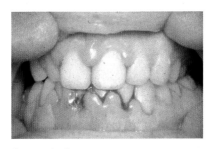

Fig 2.87: Bleeding gums

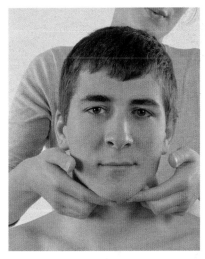

Fig 2.88: Feeling for neck lymph nodes

How do you differentiate between an enlarged spleen and a kidney?

Spleen	Kidney
Notch present	No notch present
Dull to percussion	Resonant to percussion
Cannot get between the ribs and spleen	Can get fingers over the kidney
Moves down on inspiration	Does not move with breathing

Hepatomegaly

Usually smooth and non-tender in haematological disease. Common haematological causes include lymphoma and leukaemia.

Moderate (3-5 finger breadths)	Massive (Greater than 5 finger breadths)
Lymphoma	Chronic myeloid leukaemia
Chronic leukaemia	Myelofibrosis

Haemarthrosis (bleeding into the joints) can cause deformity, swelling, tenderness, and restricted joint movement. It is often associated with infection, but can also be associated with congenital bleeding disorders; e.g. haemophilia A and B.

Legs

- Peripheral circulation and any associated gangrene (toes)
- Oedema (from lymphatic obstruction)
- Thrombocytosis (elevated platelets) can lead to peripheral arterial thrombosis, leading to acute limb ischaemia

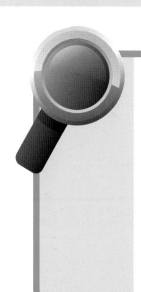

PRESENT YOUR FINDINGS...

'Mrs Hutchison is comfortable at rest. She is cachectic, sweating and has a temperature of 38°C. She has moderate hepato-splenomegaly. There is also evidence of bilateral leg oedema with palpable inguinal and axillary lymph nodes, which are smooth and non-tender.

This is consistent with a possible diagnosis of lymphoma.'

Station 23: EYE EXAMINATION

Mrs Baker is an 80 year-old lady and lifelong smoker. She has noticed that her left eyelid has become droopy. Please examine her eyes. You do not need to examine her fundi.

- Introduce yourself, explain what you would like to do, and seek permission

Inspection

- Look for the presence of glasses, any asymmetry between the eyes, ptosis, proptosis, lid lesions, red eyes or signs of systemic disease e.g. xanthelasma

Visual Acuity

- Test each eye in turn, with glasses kept on
- Test distance vision using a Snellen chart at 6m
- *'Please cover one eye and read the letters on the chart'*
- Acuity of 6/12 = that line on the chart was read from 6m, whereas a healthy eye could read it from 12m
- Vision improving with a pinhole suggests a refractive error
- Test near vision at ~30cm asking the patient to read small text

If unable to see the Snellen chart, test:
- *Counting fingers*
- *Hand movements*
- *Perception of light*

Causes of a Red Eye

- *Conjunctivitis*
- *Episcleritis*
- *Scleritis*
- *Keratitis or corneal abrasion*
- *Corneal foreign body*
- *Dry eyes*
- *Subconjunctival haemorrhage*
- *Acute angle-closure glaucoma*
- *Anterior uveitis*

Visual Fields

- Sit facing the patient. *'Cover one eye and keep looking at my nose. I'm going bring my pen in from the edges of your vision and I want you to say yes when you first see it'*
- Shut your eye too, the opposite one from theirs. Bring a small object (ideally red) or pen in from the periphery in each quadrant. Compare your field with theirs.

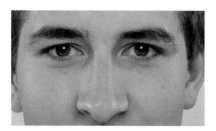

Fig 2.89: Inspection of eyes

Pupillary Reflexes

- Assess size, shape and symmetry
- With a pen torch, test reaction to light (direct and consensual) and to accommodation
- Test for a relative afferent pupillary defect (RAPD). This is due to damage to the optic nerve (e.g. optic neuritis), which forms the afferent limb of the pupillary light reflex
  - Test using the 'swinging light test': when a torch is shone alternately in each eye in close succession
  - Shining a torch in the normal eye (stimulating the normal optic nerve) produces full constriction in the normal eye (direct reflex) and in the abnormal eye (consensual reflex)
  - After this, immediately shining a light in the abnormal eye (stimulating the damaged optic nerve) produces an apparent dilatation of both eyes. This is because the same stimulus through the damaged optic nerve is weaker than through the normal optic nerve

Eye Movements

- *'Keep your head still; follow my pen with your eyes. Let me know if you see double'*
- Look for nystagmus (note its direction and the number of beats) and diplopia
- Assess the completeness of eye movements - if one eye fails to move in one direction, can you relate this to a cranial nerve deficit? The extraocular muscles are supplied by CN III (medial, inferior and superior recti, plus inferior oblique), IV (superior oblique) and VI (lateral recti)

Fundoscopy

- See station 5.7
- *'To conclude the examination, I would like to perform fundoscopy to examine the retina'*

In some cases, it may be appropriate to say that you think slit lamp examination and measurement of intraocular pressure are required; this would normally be performed by an ophthalmologist.

Horner's Syndrome

- *Miosis*
- *Partial ptosis*
- *Anhydrosis*

Due to damage to the sympathetic supply to the pupil. Can be caused by lesions in the brainstem, spinal cord, neck or cavernous sinus, e.g:

- *Pancoast's tumour*
- *Syringomyelia*
- *Internal carotid artery aneurysm*

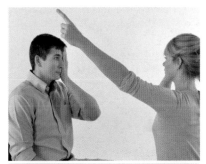

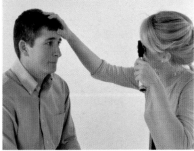

Fig 2.90: Visual fields assessment (top): ensure that you cover your eye directly opposite the eye not being tested (e.g. cover your right eye if testing the patient's right eye), fundoscopy (bottom): testing for red reflex

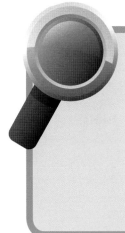

PRESENT YOUR FINDINGS...

'Mrs Baker has a left sided partial ptosis, as she had noticed. Her pupil is miotic, approximately 1mm smaller than the right, but reacts normally to light and accommodation. Her visual acuity, visual fields and eye movements are normal, with no diplopia or nystagmus.

This is consistent with a diagnosis of a left Horner's syndrome.

I would like to ascertain whether she has anhydrosis on the affected side. Causes of Horner's Syndrome include a Pancoast's tumour, and with her smoking history, I would like to examine Mrs Baker's chest and order a chest X-ray.'

Station 24: EAR EXAMINATION

Mrs Mason is an 82 year-old lady who is finding it increasingly difficult to hear. Please examine her ears and present your findings.

The Ear examination can be divided into four components:

1. Examination of the external ear (visual inspection)
2. Examination of the auditory meatus and tympanic membrane (Auriscope)
3. Examination of hearing (Whisper Test, Rinne's Test and Weber's Test)
4. Examination of the facial nerve (since it runs through the middle ear). This is described under neurological examination

Before Starting the Examination

- Explain the procedure and gain consent
- Ask if the patient has any pain or tenderness in the ear (if pain is present, reassure the patient that you will be gentle)
- Ask if the patient has a good or bad side. Always examine the good side first

1. Examination of the External Ear

- Inspect the pre-auricular area for an endaural incision scar (suggests previous ear surgery)
- Inspect the pinna and comment on any lesions seen
- Inspect the post-auricular area for a post-auricular incision scar (suggests previous surgery to the ear i.e. you may find a mastoid cavity)
- Palpate the mastoid area for tenderness (mastoiditis) and the post-auricular area (evidence of cochlear implant: the 'BAHA' abutment of a cochlear implant may be palpated here)

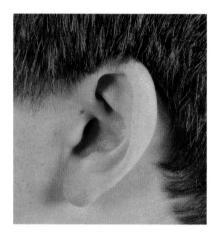

Fig 2.91: External ear inspection

2. Examination of the Auditory Meatus and Tympanic Membrane

- Select the appropriate size speculum. There are normally two types. Use the larger (4mm) as it is safer (less likelihood of damaging canal/drum) and you can see more. A 3mm speculum may be necessary in paediatrics or for a small ear canal
- Turn the light source of the auriscope to full brightness and test that it is bright enough
- Grip the auriscope like a pencil. For the right ear use the right hand, and for the left ear use the left hand
- Hold the auriscope correctly by placing your little finger on the patient's zygoma. This acts as an anchor, preventing damage to the inner ear if sudden movement of the patient's head should occur
- Elevate the pinna upwards and backwards with your free hand. You may also need to get the patient to tilt their head away from you
- Put the speculum on the back of the tragus, under direct vision, and then slowly insert the speculum whilst looking through the eye-piece
- Comment on the ear canal (wax, signs of infection) and the tympanic membrane. A healthy drum is translucent and pinky-grey; if it is normal just say so. If it is abnormal, describe the location and nature of the pathology according to whether it is in the pars flaccida or pars tensa. If it is in the pars tensa, describe what quadrant it is in (e.g. antero-inferior, postero-superior). In general the tympanic membrane is a circle with a 1cm diameter; try to describe the size of a perforation, if there is one

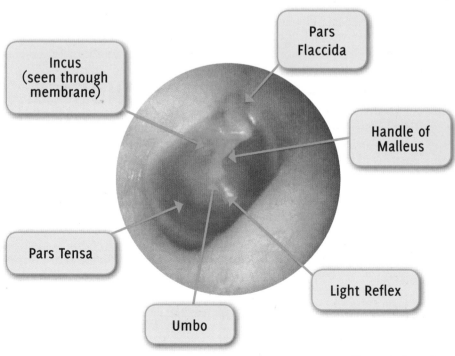

Incus (seen through membrane)

Pars Flaccida

Handle of Malleus

Pars Tensa

Light Reflex

Umbo

Fig 2.92: Anatomy of ear

3. Examination of Hearing (Whisper Test, Rinne's Test and Weber's Test)

Whisper Test

- This is a crude bedside method of establishing hearing levels
- Sit to the side of your patient (remember to start with the good side first)
- With one hand, obscure the entrance to the contralateral ear canal and rub gently (do this by pushing the tragus in to the canal). This will muffle

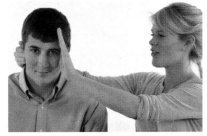

Fig 2.93: Whisper test

this ear and ensure that you are only testing one ear at a time
- With the other hand, cover the patient's eyes (so that they cannot lip read)
- Ensure that you are at full arm's length
- Whisper a combination of a number and a letter (e.g. 'N4') and ask the patient to repeat what you are saying. Get increasingly louder until they can hear you

'Rinne's Tuning Fork Test'

- Tap a 512Hz tuning fork on your elbow (not on a piece of furniture). Check that you have made the tuning fork ring by placing it next to your own ear first
- Place it on the bony mastoid process behind the patients ear and then in front of the ear
- Ask where they hear it loudest: in position 1, on the mastoid process, or position 2, in front of the ear

When holding the tuning fork on a bony process, always support the other side of the head with your free hand. When holding the tuning fork in front of the ear, make sure the two prongs are upright pointing toward the ceiling, and in line with the ear canal's entrance

Interpretation of Rinne's test:

1. **Normal Hearing or Sensori-neural Deafness:** "Rinne's positive". Air conduction is greater than bone conduction (louder in front of ear than on mastoid process)
2. **Conductive Deafness:** "Rinne's negative". Bone conduction is greater than air conduction (louder on mastoid process than in front of ear)

Weber's Tuning Fork Test

- Tap the tuning fork as before and place the base on the vertex of the head or forehead. Support the patient's head with your other hand
- Ask the patient the following; *"In which ear do you hear the sound loudest, left, right or in the middle?'*

Interpretation of Weber's Test:

1. **Normal (or Symmetrical Loss):** Sound heard in the midline, equally in both ears
2. **Sensori-neural Deafness:** Sound loudest in the less affected ear
3. **Conductive Deafness:** Sound loudest in affected ear

Always say that, in order to assess the patient's hearing fully, you would like to perform a "Pure tone audiogram" and a "Tympanogram". Be confident in interpreting common patterns of hearing loss such as presbycusis (age-related hearing loss)

Stop and think in order to put together the results of both tests. For example a patient with otosclerosis in the right ear (a fusion of the stapes, therefore a conductive hearing loss) will have a Rinne's negative test in the right ear, Rinne's positive in the left ear, and Weber's will lateralize to the right.

4. Examination of the Facial Nerve

- Quickly check for facial nerve integrity by getting the patient to make a few faces at you. Making the patient laugh is always a nice note to end on

Some Common Ear Pathology and Presentation of Associated Auroscopy Findings

1. *Perforation*

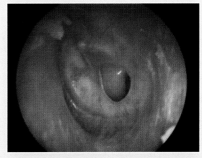

2. *Mastoid Cavity*

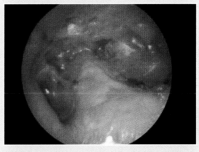

3. *Tympanosclerosis*

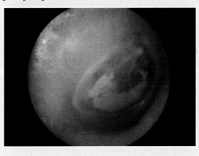

1. Perforation (see 'present your findings')

2. Mastoid Cavity: *'On examination of the external auditory meatus and tympanic membrane, I can see that this is a dry ear with no signs of infection or bleeding. There is an obvious cavity in the supero-posterior aspect of the ear canal that is consistent with a mastoid cavity, perhaps indicating previous surgery for a Cholesteatoma. The tympanic membrane is intact with a positive light reflex. I would like to perform a Pure Tone Audiogram in order to see if there is any conductive hearing loss, which can occur due to ossicular erosion with Cholesteatomas'*

3. Tympanosclerosis: *'On examination of the external auditory meatus and tympanic membrane, I can see that this is a dry right ear. There is opacification of the tympanic membrane consistent with Tympanosclerosis. I would like to perform a tympanogram in order to see if there is reduced motility of the drum, and a pure tone audiogram to see if there is any associated conductive hearing loss.'*

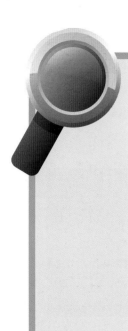

PRESENT YOUR FINDINGS...

'Mrs Mason is an 85 year-old lady presenting with hearing loss.

On examination of the external ear, there are no pinna lesions or deformities, no mastoid tenderness, no evidence of previous ear surgery. She wears no hearing aids or implant devices. On examination of the external auditory meatus and tympanic membrane, she has bilaterally dry ears with no mastoid cavities; her right tympanic membrane looks healthy and normal, however her left ear has a 10% central perforation in the posterio-inferior quadrant. This ear was Rinne's negative suggesting conductive hearing loss. There was no lateralisation on Weber's test. Whisper testing was normal in both ears.

These findings are consistent with a left tympanic membrane perforation. Causes for this may be 1. Perforation secondary to acute otitis media, 2. A complication of grommet insertion 3. Baro-trauma.

To fully assess the patient's hearing I would like to perform a Pure Tone Audiogram and a Tympanogram.'

Station 25: NEWBORN BABY EXAMINATION

You are the junior doctor covering the postnatal ward. You routinely perform a baby check on baby Barton, who is 12 hours old. He is the first child of a 36 year-old woman, and was delivered by normal vaginal delivery. Combined antenatal screening was not undertaken. Before seeing the baby, the midwife has called your attention to the baby's facial features.

The newborn check is conducted for every child after 6 hours of age. The aim is to examine and identify clinical concerns, with particular attention to problems that require immediate or timely intervention. The check is repeated by the GP at six weeks of age. The examination is a head to toe examination, but like all paediatric examinations it is best performed opportunistically. For example, if the baby is quiet or asleep, auscultate the precordium first, as you will struggle to examine this once the baby begins to cry. A systemic approach to examination follows:

Head

- **Shape:** common findings include caput and cephalhaematoma, which are swellings or bruises caused by pressure from the cervix or ventouse delivery respectively. It is important to ensure the swelling does not cross the suture lines. Examine sagittal and coronal suture lines
- **Size:** measure and plot the head circumference. Do this by measuring the longest distance around the head from the occiput, and repeat twice, taking the longest measurement
- **Fontanelles:** ensure normal size and shape of both anterior and posterior fontanelles
- **Face:** examine for abnormal facial features, for example, hypertelorism (widely spaced eyes) and micrognathia (small chin), which may be consistent with an underlying syndrome
- **Eyes:** absence of red reflex warrants further investigation to exclude cataracts or retinoblastoma
- **Mouth:** ensure normal shape with no cleft lip. Examine below the tongue to exclude tongue-tie. Insert a cleaned little finger tip to palpate the palate for clefts and assess suck reflex
- **Ears:** examine to ensure normal position (the superior aspect of the ear should be the same height as the eyes), and exclude auricular skin tags and sinuses

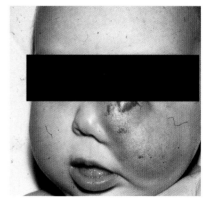

Fig 2.94: Haemangioma

Cardiovascular

- **Precordium:** palpate for heaves/thrills, auscultate for heart sounds and murmurs (apex, left sternal edge, pulmonary and aortic areas). Measure heart rate and rhythm (normal 100-140 per minute)
- **Pulses:** palpate femoral pulses, as weak or absent femoral pulses may be the only sign of coarctation of the aorta
- **Colour:** ensure no cyanosis. Consider pulse oximetry if uncertain. Many centres advocate routine pulse oximetry although this is currently not universally accepted

Respiratory

- **Chest:** examine for deformity such as pectus excavatum or accessory nipples
- Auscultate chest. Ensure no signs of distress are present and measure respiratory rate

Skin

- Skin should be examined over the entire body
- **Birthmarks (Naevi):** common birthmarks include haemangioma and Mongolian blue spots
- **Rash:** it is common for babies to have erythema toxicum (a benign rash characterised by erythematous macules with overlying white/yellow papules). Exclude more worrisome rashes such as petechiae

Abdomen

- **Palpation:** ensure no organomegaly or masses
- **Herniae:** common sites include umbilical (which are extremely unlikely to strangulate) and inguinal (which can strangulate and require surgical referral)
- The umbilical stump normally dries and separates over 5-10 days. This is a possible site of early infection characterised by spreading erythema
- **Anus:** examine externally, should be patent. Bowels should open within 24 hours of birth

Genitalia

- Inspect to ensure no ambiguity – if any doubt do not assign gender until reviewed by a senior colleague and relevant investigations are performed
- In boys ensure both testes are descended and the penis is normal without hypospadias

Musculoskeletal

- **Hands / feet:** inspect for polydactyly (accessory digits) and syndactyly (fused digits), as well as looking at the pattern of palmar creases (simian crease associated with Down syndrome). Examine the feet for talipes and determine whether this is positional (can be moved to correct anatomical position) or fixed (cannot be moved)
- **Spine:** should be straight without scoliosis. Sacral dimples or tufts of hair may indicate spinal fistulae or cord tethering
- **Hips:** examination is to exclude developmental dysplasia of the hip
- **Barlow:** adduct the hip and apply pressure posteriorly on the hip. If the hip moves posteriorly with a clunk, it is dislocatable
- **Ortolani:** stabilise the pelvis by firmly holding the symphysis pubis and coccyx between thumb and middle finger of one hand. Then, with the baby's hips and knees flexed, and the index finger of your other hand on the greater trochanter, abduct the baby's hip. A palpable clunk signifies relocation of a posteriorly dislocated hip

Neurological

- **Reflexes:** perform the Moro by gently allowing the head to drop back a few centimetres whilst holding the baby supine. The baby will spread both arms
- Pull baby to sit from lying position, and assess degree of head lag. Hold the infant in vertical suspension to assess tone. Allow the feet to touch the floor to elicit the stepping reflex
- Examine in ventral suspension for tone (this allows inspection of the spine)
- Be aware of possibility of Erb's palsy (waiters tip) after shoulder dystocia. May also present as an asymmetrical Moro reflex

The newborn screening programme is not limited to physical examination. It is important to be aware that the Guthrie card (blood spot) is collected by the midwife or health visitor in the first week of life. This is a biochemical screening process that looks for markers of diseases including neonatal hypothyroidism, cystic fibrosis, sickle cell disease, phenylketonuria, and medium-chain acyl-CoA dehydrogenase deficiency.

> 'Practical tip on the Moro. Be really careful performing this, and do it over a bed. Years ago in Dublin exams a baby had a really exaggerated Moro and "leapt" out of the candidate's hands and fell on the floor. The candidate failed simply because the baby was not safe at all times. I tell my students this anecdote, and then suggest in exams they ask "Would you like me to perform the Moro reflex?" It startles the child, and can result in crying. Most examiners will decline your considerate offer.'
>
> **Patrick Byrne**
> GP and Physician in General Medicine
> Belford Hospital, Fort William

Examination

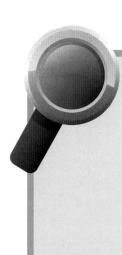

PRESENT YOUR FINDINGS...

'Baby Barton, born by SVD, with no antenatal or delivery concerns noted, is now 12 hours old.

On examination, there is evidence of hypertelorism, epicanthic folds, upslanting palpebral fissures, a flattened nasal bridge and macroglossia. With regard to breathing, he has good bilateral air entry, and a respiratory rate of 50. Heart sounds are normal, with no thrills or heaves. Peripheral pulses are normal, and he is pink. Reflexes are normal, there is a good cry, but tone is reduced throughout. Baby Barton also has single palmar creases, with short broad hands. Examination is otherwise unremarkable.

In summary, this baby has features that might suggest Down Syndrome.

After appropriate counseling, genetic karyotyping will be required, and if Down syndrome is confirmed, multidisciplinary team follow-up will be required to monitor growth and development.'

What is the management of suspected dysplasia of the hip?

An ultrasound scan of the hip should be performed, and if positive, this may require physiotherapy review, and further treatment; for example a Pavlik harness

What cardiac complications are associated with Down syndrome?

AVSD (atrioventricular septal defect) is the most common cardiac complication, but it is also commonly associated with ASD (atrial septal defect) and VSD (ventral septal defect)

The diagram below summarises the detailed explanation above to allow visualisation of the head to toe approach. This helps to ensure that no aspect of the examination is overlooked.

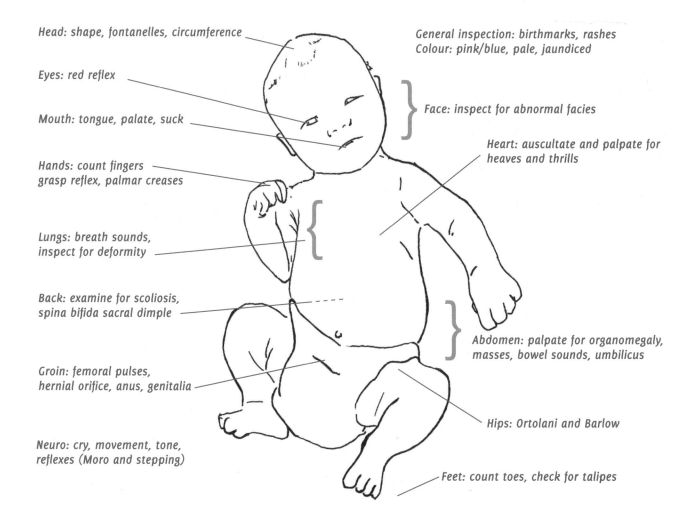

Head: shape, fontanelles, circumference

Eyes: red reflex

Mouth: tongue, palate, suck

Hands: count fingers grasp reflex, palmar creases

Lungs: breath sounds, inspect for deformity

Back: examine for scoliosis, spina bifida sacral dimple

Groin: femoral pulses, hernial orifice, anus, genitalia

Neuro: cry, movement, tone, reflexes (Moro and stepping)

General inspection: birthmarks, rashes
Colour: pink/blue, pale, jaundiced

Face: inspect for abnormal facies

Heart: auscultate and palpate for heaves and thrills

Abdomen: palpate for organomegaly, masses, bowel sounds, umbilicus

Hips: Ortolani and Barlow

Feet: count toes, check for talipes

3 Orthopaedic Examinations

Before dealing with individual joints, here are some general principles that are applicable to all orthopaedic examinations:

1. Do not cause the patient additional pain
2. Expose the joint and surrounding structures adequately
3. Always examine the 'normal' limb, comparing it with the 'abnormal' limb
4. Always assess the joint above and below the 'abnormal' one
5. Assess active before passive movements
6. Use standard terminology when describing deformities and movements

This chapter contains notes on the following scenarios:

3.1 Thoraco-Lumbar Spine Examination

3.2 Cervical Spine Examination

3.3 Hand Examination

3.4 Shoulder Examination

3.5 Hip Examination

3.6 Knee Examination

3.7 Gait Arms Legs Spine (GALS) Examination

LOOK	... for deformity, swelling, erythema, scars, sinuses and muscle wasting. Each joint may have other specific features to be assessed
FEEL	... when palpating a joint, one should always assess for tenderness (bony and soft tissue) and warmth
MOVE	... assess the range of movements possible at the joint, first by asking the patient to perform the movement themselves (active movement); second, with the examiner facilitating the movement (passive movement)
SPECIAL TESTS	... are unique to the joint being examined; for example, Lachman's test when examining the knee to assess the integrity of the anterior cruciate ligament
DISTAL NEUROVASCULAR INTEGRITY	... compromise to either of these requires urgent management

Term	Definition
Flexion	Bending from the neutral position at a joint
Extension	Straightening to the neutral position at a joint
Adduction	Movement towards the midline of the body
Abduction	Movement away from the midline
Internal Rotation	Turning of a limb about its axis of rotation toward the midline of the body
External rotation	Turning of a limb about its axis of rotation away from the midline of the body
Varus	The part distal to the joint is deviated medially
Valgus	The part distal to the joint is deviated laterally

Study Action Plan

- Practice, practice, practice is the key to learning orthopaedic examination
- In order to get the most out of seeing patients with real clinical signs, ensure that you have practiced the routines on healthy volunteers until they are second nature
- Practicing on healthy volunteers also allows you to understand what is a normal range of movement for each specific joint
- Practicing in groups of three is ideal: one person to examine, one to be examined, and a third to time the examination as well as to provide a critique

Station 1:
THORACO-LUMBAR SPINE EXAMINATION

Mr Lasèugue is an 85 year-old gentleman who has recently developed back pain. He is known to have prostate cancer. Please examine his thoraco-lumbar spine.

Look

- Ask the patient to remove clothing so the entire back can be inspected
- Observe the patient's gait (if already sitting, ask the patient to stand up and walk to the door and back)
- With the patient standing, look at the back from the side and behind
- Look for café au lait spots (neurofibromatosis), fat pad or hairy patch (spina bifida), winged scapula, and scarring from previous surgery
- Look for muscle spasm
- Look for asymmetry
- Check whether the shoulders, hips, knee and ankles are parallel
- Assess both the thoracic and lumbar curvatures
- Increased thoracic kyphosis is a feature of osteoporosis and advanced ankylosing spondylitis
- Flattening or reversal of lumbar lordosis is a common finding in prolapsed intervertebral disc, osteoarthritis of the spine, infections of the vertebral bodies and ankylosing spondylitis
- Look for lateral curvature (may be a sign of scoliosis)
- Ask the patient to stand with their back against the wall. The heels, pelvis, shoulders and occiput should all be able to touch the wall simultaneously (Fig 3.1). In patients with ankylosing spondylitis or increased thoracic kyphosis this may be difficult or impossible

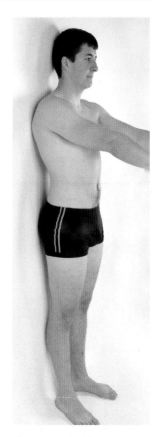

Fig 3.1: Assessing the curvature of the spine. Note the position of the heels, pelvis, shoulders and occiput

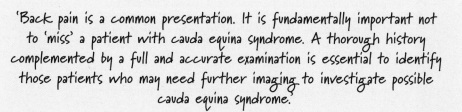

'Back pain is a common presentation. It is fundamentally important not to 'miss' a patient with cauda equina syndrome. A thorough history complemented by a full and accurate examination is essential to identify those patients who may need further imaging to investigate possible cauda equina syndrome.'

Mark Rodrigues,
Orthopaedic SHO (2011)
Edinburgh Royal Infirmary

Feel

- With the patient standing, palpate the spinous processes from T1 to the sacrum and the sacroiliac joints for tenderness
- Palpate the paraspinal musculature

Percussion

- Lightly percuss the spine, starting at the top of the neck, going down to the sacrum; significant pain is associated with infection, malignancy, and fractures

Move

- Flexion, extension and lateral flexion are movements of the lumbar spine
- Rotation occurs in the thoracic spine

Flexion

- Ask the patient to try to touch their toes (keeping their legs straight)
- Watch closely for curvature of the spine, smoothness of movement and any restriction, remembering that hip flexion can compensate for a stiff lumbar spine

Measure flexion through the modified Schober method (fig 3.2):

- Locate the dimples of Venus (which overlie the sacroiliac joints)
- Using a tape measure, mark 10 cm above the dimples of Venus with a pen (Point A) and 5 cm below (Point B)
- Anchor the top of the tape with a finger at Point B and ask the patient to flex forward as far as they can
- The distance between Point A and Point B increases with lumbar flexion. Measure the change in this distance with the above manoeuvre
- This is normally 6-7cm; anything less than 5cm is suggestive of spinal pathology

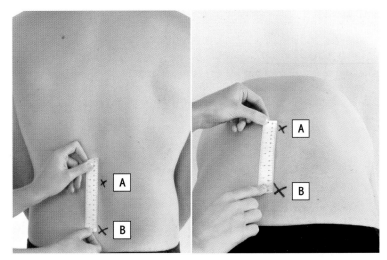

Fig 3.2: Modified Schober method for assessing flexion

Extension

- Ask the patient to arch their back, assisting them by steadying the pelvis. The normal extension is 30°

Lateral Flexion

- Ask the patient to slide their hands down the side of each leg in turn, the left hand down the left leg, and then the right hand down the right leg. Ensure that the legs are straight; the normal lateral flexion is 30°

Rotation

- With the patient seated, ask them to twist their shoulders around to each side
- Rotation is measured between the plane of shoulders and the pelvis; the normal rotation is 40°

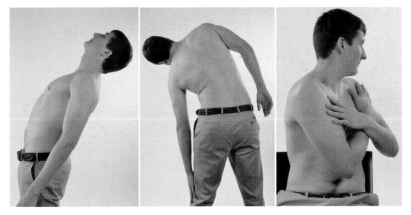

Fig 3.3: Assessing extension, lateral flexion and rotation (from left to right)

Special Tests: Root Compression Tests

Straight Leg Raise (Assesses L4, L5, S1 nerve roots i.e. L4/5, L5/S1 and S1/S2 disc spaces)

- With the patient lying on their back, maximally flex their hip whilst keeping the leg straight
- The test is only positive if the patient experiences pain going down the entire lower limb, past the knee; frequently there will be pain and tightness that affects the posterior thigh only – this is not a positive test
- Measure the angle between the bed and the leg (normal is 80-90° hip flexion)

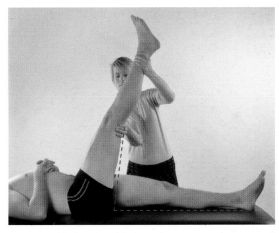

Fig 3.4: Straight leg raise with the angle to measure demonstrated

Tibial Stretch Test (Assesses L4-S3 nerve roots)

- With the patient lying supine, passively flex the knee to 90° and then flex the hip to 90°, before extending the knee (keeping the hip flexed to 90°)
- Apply pressure over both of the hamstring tendons in one leg; observe for pain; and then apply pressure over the middle of the popliteal fossa (where the tibial nerve runs)
- Pain when the nerve is pressed, BUT NOT when the hamstring tendons are pressed, is a positive result

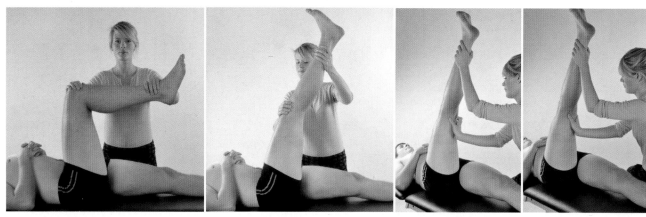

Fig 3.5: Tibial stretch test: (left to right) flexing the knee and hip, straightening the knee, pressure over the hamstring tendons, pressure over the tibial nerve

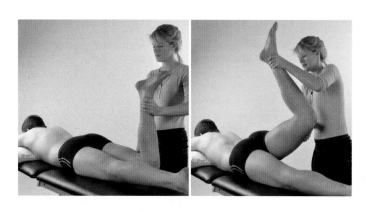

Femoral Stretch Test (Assess L2-4 nerve roots)

- With the patient lying on their front, flex the knee to 90° and maximally extend the hip
- Pain in the back or radiating down the anterior thigh is a positive result

Fig 3.6: Femoral stretch test

Neurovascular Assessment

- Neurological assessment of the lower limbs, assessing dermatomes, myotomes and reflexes
- Rectal examination to assess anal tone and saddle anaesthesia

Nerve Root	Dermatome	Myotome	Reflex
L2	Medial upper thigh	Hip flexion	Nil
L3	Medial lower thigh	Knee extension	Knee
L4	Medial calf	Ankle dorsiflexion	Knee
L5	1st dorsal webspace, lateral calf and dorsum of foot	Great toe dorsiflexion	Nil
S1	Lateral sole of foot and postero-teral calf	Plantar flexion	Ankle

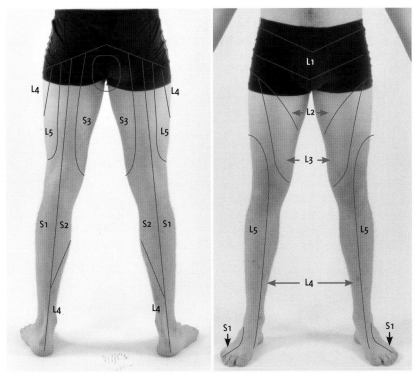

Fig 3.7: Lower limb dermatomes

Orthopaedics

Other Joints

The hips, shoulders and cervical spine should also be examined

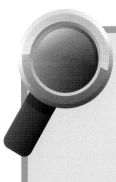

PRESENT YOUR FINDINGS...

'This gentleman has tenderness over his lumbar spinal and paraspinal muscles to palpation and percussion. He has a decreased range of hip flexion and extension bilaterally. Straight leg raise is positive at 65° flexion. Neurologically, he has hypoaesthesia over the L4-S1 dermatomes and flaccid weakness of ankle and toe dorsiflexion and plantar flexion bilaterally. Both ankle reflexes are absent. In addition, he has perianal hypoaesthesia on PR examination with normal anal tone.

These findings are consistent with a diagnosis of cauda equina syndrome, most likely secondary to prostatic cancer bone metastasis.

This is a medical emergency, requiring an urgent MRI, steroid therapy, and consideration for further neurosurgical/oncological intervention'

How would you manage this patient?

Cauda equina syndrome is an oncological emergency requiring early diagnosis and treatment.

Initial management involves:

- Analgesia
- Oral dexamethasone
- Urgent MRI spine
- Early discussion with oncology and neurosurgery with the possibility of neurosurgical decompression or palliative radiotherapy

Station 2: CERVICAL SPINE EXAMINATION

Mr Smith is an 85 year-old gentleman who fell off a ladder. He is complaining of some neck pain. Please examine his cervical spine.

Look

- Ask the patient to remove enough clothing to expose the neck and upper thorax
- Inspect from front, side and back
- Posture/position of neck
- Loss of normal lordosis (commonly due to muscle spasm)
- Muscle wasting
- Scars
- Lumps

Feel

- **Spinous Processes:** Palpate along the midline for tenderness starting from the occiput and moving downwards; the cervical spine from C2 downward is palpable; C7 and T1 spinous processes are the largest
- **Facet Joints:** Move your fingers 2.5cm lateral to the spinous processes to palpate facet joints for tenderness; **the facet joints between C5 and C6 are those that are most often involved in osteoarthritis** (in the cervical spine) and may be painful on palpation
- Palpate the paraspinal muscles and trapezius muscles for tenderness
- **Supraclavicularly:** Palpate for a cervical rib (overdevelopment of the seventh cervical vertebra can affect the subclavian artery and first thoracic nerve)
- **Crepitus:** Spread your hands on each side of the neck and ask the patient to flex and extend their spine

> 'Examining a potentially unstable cervical spine can have dire consequences. In such cases the patient should have inline neck immobilisation, and only once the cervical spine has been 'cleared' by an experienced doctor using X-rays and examination should the immobilisation be removed.'
>
> **Mark Rodrigues**
> *Orthopaedic SHO (2011)*
> *Edinburgh Royal Infirmary*

Move

Assess with patient sitting in chair:

- **Flexion:** Should be able to touch chin to chest (80°); chin-chest distance can be measured
- **Lhermitte's Test:** Electric shock-like sensation in the spine or limbs on neck flexion; can be caused by multiple sclerosis, myelopathy from cervical spondylosis, vitamin B12 deficiency or whiplash injury
- **Extension:** Make sure patient is seated; the plane of the nose and forehead should normally be nearly horizontal (normal 50°)
- **Rotation:** Chin normally falls just short of the plane of the shoulders (normal 80°)
- **Lateral Flexion:** Should nearly be able to touch the ear on shoulder (normal 45°)

Passive movements can be assessed gently if there are reduced active movements

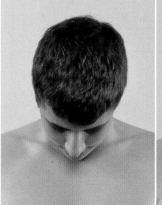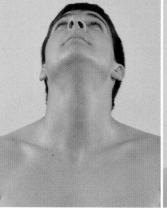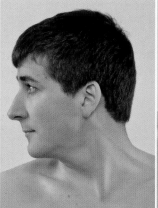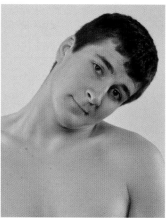

Fig 3.8: Neck movements (from left to right) flexion, extension, rotation and lateral flexion

Orthopaedics

Neurovascular Assessment/Cord Compression

- Examine the limbs, paying particular attention to lower motor neuron signs in the upper limbs (e.g. hypotonia, wasting, fasciculations, hyporeflexia) and upper motor neuron signs in the lower limbs (hypertonia, weakness, upgoing plantars, hyperreflexia)
- Perform rectal examination to assess the anal tone, palpate/percuss for a bladder and examine for saddle anaesthesia if concern over cord compression

Nerve Root	Dermatome	Myotome	Reflex
C5	Over deltoid	Shoulder abduction	Biceps, supinator
C6	Thumb and radial aspect of forearm (dorsal and palmar)	Elbow flexion (also C5)	Biceps, triceps, supinator
C7	Palmar and dorsal surface of middle finger	Elbow extension (also C8)	Triceps
C8	Palmar surface of little finger; ulnar aspect of forearm; dorsal surface of little finger	Finger flexion	Nil

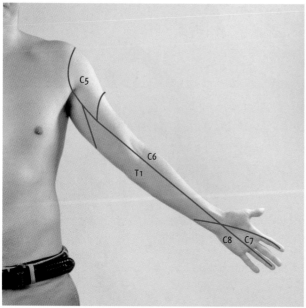
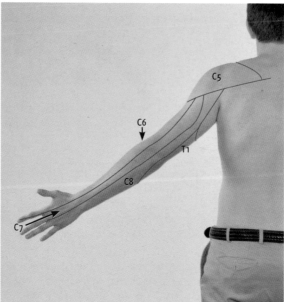

Fig 3.9: Upper limb dermatomes

Cervical Rib/Thoracic Outlet Syndrome

- Inspect the hands: may be perishingly cold, discoloured and atrophic
- Palpate radial pulse; then apply traction to arm for several seconds; reduction of radial pulsation after this manoeuvre suggests the presence of a cervical rib

Other Joints

- The shoulders should be examined as shoulder pain can be referred to the neck and vice versa

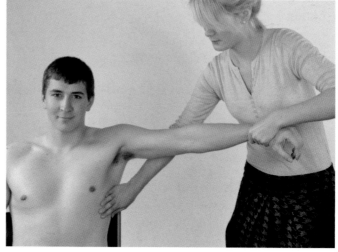

Fig 3.10: Applying traction to the arm (whilst palpating the radial pulse) to assess for a cervical rib

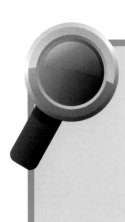

Orthopaedics

PRESENT YOUR FINDINGS...

'Mr Smith has a hard collar and in line immobilisation in situ. I have not assessed active and passive movements as the cervical spine has not been cleared. He has no neurological deficits in any limb.

Given the mode of injury and tenderness, I am concerned that Mr Smith has sustained a cervical spine fracture.

In line with ATLS guidelines, he requires AP and lateral X-rays of his cervical spine, including an odontoid peg view. The films must include the upper border of T1 in order to be adequate. Further imaging such as CT or MRI, plus discussion with neurosurgeons or orthopaedics may be required.'

How would you manage a patient with a possible unstable cervical spinal fracture?

Cervical spine injuries can result in devastating neurological sequelae.

Initial management involves:

- Inline triple immobilisation
- Analgesia
- AP and lateral X-rays of the cervical spine (C1-T1) and a peg view
- Discussion with neurosurgeons/ orthopaedics (depending on the results of XR)
- Further imaging (CT/MRI) may be required

Station 3: HAND EXAMINATION

Mr Payne is a 50 year-old gentleman who has been suffering from arthritis for the last 10 years. He is finding it progressively more difficult to write and to carry out household tasks with his hands. Please examine his hands and present your findings.

Look

- Stand back and look at the patient; there may be evidence of systemic disease, or systemic effects of rheumatological treatments. For example, are they Cushingoid due to long-term steroid use?
- Ask the patient to roll up their sleeves above their elbows and put their hands on a pillow in front of you. Look for rheumatoid nodules
- Look for a tremor with the patient's hands outstretched
- Assess resting posture; is there evidence of nerve damage, such as muscle wasting?
- Remember to look at the outer part of the ear for gouty tophi, and to look behind the ears for psoriasis (normally done after completing examination of the hands)

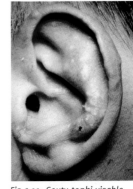

Fig 3.11: Gouty tophi visable on general inspection

With the patient's *palms down*, look for:

- Swelling and deformity
- Radio-carpal subluxation, ulnar deviation at the metocarpophalangeal (MCP) joints
- Swan neck deformity (flexion at MCP and distal interphalangeal (DIP) joints, extension at proximal interphalangeal (PIP) joint)
- Boutonniere deformity (extension at MCP and DIP joints, flexion at PIP joint)
- Z-shaped deformity of the thumb (flexion at MCP joint, hyperextension at IP joint), mallet finger (involuntary flexion of the distal phalanx of a finger), Heberden's (DIP) or Bouchard's (PIP) nodes
- Muscle wasting and scars
- Thinning and bruising of skin due to steroid use
- Nail changes – in psoriasis: pitting, onycholysis (detachment of nail from nail bed, which starts distally), nail fold infarcts

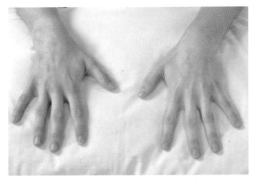

Fig 3.12: Palms down. Using a pillow to rest the patient's hands on is often the most comfortable way to inspect them

- Decide whether changes are symmetrical or asymmetrical
- Do changes mainly involve small joints (PIPs, DIPs, or MCPs) or wrists?

Ask patient to turn hands over with *palms up*, look for:

- Problems turning the hand are associated with radio-ulnar joint abnormality
- Palmar erythema
- Muscle wasting: if present, is it in both thenar and hypothenar eminences?
- If only the thenar eminence, this suggests median nerve damage, and possible carpal tunnel syndrome
- If only the hypothenar eminence, this suggests ulnar nerve damage
- Scars from carpal tunnel release operation in wrists or surgery for rheumatoid arthritis

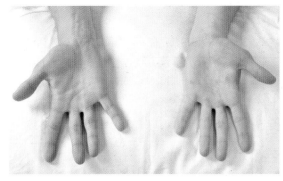

Fig 3.13: Palms up inspection

Feel

With the patient's *palms up*:

- Temperature
- Feel for radial pulses together
- Feel for bulk of thenar and hypothenar eminences
- Feel for tendon nodules and Dupuytren's contracture (fixed flexion contraction of hands, caused by thickening of the palmar aponeurosis)
- Assess medial and ulnar nerve sensation by gently touching over thenar and hypothenar eminences – is sensation present and equal? (See below for a full neurological assessment of the hand)

> 'Patients with rheumatoid arthritis often have painful hands. Be sure not to cause the patient any harm during your examination — ask the patient to turn their hands over themselves rather than doing it for them'
>
> ### Mark Rodrigues
> *Orthopaedic SHO (2011)*
> *Edinburgh Royal Infirmary*

Ask patient to turn hand over, with *palms down:*

- Using the back of your hand, assess the temperature at patient's forearm, wrists, and MCP joints
- **Ask whether there is any pain,** then whilst looking at the patient's face, gently squeeze across a row of MCP joints, assessing for tenderness
- Bimanually palpate any MCP, PIP, or DIP joint that appears swollen. This should be done by having your thumbs above and index fingers below the joint
  - Are there any signs of active synovitis? Does the joint feel warm, swollen, tender and rubbery?
- Are there hard, bony swellings?
  - Bouchard's nodes (PIP) and Heberden's nodes (DIP)
- Bimanually palpate the wrists, asking about pain first and looking at patient's face while examining
- Run your hand up the patient's arms to their elbows, looking for rheumatoid nodules or psoriatic plaques

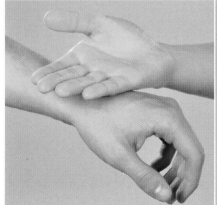
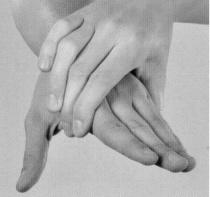
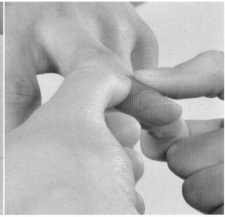

Fig 3.14: Feeling the hands for temperature   *Fig 3.15: Feeling for tenderness*   *Fig 3.16: Bimanually palpating the PIP joint*

Orthopaedics

Move

- Ask patient to straighten fingers fully
- Ask the patient to make a fist
- Ask patient to abduct and adduct fingers and touch the tip of each finger with their thumb (opposition)
- Assess wrist extension and flexion e.g. ask the patient to make the prayer and reverse prayer signs
- Then assess wrist flexion and extension passively
- Assess ulnar and radial deviation of the wrist. To assess ulnar deviation, stabilise the forearm with one hand, and then, while

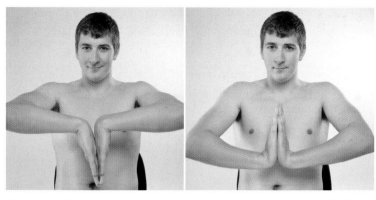

Fig 3.17: Assessing active movement. Assess flexion with the reverse prayer sign (left) and wrist extension with the prayer sign (right)

grasping the metacarpals from the radial side with the other hand, apply traction in the ulnar direction. Do the opposite for radial deviation. Ulnar deviation should be greater than radial

- Assess supination and pronation

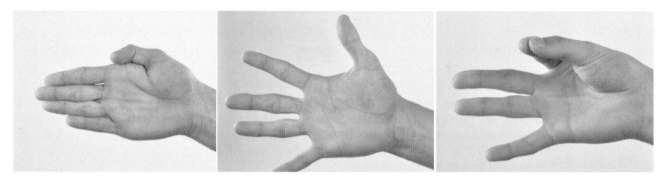

Fig 3.18: Assessing active movement (from left to right) adduction, abduction and opposition

Function

Ask the patient to:

- Grip 2 of your fingers to assess power grip
- Pinch your finger to assess pincer grip
- Pick up a small object such as a coin
- Flex and extend at the elbows. Can they bring their hands to their mouth?
- Put their hands behind their head
- Put their hands over their spine

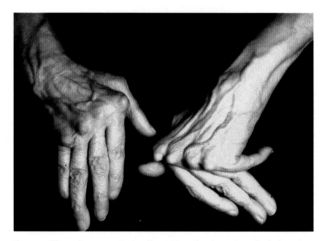

Fig 3.19: Bilateral symmetrical arthropathy, showing: ulnar deviation of the fingers, swelling of the MCP joints, guttering/muscle wasting (between extensor tendons over the metacarpals)

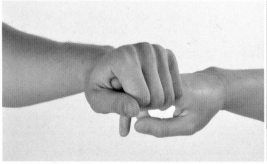
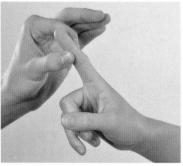
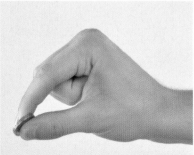

Fig 3.20: Testing function (from left to right) power grip, pinch grip and precision grip

Orthopaedics

Special Tests (Depending on clinical context)

Phalen's Test

- Hold the wrist in forced flexion for 60 seconds (reverse prayer position)
- Paraesthesia in the distribution of the median nerve is suggestive of carpal tunnel syndrome

Tinel's Test

- Percuss over the carpal tunnel (the skin crease over the ventral aspect of the wrist)
- Paraesthesia in the distribution of the median nerve is suggestive of carpal tunnel syndrome

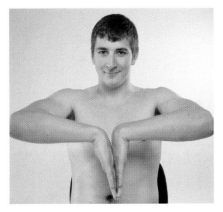

Fig 3.21: Phalen's Test

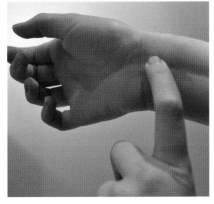

Fig 3.22: Tinel's Test

Assessing Tendons

Suspect a tendon injury if the patient is unable to perform the following tests:

Flexor digitorum profundus	Ask the patient to flex their DIP joint whilst keeping the PIP joint, MCP joint and wrist joint extended	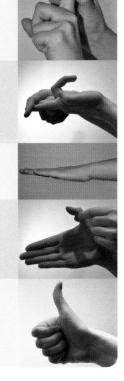
Flexor digitorum superficialis	Hold the non test fingers fully extended and ask the patient to flex the PIP joint you are examining	
Extensor digitorum	Ask the patient to extend their fingers whilst their wrist is held in the neutral position	
Flexor and extensor pollicis longus	Ask the patient to flex and extend their IP joint of the thumb whilst holding the proximal phalanx of the thumb	
Extensor pollicis brevis	Ask the patient to extend their thumb like a hitch-hiker	

Assessing Nerves

Assess nerves systematically. Some of the examination, such as inspecting for muscle wasting and posture, should have already been performed in the 'Look' part of the examination. Assess sensation for each nerve before moving on to assessing the motor function.

	Radial Nerve	**Median Nerve**	**Ulnar Nerve**
Muscle wasting	None – no intrinsic muscles are supplied by the radial nerve	Thenar eminence	Small muscles of hand (except thenar eminence)
Sensation	1st dorsal webspace	Radial border of the index finger	Ulnar border of the 5th finger
Motor Supply	Triceps brachii, anconeus, brachioradialis, extensor carpi radialis longus **Deep branch:** Extensor carpi radialis brevis, supinator **Posterior interosseous:** Extensor digitorum, extensor digiti minimi, extensor carpi ulnaris, extensor pollicis brevis, extensor pollicis longus, extensor indicis and abductor pollicis longus	Supplies the 'LOAF' muscles of the hand (lateral 2 lumbricals, opponens pollicis, abductor pollicis brevis and flexor pollicis brevis) plus all of the flexors of the forearm (except flexor carpi ulnaris, and the ulnar part of flexor digitorum profundus)	Supplies all muscles of the hand except 'LOAF' plus flexor carpi ulnaris and the ulnar part of flexor digitorum profundus
Posture	Wrist drop	Hand of Benediction. Proximal lesion of the median nerve result in the Hand of Benediction when the patient **tries to make a fist** The patient is **unable to flex the MCP, PIP or DIP** joints of the **index and middle fingers** due to loss of the **lateral 2 lumbricals;** the ring and little finger can flex at these joints	Claw hand **Occurs at rest** Loss of innervations of the **medial 2 lumbricals** results in **extension at the MCP joints of the ring and little fingers** due to unopposed action of the extensor digitorum If the lesion is at the wrist, some flexion will be observed at the PIP and DIP joints because the innervations of the medial half of flexor digitorum profundus is intact If the lesion is at the elbow, the claw will be less marked due to paralysis of the medial half of the flexor digitorum profundus, with resultant loss of flexion at the PIP and DIP joints

The difference between the Hand of Benediction and the Claw hand can be confusing.

Remember:

1. The Hand of Benediction only occurs when the patient tries to make a fist, whereas the claw hand occurs at rest

2. There is flexion at the MCP joints of the ring and index fingers in the Hand of Benediction, whereas the MCP joints of these fingers are extended in the claw hand

3. If you are still having difficulty, don't worry. The rest of the neurological signs should help differentiate between median and ulnar nerve lesions

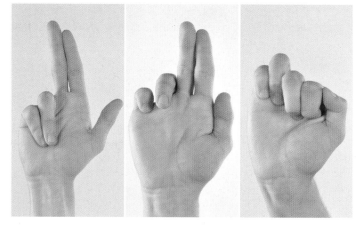

Fig 3.24: From left to right. 1. The hand of Benediction occurring when trying to make a fist (Note the 4th and 5th MCP joints are flexed). 2. The claw hand occurring at rest (Note the 4th and 5th MCP joints are extended. 3. The claw hand when trying to make a fist (Note the 4th and 5th MCP joints remain extended)

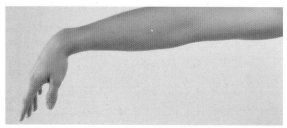

Fig 3.23: Wrist drop due to a radial nerve lesion

Orthopaedics

Radial Nerve	Ask the patient to extend their fingers against resistance, (and then their wrist) with their arm flexed to 90 degrees at the elbow and pronated Ask patient to extend their thumb against resistance	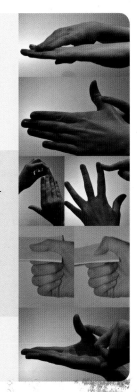
Ulnar Nerve	Assess finger adduction by asking the patient to hold a piece of card between their extended fourth and fifth fingers (left); assess finger abduction by asking the patient to abduct their extended index finger against resistance (right) Froment's sign: grip a piece of card between adducted thumb and palm; a positive Froment's sign is when the IP joint flexes as the patient tries to compensate for a weak thumb adductor with flexor pollicis longus, which is innervated by the median nerve. A negative test (left), shows NO significant flexion of the PIP, unlike a positive test (right)	
Median Nerve	Abduct thumb against resistance	

Other Joints

- The elbow should also be examined because pain in the elbow can be referred to the hand. Pathology at the elbow, such as rheumatoid nodules, can be related to pathology in the hand and also limited function of the elbow indirectly limits the function of the hand

> 'The radiological features of osteoarthritis and rheumatoid arthritis are applicable for any joint'
>
> **Mark Rodrigues**
> *Orthopaedic SHO (2011)*
> *Edinburgh Royal Infirmary*

What clinical features differentiate osteoarthritis and rheumatoid arthritis?

	Rheumatoid Arthritis	**Osteoarthritis**
Typical Joints Affected	MCP Joints	DIP and PIP joints and CMC (carpometacarpal) joint of thumb
Palmar Features	Wasting of thenar eminence Palmar erythema Z thumb deformity Reduced range of movement Boutonniere and Swan-Neck deformities Raised temperature	Disuse atrophy Reduced range of movement Normal temperature
Dorsal Features	Wrist subluxation Soft tissue swelling – spindling of joints and loss of valley between knuckles Wasting of intrinsic muscles (guttering)	Squaring of carpometacarpal joints Bouchard's nodes (PIP) Heberden's nodes (DIP) Crepitus
Radiological Features	Loss of joint space Erosions Periarticular osteoporosis Deformity Soft tissue swelling	Loss of joint space Subchondral sclerosis Bone cysts Osteophytes

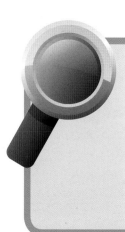

PRESENT YOUR FINDINGS...

'There is a bilateral symmetrical polyarthropathy affecting the small and large joints of both hands, predominantly the proximal interphalangeal and the distal interphalangeal joints. There is evidence of active inflammation, and functional impairment. There is also pitting of the nail beds and psoriatic plaques over the flexor surface of the elbows.

This is consistent with the diagnosis of psoriatic arthritis.

I would like to examine the rest of the skin, all of the other joints, and formally assess function'

Station 4: SHOULDER EXAMINATION

Mr O'Humeral is complaining of pain in and around his right shoulder. Please examine his shoulder.

Look

- Expose the upper limbs, neck and chest
- Assess each shoulder from standing in front, to the side and behind the patient, starting with the normal shoulder
- Look for deformity, swelling and scars
- Assess the muscle bulk of the deltoid, supraspinatus and infraspinatus, looking for muscle wasting
- Look at the scapula for winging

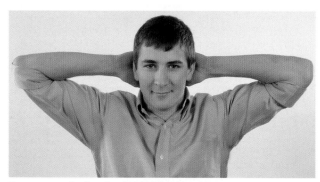

Fig 3.25: Assessing function: hands behind head

Feel

- Starting at the sternoclavicular joint, palpate the clavicle to the acromioclavicular joint for tenderness, temperature, swelling and deformity
- Palpate the acromion and coracoid for tenderness, before moving on to the scapular spine and biceps tendon
- Extending the shoulder brings the supraspinatus tendon anterior to the acromion, allowing it to be palpated

Move

- First, assess shoulder function by asking the patient to put their hands behind their head, reaching high up on the back and performing circular 'stirring' movements with each upper limb

Determine the range of active and then passive movements:

- Flexion (0-180°) and extension (0-60°)
- Abduction, whilst palpating the inferior pole of the scapula with your hand to assess the proportion of movement occurring at the gleno-humeral joint versus the amount coming from the scapular rotating (normal 0-150°)
- External rotation – ask the patient to flex their elbow to 90°, holding it in to the side of their body, with the fist pointing forward; then ask them to rotate their arm outwards (normal 0-90°)
- Internal rotation – ask the patient to rotate their arm across their back and then walk their thumb up their vertebrae; record the highest vertebra that the thumb can touch (normal mid thoracic)

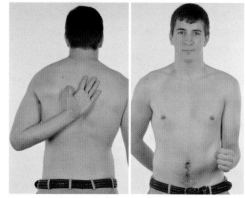

Fig 3.26: Assessing function: (from left to right) reaching up the back and making stirring movements

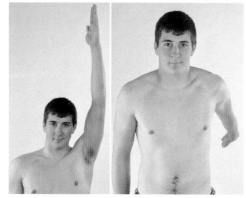

Fig 3.27: Shoulder flexion and extension

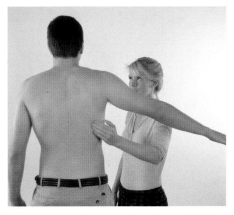
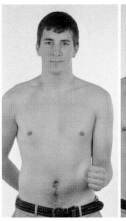
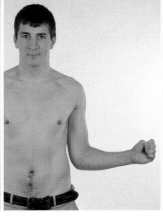
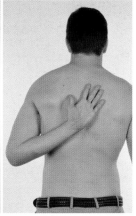

Fig 3.28: Abduction, with the examiner palpating the lower pole of the scapula

Fig 3.29: External rotation (left/middle) and internal rotation (right)

Special Tests

Impingement

- Passively abduct the shoulder
- Once it is fully abducted, let go, and ask the patient to adduct it slowly
- Pain between 60-120° implies a painful arc
- Pain during this manoeuvre is almost pathognomic of supraspinatus tendinitis

Acromioclavicular joint pathology (Scarf Test)

- Ask the patient to flex their shoulder AND elbow to 90° and place the hand on the opposite shoulder
- Apply a posteriorly directed force over the flexed elbow
- Pain indicates acromio-clavicular joint pathology

Rotator cuff

- Each of the 4 muscles forming the rotator cuff needs to be assessed. In the following tests, loss of power suggests a tear, whereas pain implies tendonitis
- **Supraspinatus:** Assess the first 15° of shoulder abduction against resistance. (Jobe's test is shoulder abduction against resistance with the thumb pointing down to the floor)
- **Infraspinatus and Teres Minor:** Assess external rotation against resistance; this test is more specific if the shoulder is flexed to 30° before externally rotating it (this diminishes the contribution of deltoid)
- **Subscapularis:** Test internal rotation against resistance by asking them to lift their hands off their back whilst you try to keep them there (Gerber's lift off test)

> 'There are over 100 clinical tests involving the shoulder, many of which test the same thing! This often leads to confusion. It is best to learn a few selected tests well. The following tests cover the main pathologies affecting the shoulder'
>
> **Mark Rodrigues**
> *Orthopaedic SHO (2011)*
> *Edinburgh Royal Infirmary*

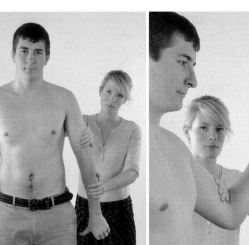
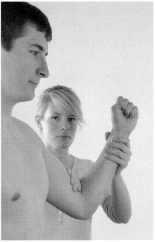
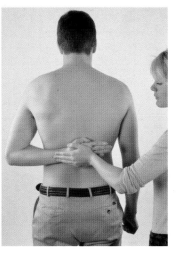

Fig 3.30: Assessing the rotator cuff: (Left to right)
Supraspinatus – Jobe's test (left) infraspinatus and teres minor (middle) subscapularis (right)

Bicipital tendonitis

- Supinate the forearm then flex the shoulder against resistance. As for the rotator cuff muscles, loss of power suggests a tear whereas pain suggests tendonitis

Winged scapula

- Ask the patient to push forcefully against a wall with the palms of both hands, whilst standing facing the wall. Look at their back for a 'winged scapula' (The scapular protrudes from the back in an abnormal way)
- This suggests damage to the long thoracic nerve supplying the serratus anterior

Shoulder apprehension test

- Stand behind the patient and ask them to abduct their shoulder to 90°, flex their elbow to 90° and externally rotate so the fingers are pointing towards the ceiling
- Put one of your hands over their shoulder and with your other hand, hold their elbow
- Push forward on their shoulder and pull back on the elbow
- Apprehension to this manoeuvre is a positive test, suggesting previous dislocation

Neurovascular Assessment

- Assess sensation at the regimental badge area – the skin covering the inferior region of the deltoid muscle (axillary nerve)
- Assess dermatomes and myotomes (C5-T1) (See station 3.2 cervical spine examination)
- Palpate the radial pulse; if not present, palpate the brachial pulse; ensure the hand is warm and well perfused

Other Joints

- Examine the neck and elbow as pain from these joints may be referred to the shoulder

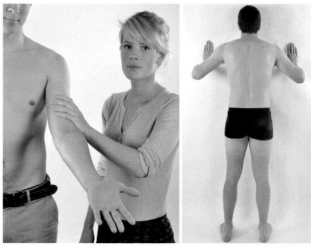

Fig 3.31: Assessing for bicipital tendonitis (left), testing for a 'winged scapula' by asking the patient to push against a wall and observing for abnormal protrusion of the scapulae (right)

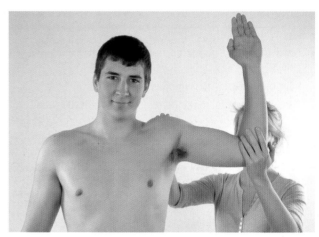

Fig 3.32: The shoulder apprehension test

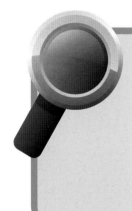

PRESENT YOUR FINDINGS...

'Mr O'Humeral's right shoulder is tender over the acromion. There are no signs of infection in the joint. Active abduction is difficult for the patient to initiate due to pain, but there is a full range of movement for passive abduction. In addition, there is a painful arc between 70-120°. The other movements at the shoulder are normal, including the other rotator muscles. The left shoulder is normal, as is examination of the elbow and neck.

These findings are in keeping with a diagnosis of chronic tendinitis/impingement syndrome.'

Station 5: HIP EXAMINATION

Mr Trendelenburg has recently fallen. His left lower limb looks shorter than his right, and it is also looks rotated. Please examine his hips.

Look

- Expose both hips
- With the patient lying as flat as possible, inspect legs and compare both sides
- Is there an obvious flexion deformity of the hip?

Look for leg length disparity:

- **True length:** measure from the anterior superior iliac spine to the medial malleolus on both legs
- **Apparent length:** compare with the distance from the umbilicus to the medial malleolus
- If there is a true leg length discrepancy, ask the patient to flex their knees (if able) whilst keeping their heels together; this allows you to see whether the shortening is below or above the knee
- If the abnormality is above the knee, place your thumbs on the anterior superior iliac spines, and with your fingers, feel for the tops of the greater trochanters to assess whether the pathology is proximal to the trochanters
- Look for scars overlying the hips, muscle wasting, swelling
- Look at the foot to identify any rotation of the lower limb

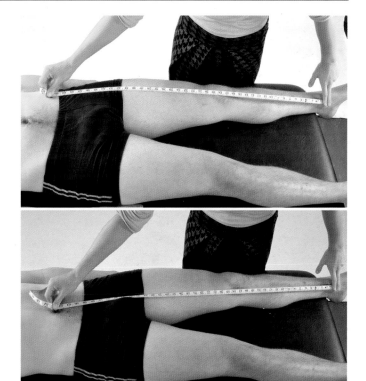

Fig 3.33: True leg length measurement (top), apparent leg length measurement (bottom)

Causes of True Leg Shortening

Pathology proximal to the greater trochanter (i.e. hip)	Pathology distal to the greater trochanter (i.e. femur and tibia)
Fractured neck of femur	Fractures
Post hip arthroplasty	Osteomyelitis
Hip dislocation	Septic arthritis
Arthritis	Epiphyseal injury
Slipped upper femoral epiphysis	Polio
Perthes' disease	Rare conditions (e.g. hemihypertrophy)

Note: apparent leg shortening is commonly caused by pelvic tilt

Feel

- Ask the patient if they have any pain currently and where it is (be extra cautious when examining these areas and remember to watch the patient's face for signs of distress)
- Palpate the hip joint; tenderness over the greater trochanter occurs in trochanteric bursitis
- Feel the temperature (it is difficult to detect any changes as the hip is a deep joint)

> 'Use common sense when examining patients; if they are lying on a couch assess the gait at the end of the examination, whereas if they are standing or sitting, gait can be examined at the start, as can Trendelenburg's Test'
>
> **Mark Rodrigues**
> *Orthopaedic SHO (2011)*
> *Edinburgh Royal Infirmary*

Move

Assess active movements:

- Ask the patient to flex their knees to 90°. Then ask the patient to flex their hip fully, followed by extending both the knee and the hip simultaneously (normal 0-120°)
- Lift the patient's leg from the couch and then ask them to abduct (normal 45°) and adduct (normal 25°) (active)

Assess passive movements:

- With the lower limbs straight, gently roll the entire lower limb externally and internally to roughly assess rotation
- Flex the hip and knee to 90°; from this position, test internal rotation by moving the foot laterally (normal 45°); test external rotation by moving the foot medially (normal 45°)
- Stabilise the pelvis with one of your arms; extend the leg; abduct (normal 45°) and adduct (normal 25°) the lower limb using your other hand
- Ask patient to roll onto their side (if possible) to assess extension

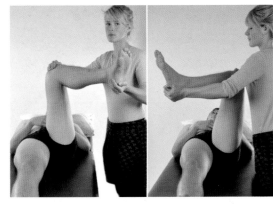

Fig 3.34: Internal rotation (left) external rotation (right)

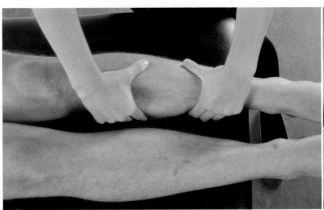

Fig 3.35: Internal rotation (left), external rotation (right) (more crudely measured than in Fig 3.34)

Special Tests

Thomas' Test

- Place one of your hands under the lower back (to ensure that the resting lordosis is removed)
- Fully flex the non-test hip with your other hand until the lumbar spine touches the fingers of the hand under the back
- Look at the opposite leg; if it is lifted off the couch as a result of this manoeuvre, there is a fixed flexion deformity in that hip
- A positive test implies a hip flexion contracture

> 'Thomas' test can be performed when assessing passive hip flexion. This will make your examination sequence more polished'
>
> **Mark Rodrigues**
> *Orthopaedic SHO (2011)*
> *Edinburgh Royal Infirmary*

Trendelenburg's Test

- With the patient standing, crouch in front of them, and gently place one of your hands on each anterior superior iliac spine, so that you can monitor the movement of the pelvis
- Ask the patient to stand on each leg in turn
- In a negative test, the pelvis remains level (or the unsupported side may rise)
- In a positive test, the pelvis will dip on the unsupported side (due to failure or weakness of the hip abductors on the opposite side)

NOTE: There is another Trendelenburg test that assesses the competency of valves in superficial and deep veins of the legs (see station 2.14)

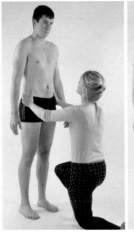
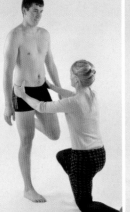
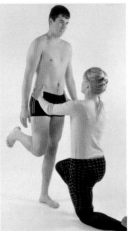

Fig 3.36: A negative Trendelenburg's Test

Orthopaedics

Standing and Gait (if able)

- This can be done at the start or the end of the examination

From the front, assess whether:
- The shoulders are parallel to the ground
- There is a pelvic tilt
- The hips, knees and ankles are aligned properly

Ask the patient to walk across the room, while you look for:
- Antalgic gait (limping)
- Trendelenburg gait (pelvis tilting away from affected hip, trunk tilting towards affected hip)

Neurovascular Assessment

- Assess sensation along the dorsum and sole of the foot (i.e. branches of the sciatic nerve) and the anterior and medial thigh and medial calf (i.e. branches of the femoral nerve)
- Palpate for the dorsalis pedis and posterior tibial arterial pulses

Other Joints

- The spine and knee should also be examined

What are the surgical options for the management of a neck of femur fracture?

The type of operation depends on the type of fracture and the level of functioning of the patient

- Extra capsular fractures: generally managed with dynamic hip screws
- Subtrochanteric fractures: generally managed with an intermedullary nail

For intra capsular fractures:
- If undisplaced (in a young patient): cannulated screws
- If displaced or (undisplaced in an older patient): Hemi-arthroplasty (limited premorbid mobility) or total arthroplasty
- In a young patient, reduction and cannulated screw fixation can also be considered for a displaced intracapsular fracture

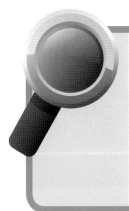

PRESENT YOUR FINDINGS...

'Mr Trendelenburg is in obvious discomfort. He has a shortened and externally rotated left lower limb. He is tender over the greater trochanter and is unable to move his left lower limb due to pain. The limb is distally neurovascularly intact. The right lower limb is normal.

This is consistent with a diagnosis of a fractured left neck of femur.

This patient requires analgesia, plus AP pelvis and lateral left hip X-rays to confirm the diagnosis'.

Station 6: KNEE EXAMINATION

Mr Smith is a 65 year-old gentleman who is suffering from pain and stiffness in his knees. Examine the knee joints and tell the examiner about any positive clinical findings as you come across them.

Look

- Look around the bedside for any clues such as braces (which may suggest polio) or walking aids
- Expose the patient's knees and thighs

With the patient standing, look (from front, side, and back):

- **Alignment:** only truly assessed while standing and weight bearing. Look for varus (bow-legged) or valgus (knock-knees) deformities

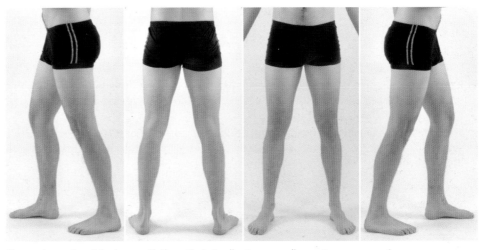

Fig 3.37: Inspection of the knees with the patient standing to assess alignment

With the patient lying down, look for:

- **Scars:** anterior cruciate ligament repair, knee replacement, arthroscopy
- **Swelling:** effusion, infection, arthritis, Baker's cyst
- **Wasting:** quadriceps wasting secondary to disuse
- **Skin changes:** psoriasis, erythema

> 'Use only one finger/thumb at a time to palpate for tenderness. If you use both hands simultaneously and the patient complains of pain you cannot be sure which site is the painful site and will have to inflict more discomfort to confirm the tender area'
>
> **Mark Rodrigues**
> *Orthopaedic SHO (2011)*
> *Edinburgh Royal Infirmary*

At this stage, the following assessments can also be made:

- **Posterior Sag:** Assess from the side with the patient supine; ask the patient to flex both their hips and knees to 90°; support their ankles, making sure they are equidistant from their buttocks. Look at the tibial tuberosities; in a positive test, the tibia is not in front of the femur (i.e. it is shifted towards the bed) - this suggests posterior cruciate ligament laxity

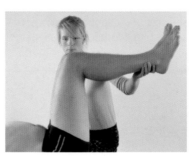

Fig 3.38: Assessing for a posterior sag

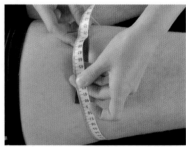

Fig 3.39: Measuring mid-thigh circumference

- Measure thigh circumference 15cm above the tibial tuberosity, to assess for muscle wasting (it is important to measure at the same site on both thighs i.e. 15cm above the tibial tuberosity)
- **Assess gait:** Look especially for an 'antalgic gait', a limp adopted to avoid pain by reducing weight-bearing time on the affected side; also the use of walking aids can be assessed

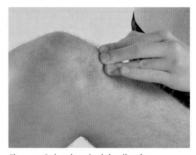

Fig 3.40: Palpating the joint line for tenderness

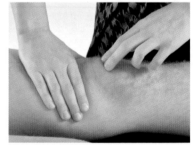

Fig 3.41: Assessing for an effusion: the patella tap

Feel

- While the knee is straight, palpate for tenderness along the patella borders
- Feel the temperature (using the back of hand); compare it to mid-thigh or mid-calf as well as comparing both sides
- Flex the knee to 90° and feel along the joint line, which is located level with the inferior pole of the patella; begin at the femoral condyles, move down to the base of the patella and then down to the tibial tuberosity
- Feel for any swelling in the popliteal fossa (Baker's cyst)

A knee effusion may be detected in several ways; for the following tests, have the patient supine, with knees extended:

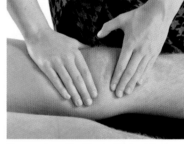

Fig 3.42: Assessing for an effusion: the sweep test

- Look for loss of dimple medial to knee cap
- **Patella Tap:** Milk fluid down out of the suprapatellar pouch and occlude the pouch with one of your hands; attempt to tap the patella. If a tap is elicited, this is a positive test (the suprapatellar pouch is an extension of the synovial sac, between the quadriceps tendon and the femur)
- **Sweep Test:** With one of your hands, firmly stroke along the medial side of the knee joint, distal to proximal; this should shift synovial fluid. Quickly repeat along the lateral side of the knee, proximal to distal; if the fluid bulges on the medial side, this is a positive test

Move

- It is important to elicit a range of active movements first so that pain is not inflicted by over-zealous passive movements
- Ask the patient to flex and extend the knee as much as possible. Is movement limited? What is it limited by – pain or stiffness? Is the knee hyperflexible?
- Ask the patient to raise their extended lower limb up off the bed (one leg at a time) to assess the integrity of the extensor mechanism. Inability to maintain full knee extension indicates an extensor lag is present secondary to disruption of the extensor mechanism or quadriceps weakness

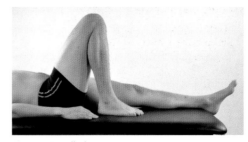

Fig 3.43: Knee flexion

- If there is a flexion deformity? Is it fixed (i.e. does it persist on lifting the opposite heel)?
- Assess passive knee flexion and extension by flexing and extending the leg yourself with the patient relaxed (while feeling for crepitus over the patella) (normal 0-140°)

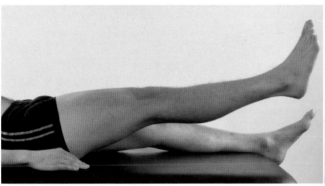
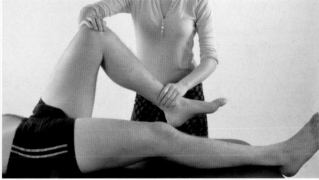

Fig 3.44: Knee extension and assessment of the integrity of the extensor mechanism (left), feeling for crepitus whilst flexing the patient's knee (right)

Special Tests

Patellar Apprehension Test

- This assesses for a patella dislocation that may have spontaneously relocated
- With the knee fully extended, apply a lateral force to the patellar whilst flexing the knee slowly
- Observe for apprehension by looking at the patient's face; resistance to flexion is a positive result

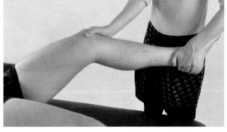

Fig 3.45: The patellar apprehension test

Anterior Cruciate Ligament

Anterior Draw Test

- With the patient supine and the test knee flexed to 90°, grip the upper tibia with both of your hands, with your thumbs on the tibial tuberosity and your fingers at the back of the leg
- Sit on the patient's foot – remember to ask them if it is okay before you do this, as you do not want to cause the patient pain!
- Ask the patient to relax their muscles and check the hamstrings are relaxed with your hands
- From the above position, pull the tibia firmly towards you, looking for significant movement of it away from the femur

Lachman's Test

- Flex the knee to 20°; with one hand, hold the patient's lower leg (behind proximal tibia), with the other hand the upper leg (grasping femur) and attempt to glide the joint surfaces forwards and backwards across each other
- There should be no gliding if the knee is stable
- This test is more sensitive than the anterior drawer test

Posterior Cruciate Ligament

Posterior Draw Test

- This test is similar to that for the anterior cruciate ligament; however, push the tibia away from you, not towards you

The patient may also have a posterior sag (as previously described)

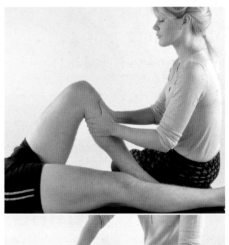
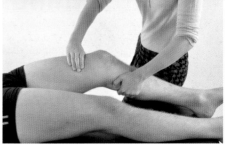

Fig 3.46: Testing the anterior cruciate ligament. Top: Anterior drawer test. Bottom: Lachman's test

Medial and Lateral Collateral Ligaments

- Fully extend the knee
- Place the distal tibia of the leg being tested between your elbow and side
- Hold the knee joint with your hands on either side of it
- Apply valgus strain, by moving the distal tibia (outward pressure) to assess medial collateral ligament
- Apply varus strain, by moving the distal tibia (inward pressure) to assess lateral collateral ligament
- If the above is unstable, then there is likely to be damage to other ligaments in addition to the collateral ligaments
- If the above is stable, repeat with the knee flexed to 30° to assess minor median and lateral collateral laxity

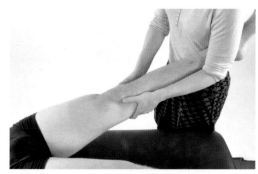

Fig 3.47: Position for testing the collateral ligaments

Meniscal Tears (McMurray's Test)

To test the medial meniscus:

- Flex the patient's knee to 90°
- Place your fingers on medial joint line
- Externally rotate the foot whilst simultaneously abducting the hip (i.e. applying a varus stress to the knee)
- Slowly flex and extend the knee while feeling over the joint for a clunk/click

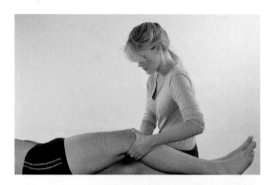

To test the lateral meniscus:

- Flex the patient's knee to 90°
- Place your fingers on the lateral joint line
- Internally rotate the foot whilst simultaneously adducting the hip (i.e. applying a valgus stress to the knee)
- Slowly flex and extend the knee while feeling over the joint for a clunk/click

NOTE: this test can be extremely painful if there is a genuine meniscal injury

Neurovascular Assessment

- Test sensation along the dorsum and sole of the foot
- Palpate popliteal, dorsalis pedis and posterior tibial pulses

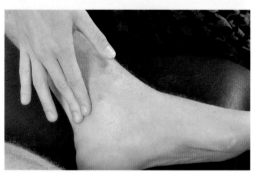

Fig 3.48: Popliteal pulse (top), posterior tibial pulse (bottom)

Other Joints

- The ankle and hip should also be examined

PRESENT YOUR FINDINGS...

'This gentleman who presents with a 3 year history of gradually worsening knee pain has a varus deformity of both knees. There is patello-femoral crepitus and a decreased range of movement in both knees, more marked on the left knee. He also requires a walking aid.

This is consistent with a diagnosis of osteoarthritis.'

How would you treat osteoarthritis of the knee?

- Conservative: Weight loss, stop smoking, icepacks, physiotherapy (strength), walking aids
- Medical: NSAIDs, simple analgesia, intra-articular steroids
- Surgical: Total knee replacement

Station 7: GAIT, ARMS, LEGS AND SPINE (GALS) EXAMINATION

Mrs Georgeson is a 45 year-old woman who has increasingly stiff joints. Please perform a GALS screen on her and present your findings.

Screening Questions

1) Do you have any pain or stiffness in your muscles, joints or back?
2) Can you dress yourself completely without any difficulty?
3) Can you walk up and down stairs without any difficulty?

Gait

Ask the patient to walk a few steps, turn and walk back. You are looking for:

- Symmetry
- Smoothness
- Ability to turn quickly

With the patient standing in an anatomical position, inspect from:

Front

- Shoulder bulk and symmetry
- Quadriceps bulk and symmetry
- Forefoot abnormalities

Behind

- Shoulder muscle bulk and symmetry
- Spinal alignment
- Gluteal muscle bulk and symmetry
- Popliteal swelling
- Calf muscle bulk and symmetry
- Hind foot abnormalities

Side

- Cervical lordosis
- Thoracic kyphosis
- Lumbar lordosis
- Knee flexion/extension

> 'Try to present your findings in a systematic manner; use the same structure as you did to perform the examination e.g. look, feel, move, special tests, distal neurovascular integrity. Be selective in what you present; present positive findings first, but also mention important negative findings'
>
> **Mark Rodrigues**
> *Orthopaedic SHO (2011)*
> *Edinburgh Royal Infirmary*

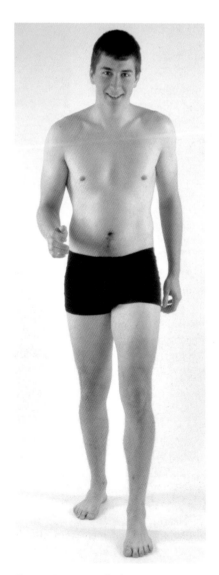

Fig 3.49: Assessment of gait

Arms

- Ask the patient to put their hands behind their head; this assesses shoulder abduction, external rotation, and elbow flexion
- With the patient's hands held out, palms down and fingers outstretched, observe the back of the hands for swelling and deformity
- Ask the patient to turn their hands over and look for muscle bulk and symmetry
- Ask the patient to make a fist
- Ask the patient to squeeze your fingers and assess grip strength
- Ask the patient to bring each finger in turn to meet the thumb; this assesses fine precision pinch
- Gently squeeze across metacarpo-phalangeal joints for tenderness suggesting inflammation; be sure to tell patient first and watch their face for pain!

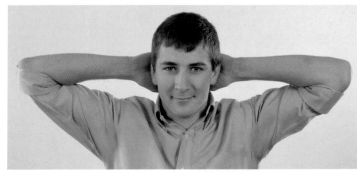

Fig 3.50: Hands behind head position

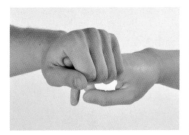

Fig 3.51: Grip strength

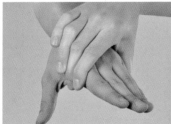

Fig 3.52: Squeezing across metacarpo-phalangeal joints

Legs

- Ask the patient to lie on the couch
- Assess passively flexion and extension of both knees whilst feeling for crepitus
- With the patient's hips and knee flexed to 90°, hold the knee and ankle, and assess the internal rotation of both hips
- Perform a patellar tap to check for effusion (as detailed previously)
- From the end of couch, inspect the feet for swelling and deformities
- Gently squeeze across the metatarso-phalangeal joints for tenderness suggesting inflammation; be sure to tell patient first and watch their face for pain!

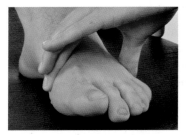

Fig 3.53: Assessing for MTP tenderness

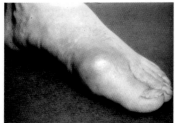

Fig 3.54: Swelling of the 1st MTP in acute gout. This is likely to be tender

Spine

- With the patient standing, inspect spine from behind for scoliosis
- Assess lateral flexion of the cervical spine; ask the patient to tilt their head to each side, left then right, bringing the ear towards shoulder
- Assess the temporo-mandibular joint; ask the patient to open their mouth and move their jaw from side to side
- Ask the patient to bend and touch their toes
- Assess lumbar spine flexion by placing 2 of your fingers on the lumbar vertebrae; your fingers should move apart on flexion and back together on extension

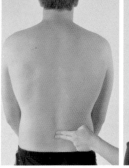 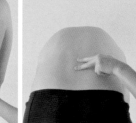

Fig 3.55: Crudely assessing lumbar spine flexion

Fig 3.56: Assessing the temporo- mandibular joint

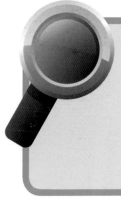

PRESENT YOUR FINDINGS...

'Mrs Georgeson has early morning pain and stiffness affecting the small joints of her hands. She is having difficulty with dextrous tasks, such as buttoning shirts. On examination, there is prominent deformity of the metacarpo-phalangeal joints with ulnar deviation of the fingers and 'Z-shaped thumbs' bilaterally. There is bilateral symmetrical joint swelling and tenderness affecting all metacarpo-phalangeal and metatarso-phalangeal joints, with reduced range of movement in her hands. Her gait, lower limb and spinal examinations are unremarkable.

This clinical picture is consistent with a diagnosis of Rheumatoid Arthritis of the hands.'

4 Communication

Successful communication rests on relevant knowledge as well as on effective patient interaction. The most important thing being assessed is your ability to communicate clearly, sensitively and succinctly. If you do not know a particular fact, you can always ask a senior doctor, or look up the information, but poor communication skills can lead to misunderstandings, and loss of patient trust.

The salient background factual information for each station is listed in the following chapter. Success relies on being able to sieve through this information, to identify that which is most important to the patient in front of you, and perhaps to add additional information based on the specific circumstances presented. As an example, in the broad area of 'Explaining an EEG to a Parent', the scenario may involve an EEG for a child with learning difficulties, and ADHD. When you are talking about the electrode stickers being placed on the child's head, the mother may remark 'he doesn't let anyone touch his face'. A large part of this consultation then becomes acknowledging this difficulty, and with the help of the mother, working on a practical solution to it. For example you might let the child put the stickers on himself, involve a play therapist, or do the EEG whilst the child is asleep.

A flexible generic framework as follows can provide a useful structure to follow. Remember to spend time gauging who your patient is, their ideas, concerns and expectations. The same word might mean different things to two different patients. There is no spiel that can be memorised on 'cystic fibrosis counselling' only a framework, to be adapted to the patient in front of you.

It is also important to ensure that you regularly check understanding. 'Chunk and check': give the information in small fragments, and make sure that the patient is following you at each stage.

Explanation Framework

Introduction

- Shake hands and introduce yourself
- Make eye contact, smile (this may not be appropriate in all situations e.g. breaking bad news)
- Ensure that you are not going to be disturbed, and that you can give the patient your full attention
- Establish a plan: *'In the next ten minutes we are going to talk about the results of your cervical smear test, and discuss any concerns you might have'*

Establish the patient's initial understanding

- Use open questions such as *'What have you been told so far about your condition?'*
  - This will allow you to act sensitively when you identify and introduce new concepts to the patient
  - This also gives an idea of the type of language the patient uses to understand medicine, helping you tailor the explanation to their vocabulary
- Ask the patient at the beginning about their questions and concerns. This way, the things most important to the patient can be explained first, getting you off on a good footing with them

Explain the procedure/test/treatment

- Check regularly that the patient understands you: *'Just to be sure I have explained everything clearly, can you tell me your understanding of what causes cervical cancer?'*
- Avoid jargon in general, especially if the patient does not initially use medical terms when talking about what they understand
- Use diagrams to illustrate complex points, for example the placenta blocking the exit of the womb in 'placenta previa'

Conclude

- Give a brief summary of what you have explained
- Offer written literature
- Ask the patient if they have any further questions, and specifically address these straight away if possible. If helpful, arrange to meet again, when the patient has had time to digest the information and discuss it with other people, such as their partner

Study Action Plan

- Unlike history taking or examination, it is difficult as a medical student to practice communication skills on patients. However, you can observe communication skills in clinical scenarios and learn from them

- If it helps, develop a framework to guide your communication: some frameworks are suggested in the text. However, remember always to adapt to each patient

- Practice with friends, not only to assess each other at how you communicate facts, but also to confirm that you identify and appropriately address patient concerns

This chapter contains notes for the following topics:

You have been asked to see Mr Cleghorn by the GI team. He has been admitted with haematemesis. He has known alcoholic liver disease. His AMT score is currently 6/10. He is refusing to have an endoscopy and says that his symptoms will improve spontaneously. Please explain the endoscopy procedure to him, and assess his capacity to consent for endoscopy.

- Assessment of capacity involves making a decision on whether the patient's mental state allows them to accept or refuse treatment
- A common mistake is to consider capacity assessments as the ability of patients to make ANY decisions – instead, capacity judgement should be made with respect to a specific question

Introduction

- Introduce yourself and establish a rapport
- Clearly explain to the patient why you are seeing them
- In this context, explain why an endoscopy is being recommended, and explore the reasons why the patient may not want to have it

Explore the Patient's Beliefs

Ask the patient questions to establish very generally their awareness level. *'What is your understanding of why you are here?'* *'How long have you been here for?'*

Since capacity is 'decision specific', you must explore the issues surrounding endoscopy:

Assess the patient's current understanding of 'endoscopy'
- *'What is your understanding of having an endoscopy?'*
- *'Do you understand why we would like to perform an endoscopy on you?'*

Explore the patient's reasons for refusing treatment. There may be legitimate concerns that you can address:
- *'Is there any aspect of the procedure that worries you?'*
- *'Do you know anyone that has had problems with it before?'* *'Have you had this procedure before?'*

Reinforce the Details of the Procedure

Procedure Information

- *'An endoscopy is a common test where a doctor looks at the gut, with a camera. We will be looking at the upper part of your gut'*
- *'An endoscope is a thin, flexible tube, about the width of your little finger, that we pass through the mouth into your gut'*
- *'We can give you something to help you relax'*
- *'We can take pictures of your gut, and take tissue samples if necessary, as well as directly treat certain problems'*

Potential Complications

- *'Most endoscopies happen without a problem. You may have a mild sore throat afterward, and may feel sleepy from the medicine we give to help you relax'*

- *'Sometimes the endoscope causes damage to the gut and we will ask you to let us know if you develop tummy pain, difficulty breathing, or feel like you may vomit'*
- *'There is also a slightly increased risk of getting a chest infection'*
- *'Very rarely, people might have a reaction to the sedative medication. This is normally due to an underlying sensitivity'*

Contextualise the Information and Explain Alternatives

- *'We are concerned that you may be bleeding from your stomach'*
- *'The best way to diagnose this, and potentially treat it, is by using this camera test'*
- *'We strongly recommend you have this procedure'*
- Explore these points in the context of the anxieties that may have become apparent from the previous line of questioning
- Explain alternatives and what the consequences of not having the procedure might be

Assessing Capacity

Capacity can be assumed if the patient can:

Understand the Information Given to Them

- This can be difficult to assess, particularly if the patient has a radically different opinion to that of the doctor
- It is useful to ask the patient to repeat back the information given to them. Ask the patient to explain what they believe the consequences of their decision will be
- The patient must also be able to retain this information long enough to be able to make a decision based on it

Show evidence of reason and deliberation, acting on a set of consistent and clear values

- An individual may legitimately refuse to give consent for a particular treatment even though it might seem unwise or irrational to their doctor. This is only as long as it is based on consistent and clear values

Communicate the decision they have made

- This is not relevant to the above patient, but would be relevant, for example, if the patient was in a coma, or had had a stroke that affected speech

Act Free of Coercion

- A patient's expressed opinion may be different when family members are in the same room, or after speaking to a relative. It may be beneficial to speak to the patient away from relatives
- Coercion may also occur from medical staff. Whether coercion has occurred may be difficult to assess in practice

The assessment should be decision specific

If a patient was, for a previous decision, deemed not to have capacity, do not assume that for subsequent decisions they still do not have capacity. The previous instance could have been due to a) transient illness that has now resolved or b) the nature of the previous decision being far more complicated.

Enhancing Capacity

If the patient does not have capacity, several techniques can be used to try and enhance it:

Using Plain Language

- This will ensure that the patient understands what is being said to them. It is important to avoid trying to push one answer on the patient

Allowing the Patient to have Family and/ or Friends Present

- Involving others in this manner can be difficult. It may sometimes conflict with ensuring that a decision is being made free of coercion

Allowing Time to Pass

- If the intervention for which consent is required is not urgent, **allow time to pass.** This may allow for any acute illness to resolve and the effect of any mind altering drugs to stop
- More generally, it will give the patient time to think over their decision. In this regard the ability to consent can be considered 'time specific'

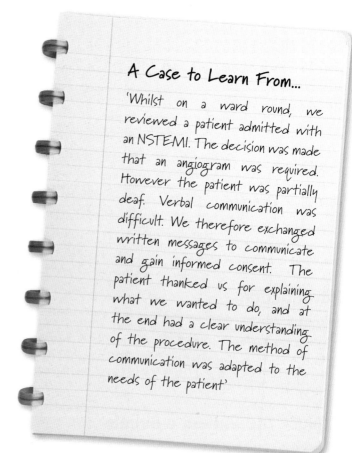

A Case to Learn From...

'Whilst on a ward round, we reviewed a patient admitted with an NSTEMI. The decision was made that an angiogram was required. However the patient was partially deaf. Verbal communication was difficult. We therefore exchanged written messages to communicate and gain informed consent. The patient thanked us for explaining what we wanted to do, and at the end had a clear understanding of the procedure. The method of communication was adapted to the needs of the patient'

If the patient does have capacity, and agrees to the procedure, ensure that they sign and date a consent form. If they do not want the procedure, and have capacity, make sure that you have a clear discussion with them about the possible consequences. Explore alternative diagnostic modalities/treatment, in the context of the patient's anxieties

If they do not have capacity, it may be necessary to treat under the 'Mental Capacity Act' or 'Adults with Incapacity Act' (Scotland)

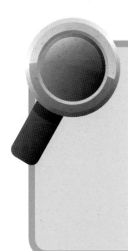

PRESENT YOUR FINDINGS...

'Mr Cleghorn has had the risks and benefits of an endoscopy explained to him, but is refusing to have one 'because it is pointless'. However, he is unable to understand the information given to him, and has not shown reason or deliberation in the decision making process. This is despite the use of plain language, and the support of his relatives.

Therefore, he does not currently have the capacity to consent to or refute endoscopy.

Given the medical urgency of the intervention, allowing time to pass, or alternative treatment/ tests are not practical options. He may require the procedure to go ahead, in his best interest after a 'Consent form 4' / 'Adults with Incapacity Act' form (Scotland) has been signed.

Mrs Fredrick has attended a GP clinic and is asking for a HIV test. Establish whether she is at low, or high risk for HIV. Please explore the risks and benefits of HIV testing.

- *'May I ask why you have attended the clinic today?'* *'Why are you considering a HIV test?'*
- *'Would you mind discussing the issues surrounding HIV testing with me?'*
- Warn the patient that you may ask some embarrassing questions, but everything will be taken in strictest confidence

Assess the Risk of the Patient

- Sexual
  - **Orientation:** must establish for males whether any same-sex relationships have occurred
  - **Type of sex:** must establish if penetrative anal intercourse, with or without condoms, has occurred since the last HIV test
  - **Number of partners and number known to be HIV positive or at high risk**
  - **Condom usage:** never, not always, always
  - **Prostitutes:** *'have you ever paid for sex?'*
  - **Sex abroad:** further details: country of origin, gender of partner, type of sex, barrier contraception
  - **Sexual assault**
- Invasive procedures in non-sterile conditions
- Other sexually transmitted infections
- Blood transfusions – overseas (and particularly from 1975-1985 in UK)
- Intravenous drug abuse
- Health problems – opportunistic infections, immunocompromised states
- *'I understand that this can be a very anxious time for you. I would put you at ...risk of having HIV.'* Give an assessment as to whether patient is at low/high risk. If the patient is at high risk, consult seniors before counselling the patient

The HIV Test

- *'What do you understand about the HIV test?'*
- The HIV test looks for antibodies against the HIV virus from a sample of blood
- AIDS is caused by the HIV virus and leads to weakness of the immune system
- There are now 4th generation 'Point Of Care' tests for HIV that are accurate from 6 weeks onwards and these may be used when HIV is suspected – HOWEVER, these tests still need to be repeated at 3 months
- Offer more in-depth counselling to discuss the implication of test results to ensure that the patient is ready for the test and prepared for the consequences
- Offer another chance to ask any questions or voice concerns
- Enquire about a support network

Antenatal HIV Testing

- With appropriate care, the risk of a baby (from a HIV positive mother) developing HIV can be reduced to less than 2% but ONLY IF the mother is diagnosed before or early in the pregnancy
- HIV is more aggressive in children
- All babies benefit from intervention
- Without treatment, 25% of HIV positive children die before they reach the age of 6
- Breastfeeding is contraindicated (unless risks outweigh the benefits, e.g. in third-world nations)

Station 3: AUTOPSY CONSENT

Mrs Parker died last week. You are talking to her daughter. The cause of death was pneumonia. A number of abdominal lesions were noted on CT scanning, which are not thought to be related to the cause of death, but are of unknown origin. The family and medical team are interested to explore this further and your consultant has asked you to get authorisation for a hospital autopsy.

Preparation

- Establish that the case does not need to be referred to the Coroner (or Procurator Fiscal in Scotland) for a medicolegal autopsy
- Ensure that you know and understand local rules for seeking authorisation for a post mortem – for example, most hospitals will require a death certificate to have been issued and others have policies requiring authorisation to be obtained by medical staff of at least FY2 grade
- Make sure that you have the relevant authorisation forms and patient information leaflets with you
- You will need someone else with you to act as a witness for your discussion; that person must be able to sign the authorisation form. This need not be a doctor and is often a nurse who may have known the family
- Give your bleep to a colleague and plan to speak to the patient's relative in a side room (or somewhere you are unlikely to be disturbed or interrupted)

Meeting with the family

Introduction

- Introduce yourself and other members of staff present
- Establish if the relative would like anyone else there and explore any immediate concerns they may have
- Attempt to find out if the deceased patient had ever expressed any views on having an autopsy

The Autopsy

- Explain why you are seeking authorisation to perform an autopsy and what questions you are seeking to answer
- The examination may reveal information that help the relatives understand the circumstances around the death
- Roughly half of the autopsies performed produce findings that are not suspected before the person died

Respecting the Deceased

- The examination will be carried out in a manner that is respectful to the deceased and family's wishes. Organs will not be retained without specific permission but, in some regions of the UK, small thumbnail pieces of tissue will routinely be retained for microscopic examination
- Explain that the autopsy examinations can be limited to one area of the body or even to one organ, but that this will prevent any comment being made on any other disease processes elsewhere
- An open 'casket' will still be possible if that is what the family or deceased patient would have wanted

'In complex cases, seek advice from a senior colleague or a pathologist regarding what may be involved in answering specific questions – for example, there is no point in obtaining authorisation for a limited examination which excludes the head when the patient may have died of a neurological condition'

William Wallace
Consultant Pathologist
Edinburgh Royal Infirmary

'Find out if there are specific questions that the family want answers to – there may have been other health issues not directly relevant to the final illness which they would like clarified – for example, that a previously diagnosed and treated malignancy has not returned'

William Wallace
Consultant Pathologist
Edinburgh Royal Infirmary

Respecting Patient/ Family Wishes

- Explain that this is not something that has to be agreed to and that permission can be refused. Be supportive of such a decision: for example, *'If you think your mother would rather have her body left in peace, then that is understandable'*
- Explain that the family can withdraw authorisation at any time up until the examination itself has started

Closing the Discussion

- Check family members' understanding of the conversation and give them the opportunity to ask questions or to take some time to think about the decision
- The relative may have specific fears and worries regarding the autopsy and you should give them another opportunity to voice these

After meeting with the family

- Having established that the family are happy to give authorisation, complete the form recording their wishes, particularly with respect to any limitations being placed on the examination, their wishes with regards to tissue retention and eventual disposal
- The form must be signed and witnessed as required
- A copy of the form should be given to the relatives, along with information booklets if they so wish
- The case notes, authorisation form and any required pathology request form should be passed to the mortuary without delay

Station 4: HERNIA REPAIR

Mr Penneck has recently been diagnosed with an inguinal hernia. Please explain to him what management options are available for him. Please explain to him the risks and benefits of surgical repair of the hernia.

- Explain that you are here to describe the surgical procedure and possible alternative management options
- Ask if the patient has read the patient information sheet regarding the procedure (if the patient has not, provide them with one)
- Describe the procedure, using diagrams if appropriate
- If you do not know the answer to any questions, then say that you will ask the doctor who will be performing the procedure and that you will get back to the patient with the answer
- Once the patient has been informed, ask them to sign and date the consent form – you should countersign and date it

Hernia Repair

Explain what a Hernia is:

- *'A hernia can be thought of as a hole or a weak spot in the wall of the tummy, where your internal organs (usually the intestine or gut) partly come out through the hole and appear under the skin causing a lump'*
- *'This can potentially cause you problems, such as pain. The gut that's sticking out can become kinked, compressed or blocked and if the blood supply is also kinked or compressed, the gut may suffer and may even burst'*

Explain what the Treatment is:

- *'We can treat this now before these problems develop by performing surgery. Surgery is the only effective treatment to repair the hernia, but hernias currently not causing any symptoms can often simply be monitored'*
- *'If you opt for surgery, this could be done as an open procedure or key-hole (laparoscopically) – depending on patient and hospital factors'*

> *'Infection and numbness are much less common after a laparoscopic repair'*
>
> **Bruce Tulloh**
> *Consultant General Surgeon*
> *Edinburgh Royal Infirmary*

Laparoscopic Repair:

- *'Using a keyhole technique, we place a camera and some surgical instruments inside your tummy through several small cuts in your belly. Any tissues sticking out through the hernia are pulled back in through the hernia "hole" and we can then repair this hole in the wall of the tummy. A patch is then put over the original site of the hernia, to help reduce the chances of this happening again'*
- *'For a key-hole repair, you will require a general anaesthetic'*
- *'In about 2% of cases, the procedure has to be converted to open surgery, using more traditional larger cuts'*

Open Surgery:

- 'A 10 cm cut is made in the groin, just above the swelling. The protruding gut is pushed back in, the hole is stitched over and a patch is placed over the site of the hole'
- 'Open repair is commonly done under general anaesthetic'

Explain what the Risks are:

- Generally regarded as a safe procedure that is very commonly done in hospital

Short Term:

- **Infection**: the mesh is a foreign body; if it gets infected, it may need to be removed and replaced
- **Bleeding**: due to damage to blood vessels or gut
- **Difficulty passing urine (postoperative urinary obstruction)**: may require a tube in the bladder to help drain urine (short-term catheter)
- **Patches of numbness in the skin**: usually resolves
- **Testicular pain (ischaemic orchitis)**: usually resolves

Long Term:

- May develop chronic pain (abdominal/scrotal) - due to nerve damage
- Recurrence of hernia - about 5% in 5 years, regardless of technique

> 'Bowel obstruction is not a risk except with a transabdominal laparoscopic preperitoneal repair (TAPP); laparoscopic repairs which are total extraperitoneal repairs (TEP) do not carry a risk of adhesion formation because the peritoneum is never entered.'
>
> **Peter Fagenholz**
> *Consultant General Surgeon*
> *Massachusetts General Hospital*

Explain what the Alternatives are:

1. No Surgery

The decision to operate is largely based on symptoms. Hernias that don't cause any symptoms can be safely monitored under follow up, without a significant risk of complications from not operating such as incarceration, strangulation, and bowel obstruction. However, once a hernia starts to cause discomfort, the risk of developing these complications increases and the risks of surgery are easier to justify.

2. Sling/Truss/Belt

When worn, these devices can be used to help stop the gut coming out of the defect in the wall of the belly. They can be helpful for symptom control, and reduce the risk of occurrence of complications.

Other General Advice

- Treat risk factors. Look for causes of raised intra-abdominal pressure (obesity, ascites, constipation, chronic coughing e.g. COPD). These won't help the hernia but might prevent it from getting any larger, or prevent any more hernias from developing
- Manage symptoms, and seek urgent medical advice if pain worsens, or if obstructive symptoms develop (vomiting, abdominal distension, constipation, abdominal pain)

You are on the phone to a ward nurse who has called you urgently about a patient. The patient started a blood transfusion 2 hours ago. The patient's temperature is now 37.7°C, blood pressure is 99/60 and the patient is anxious. Explore this further on the phone and identify what you would like the nurse to do, and what you are going to do to further manage this patient.

- Introduce yourself to the nurse with your name and job title. Confirm where they are calling from if they have not told you already
- Ascertain quickly the urgency of seeing the patient – in particular, by eliciting the Early Warning Score (depending on Local Policy) and observations: temperature, pulse, blood pressure, respiratory rate, oxygen saturations and urine output. It is important to note how these parameters have changed over time – before and during the transfusion
- An SBAR (Situation, Background, Assessment, Recommendation) format is generally used for communication from nursing staff to medical staff
- If the patient is peri-arrest, for example, if they are no longer able to maintain their airway, advise the nurse to immediately call the On-Call Emergency/ Crash Team, and attend to the patient without delay
- All patients who become unstable whilst being transfused merit a medical review – the urgency of this will depend on the patient's history and clinical status
- If the patient is not critically unwell, briefly find out more about the patient's background and the reason for blood transfusion

Clarify any clinical concerns or change in observations:

1) **Before** the **transfusion:** Why was the patient being transfused? What were they receiving? What were the observations before the transfusion?
2) At the **start** of the **transfusion**
3) At any of the **checkpoints** (15, 30, and 60 minutes) in routine monitoring of the transfusion
4) At any **other times**

This will help you establish the time course of events, and point you in the direction of a diagnosis. For example, 'Patient 1' being transfused after an acute intra-abdominal bleed, awaiting theatre, may have deteriorated due to further bleeding, whereas this is less likely in 'Patient 2', who is being transfused for long standing anaemia secondary to chronic kidney disease.

Other possible diagnosis to consider:

- **ABO Incompatibility:** potentially catastrophic and occurs in the first few minutes
- **Non Haemolytic Transfusion Reaction:** less dramatic, may occur at any time
- **Transfusion Related Acute Lung Injury (TRALI):** more likely with Fresh Frozen Plasma (FFP)
- **Volume Overload**
- **Anaphylaxis**

For all of the above, a medical review is required, and for all of them, review is required urgently.

- Clarify any management already implemented by nursing staff e.g. stopping the transfusion, giving IV fluids
- Ask whether the transfusion is still running. The transfusion may need to be stopped, but this depends on the clinical scenario. Consider a patient that had dropped their Hb from 100 to 54 after an acute bleed. Stopping the transfusion may be detrimental if haemodynamic instability is secondary to ongoing bleeding

Blood Product Administration

- Blood must be prescribed on the relevant chart – hospitals will generally have a pathway document for blood transfusions
- Each unit must be prescribed separately
- Consider whether frusemide should be given during blood transfusion (in those with poor cardiac function, where the risk of fluid overload is a concern). Tailor dose and route (intravenous/oral) of frusemide to the clinical scenario
- Ensure intravenous access
- Use a clean giving set
- Check the patient's details, check the blood pack, check the patient's wristband. This is performed by two members of the nursing/medical staff, following a protocol
- Administer each unit of red cells over 3-4 hours. A faster rate of administration may be required in an emergency
- Check baseline observations (heart rate, blood pressure, respiratory rate, temperature) and at 15, 30 and 60 minutes after starting the transfusion

Ask nurses to call the doctor if they observe:
- Changes from baseline observations
- Urticarial rash
- Features of anaphylaxis

Communication

Assume now that the patient is having a non-haemolytic febrile transfusion reaction. Whilst making your way to review the patient, you should:

Ask nursing staff to:

- Stop the transfusion, and put up IV fluids through a clean giving set
- Give oxygen if saturations are below 94%
- Check the blood pack and patient details
- Administer paracetamol orally (if already written on the drug chart)
- Take blood (if trained) for FBC, U&Es, Group and Save (to re-crossmatch) and a Coagulation Screen
- Phone the blood bank to inform them of the reaction and send the sample back to the blood bank
- Consider inserting a urethral catheter to monitor urine output

Then state *'I am going to come and see the patient'* (with an approximate estimate of time). This will depend on other clinical emergencies, but this patient must be reviewed as a clinical priority.

At the end, ensure that, together, you and the nurse have a clear idea of the plan. Ask the nurse if they have any questions or concerns. Encourage nursing staff to contact you again if there are any further questions or concerns whilst you are making your way to review the patient.

Do not hesitate to contact your senior colleagues if you require any assistance, advice or an independent review.

Management of Common Complications of Blood Transfusion

Diagnosis	Presentation	Action	Investigations and Therapy
Acute Haemolytic Reaction: **ABO incompatibility**	• Rapid spike in temperature >40°C (at start of transfusion) • Hypotensive and tachycardic • Unwell, agitated, flushed • Pain (abdomen, chest, and/ or cannula site) • Bleeding from the cannula site	• Resuscitate the patient using an ABC approach • Stop the transfusion • Check that the correct blood was given, by looking at patient ID and documentation • Inform haematologist and blood bank • Send blood transfusion bag back to lab • May require senior help, or ITU intervention	**Investigations:** • Monitor haemodynamic stability of patient • FBC, U&Es, coagulation screen, group and save • Regularly repeat bloods and routine observations • Catheterise to monitor urine output, and dipstick urine for blood **Therapy:** • Give saline, through a clean giving set
Anaphylaxis	• Bronchospasm • Cyanosis • Tachycardic and hypotensive • Swelling • Rash	• Resuscitate the patient using an ABC approach • Stop transfusion, and send blood bag back to lab • Contact an anaesthetist if the airway compromised • May require senior help, or ITU intervention	**Investigations:** • FBC, U&Es, coagulation screen, group and save **Therapy:** • Adrenaline 0.5 mg 1:1000 IM, Chlorpheniramine 10 mg IV, Hydrocortisone 200 mg IV • Nebulisers if wheezy • Fast IV fluids to treat anaphylactic shock
Non Haemolytic Febrile Transfusion Reaction	• Slow rising temperature approximately 60 minutes after transfusion commenced	• Resuscitate the patient using an ABC approach • Slow or stop transfusion • Check the correct blood has been given • May require senior help	**Investigations:** • Monitor haemodynamic stability of patient • FBC, U&Es, coagulation screen, group and save **Therapy:** • Paracetamol 1 g • IV fluids through a clean giving set

Management of Common Complications of Blood Transfusion (continued)

Diagnosis	Presentation	Action	Investigations and Therapy
Fluid Overload	• Shortness of breath • Hypoxia • Tachycardia • Raised JVP • Bibasal inspiratory crepitations	• Slow or stop transfusion	**Investigations:** • Monitor haemodynamic stability of patient • FBC, U&Es • ECG, Arterial Blood Gases, CXR **Therapy:** • Oxygen to saturations >94% • Diuretic therapy e.g. frusemide 40 mg IV
Urticarial Reaction	• Urticarial rash on skin	• Stop transfusion • Recheck blood • Send back blood to laboratory with giving set • Flush cannula with saline • Monitor urticaria progression	**Investigations:** • Group and save **Therapy:** • Chlorpheniramine 10 mg slow IV/IM

Station 6: WARFARIN COUNSELLING

Mr Jacobs is a 70 year-old gentleman recently diagnosed with atrial fibrillation. He has been sent to your cardiology clinic, with a view to potentially starting warfarin therapy. Counsel him about warfarin therapy and its implications.

Introduction

- Before commencing patients on oral anticoagulation, check with your local trust policy
- Ensure that a good history and examination has been undertaken so you ascertain whether there are any contraindications for the use of warfarin in your patient

Approach to Counselling

- Introduce yourself
- *'We recommend that you start taking a new medication called warfarin, because of your irregular heart rhythm'*
- *'Have you heard of warfarin?'*
- *'I'd like to explain how warfarin works, and why it has been recommended that you take this medication'*

Warfarin is...

- *'A medication that thins your blood, reducing the risk of blood clots forming in your heart, legs and lungs. This is why it is important to take it regularly'*

You are asked to take Warfarin because...

- *'You have been diagnosed with an irregular heart rhythm known as Atrial Fibrillation (AF). This condition can increase the risk of developing blood clots in your heart, and increase your risk of having a stroke'*
- *'However, taking warfarin will reduce the chances of you developing this problem'*

Target INR

Normal Range	*0.8-1.2*
Atrial Fibrillation	*2.0-3.0*
PE and DVT	*2.0-3.0*
Aortic mechanical valve	*2.0-3.0*
Mitral mechanical valve	*2.5-3.5*

Communication

How this medication will impact your life...

- 'Certain foods and 'natural' health products/herbal remedies can affect warfarin levels. Some increase warfarin levels (for example: ginkgo biloba) while others reduce the warfarin effect (ginseng)'
- Vitamin K decreases the effect of warfarin. Foods rich in vitamin K, such as broccoli, brussel sprouts, and green leafy vegetables such as spinach, coriander and cabbage can be taken in the usual amounts in a normal diet, but the patient should be counselled against taking large quantities of brassicas at any one time
- Alcohol may increase the effects of warfarin, so patients should be counselled adequately about keeping their alcohol intake at a safe, stable level
- Patients must also be told to refrain from activities such as contact sports. They should speak to their GP before starting any such activity
- 'If anyone is going to prescribe, advise you or recommend to you any medication or vitamin, remedy or supplement of any kind, please tell them: "I am on warfarin, will this affect it?"'

Your first dose...

- 'Will be decided by your doctor'
- 'Each patient requires a different dose and the response to warfarin therefore needs to be monitored. It is guided by a measurement known as the INR, which is a blood test taken by your doctor that measures the thinness of the blood'
- 'The INR test should be checked at least every 4 weeks, but your INR may need to be checked more frequently if it goes out of the range of blood thinness that is required to prevent clots'
- 'The dose of warfarin should be taken roughly the same time every day. We tend to advise a dose taken at 6pm as this will allow your doctor to get in touch before you take it if your blood is too thin, so that you can be advised to reduce the dose'
- 'If you miss a dose, call your GP, take the dose missed as soon as possible and do not double up the dose the next day to make up for the missed dose'
- 'Warfarin tablets come in different strength and colour of tablets - 1mg (brown), 3mg (blue) and 5mg (pink) tablets. You will be provided with a supply of all of these to allow for dose adjustment. Remember to always check the expiration date and the label before taking any medication'

Anticoagulation Book (if applicable to your local trust policy)

- 'This is your yellow anticoagulation book. It contains details of your condition, and your target INR. Use this to log your INR values, and your warfarin doses, so that you have a record of it'
- 'With this, we will also supply you with information about taking warfarin, which is worth reading'

Watch out for...

- Bleeding or severe bruising
- Prolonged nose bleeds
- Coughing up or vomiting blood
- Passing foul smelling black 'tar like' bowel motions
- Passing blood in the urine

Patients should contact their GP or NHS-24 in the event of any of the above

End the consultation by making sure that the patient has understood what you have been discussing and be sure to leave time for questions. If possible, use a sheet to summarise the main points of your discussion and file it in the notes to record the discussion.

Certain drugs will increase bleeding risk with warfarin (e.g. antiplatelet agents such as aspirin, clopidogrel and dipyramidole) but do not necessarily affect the INR. Both the oral contraceptive pill and hormone replacement therapy should be stopped in patients with venous thromboembolic events.

What is the mechanism of action of warfarin?

- Warfarin inhibits the conversion of Vitamin K from its inactive to its active form, thereby reducing the activity of Vitamin K dependant coagulation factors
- Vitamin K is necessary for the activation of coagulation factors II, VII, IX and X
- The reduction of the activated factors II, VII, IX and X causes a prolongation of the prothrombin time (PT), usually reported in "seconds" by the laboratory. The INR is derived from the PT and is used only for patients on warfarin. The longer the prothrombin time, the longer the time for clot formation, and thus the "thinner" the blood. The higher the PT, the higher the INR, and the thinner the blood

Can you think of any other indications for warfarin?

- **Therapeutic:** venous thromboembolism e.g. deep vein thrombosis, pulmonary embolus, other types of venous thrombosis; also arterial thrombosis
- **Prophylactic:** secondary prevention of venous thrombosis, prevention of cardioembolic complications (indication in atrial fibrillation, mechanical / prosthetic heart valves)

Communication

Give me some examples of drugs that can affect the INR

Decrease in INR	Increase in INR
Alcohol (chronic intake)	Alcohol (binge drinking)
Vitamin K	Cimetidine
Azathioprine	Omeprazole
Rifampicin	Amiodarone
Oral Contraceptive Pill	Levothyroxine
St John's Wort	Macrolide antibiotics
Hormone Replacement Therapy	Metronidazole

Station 7: OPIATE COUNSELLING

Mr Smith is suffering from severe pain. He has a diagnosis of inoperable pancreatic cancer. You have found it difficult to control his pain, and now feel his analgesia should be increased. Please counsel him on the risks and benefits of morphine therapy, and discuss other adjuncts to improve his symptoms

- Discuss the patient's pain with him. Find out its exact nature, and the effect on his life
- Ensure non opiate analgesia is already optimised, following the WHO pain ladder
- Ask the patient about his current medication, what else has been tried so far, and what benefits were gained from previous approaches. Ask him about other options that he might be keen to explore, and establish the patient's knowledge of morphine

Patient Concerns

It is important to establish what worries the patient might have about starting morphine. Selectively talk about the concerns of the patient in front of you. Addressing these, even if they are not rooted in fact, increases the likelihood of patient compliance. For example:

'Will I become addicted to morphine?'
This is, in practice, extremely rare when morphine is taken for the purpose of pain relief.

'Will morphine make me die sooner?'
There is absolutely no evidence for this. However, the patient may have known someone who died shortly after commencing therapy.

'If I take the morphine now, will it mean it won't work later when I really need it?'
When pain worsens, it is usually due to disease progression, not the morphine ceasing to work. In any case, morphine can be given in the quantities needed to control the pain.

- Emphasise the need for regular administration and explain about breakthrough medication (PRN dose equivalent to 1/6th of the total 24-hour dose)
- Discuss different routes of administration that may be relevant (oral/transdermal/subcutaneous) if problems are anticipated with oral medication (e.g. vomiting)

Side Effects

Constipation	• Virtually inevitable – use prophylactic laxatives • Stimulant (e.g. Senna), Softener (e.g. Lactulose)
Nausea	• Fairly common in opiate naïve patients, sometimes clears after 1 week but may recur after a dose increase • Cover with anti-emetic (e.g. metoclopromide)
Drowsiness	• Normally an acute problem, clearing within one week. If significantly drowsy, it may be a sign of opiate toxicity, and alternative opioids (e.g. fentanyl/oxycodone) should be considered
Myoclonus	• Especially seen in renal impairment • Consider reducing the dose, changing opioid, and consider administering midazolam – especially in the terminal phase
Hallucination	• May occur, especially if dose is too high, and therefore the dose can be reduced. Individuals may have vivid dreams, which is not necessarily a problem
Tolerance	• Over time patients may require a larger dose to achieve the same pain relief. Therefore, unlike with addiction, there is a rational reason for increasing analgesia. Addiction is rare in patients started on morphine for genuine pain control

Consider Opiate Choice

• MST Continus (morphine sulphate tablets) for 'regular' analgesia and Oramorph (morphine sulphate solution), for 'break through' are usually considered first line
• Alfentanil may be more appropriate in patients with renal dysfunction

Consider other Analgesic Approaches

• Discuss referral to an appropriate palliative care team (community or hospital) for further management as these teams may be able to offer more specialist support service
• Offer emotional and spiritual support through, for example, the chaplaincy or counselling services
• Relaxation techniques and creative therapies (sensory monitoring, mindful based therapy). Use of these may provide coping strategies for the patient that they can use to augment their analgesia
• Acupuncture and aromatherapy
• TENS (transcutaneous electrical nerve stimulation)

Mr Smith is about to be discharged from hospital. He was admitted after having a heart attack. Please explore why he was at risk for developing heart disease. Explore what lifestyle measures could be adopted to reduce his risk of another event.

Modifiable Risk Factors for Cardiovascular Disease

- Smoking
- Dyslipidaemia
- Hypertension
- Obesity
- Excess alcohol (>3 units/day for men; >2 units/day for women)
- Excess salt intake
- Lack of exercise
- Environmental stress

Lifestyle Advice (WAFFLES)

- **Weight:** maintain normal BMI 20-25
  - If obese – weight loss (healthy diet and exercise)
- **Alcohol:** limit consumption/drink in moderation
  - <3 units/day for men and <2 units/ day for women
- **Fruit and vegetables**
  - 5-8 portions a day
- **Fat:** reduce intake of total and unsaturated fats. Offer dietician input, and perhaps explore the possibility of cooking classes
- **Low Salt:** reduce salt intake - <6 g/day (helps reduce blood pressure)
- **Exercise**
  - Engage in regular aerobic physical exercise (brisk walking rather than weightlifting) for 30 minutes per day, ideally on most days of the week but at least for 3 days a week
- **Smoking:** STOP! Can discuss nicotine replacement therapy, referral to Quitters, support network

The scenario may specifically ask you to talk about one aspect of lifestyle advice. Here are some examples.

Explain that you would like to talk to the patient about their cholesterol levels

- *'There are 2 types of cholesterol in the body, one of which is harmful if it is present in at higher levels (LDL), the other of which is beneficial if it is present at higher levels (HDL)'*
- *'There are things you can do to lower bad cholesterol, and increase good cholesterol, and therefore protect your heart'*
- *'Medications are available to lower cholesterol, and because you've had a heart attack we recommend starting to you on such a drug'*
- Lifestyle advice – **WAFFLES** (as above)
- *'If you like, we can give you some leaflets on dietary information or put you in touch with a dietician. Increasing exercise levels can also improve cholesterol levels'*
- *'We will check your blood cholesterol levels in three months to see if these changes have helped'*

Explain that you would like to talk to the patient about their high blood pressure

- *'High blood pressure is bad because it puts you at risk of having a heart attack and also of having a stroke'*
- *'Since you've had a heart attack, we recommend using medication to lower your blood pressure'*
- Lifestyle advice – **WAFFLES** (as above), improving diet and increased exercise will also contribute to reducing blood pressure
- *'It is worthwhile getting your doctor to check your blood pressure regularly'*

Complications of Hypertension

- Neurological: stroke, transient ischaemic attack, dementia
- Cardiovascular: left ventricular hypertrophy, heart failure, ischemic heart disease, peripheral vascular disease
- Renal impairment

Explore any Difficulties in Lifestyle Change

- Patient doesn't know how/lack of support/nobody to help
- Unaware of the benefits/doesn't think it is worthwhile
- Embarrassment

Set Goals

- Offer a short term, achievable aim to the patient, and offer material for them to take away and read
- *'This is a lot to take in; do you think you could manage halving your alcohol intake and exercising twice a week? We will meet again in two months to see how you are doing'*

Communication

Station 9: DEALING WITH AN AGITATED PATIENT

Mr Gates is a 65-year-old gentleman who has come to your clinic today. He is very angry because he was supposed to receive a staging CT scan for his bowel cancer over a month ago, and hasn't heard anything about it.

General Principles

- You should place your own safety first; give clear boundaries to the patient if they are being inappropriately aggressive or rude. Do not approach the patient if it is unsafe
- Take the patient to a private location. Give your bleep to a colleague
- Remain calm and allow the patient to vent their anger if necessary without interruption. Validate their feelings, and with the patient, come up with a shared plan regarding how to address any problems that have arisen
- Apology is very important. To reinforce this, it can be done at the beginning, middle and end of the consultation. It is not necessarily an admission of guilt, or an invitation for a complaint. It merely acknowledges what has happened, and the patient's justifiable anxiety. *'I'm sorry about your scan being delayed. I know how important it is, and now that I am aware of it being delayed, I am going to find out why this has happened, and get you a firm scan date. I'm sorry again'*

Positive Indicators

- Be focussed on the patient. *'I understand that unfortunately things haven't gone exactly as we'd planned. I'm sorry. Let's sit down and talk about what has happened, and how we can improve the situation.'* Maintain good eye contact, remain calm and be empathetic
- Make sure you acknowledge and understand the patient's concerns. It may be helpful to summarise and repeat back these concerns to the patient
- Ensure that a clear, realistic plan is established to address the problem that has arisen
- Communicate this to the patient as soon as possible

Negative Indicators

- Avoid focussing the consultation around attributing blame
  'I have done nothing wrong, it's the radiologist's fault'
- Avoid being defensive *'We are very busy and trying our best'*
- Avoid criticising the patient for his approach to the situation *'You really shouldn't expect so much out of us'*
- Avoid interrupting or patronising the patient
- Avoid giving no information: even if you are not an expert, you may be able to say something useful for the patient *'I will speak to the radiology department, explain that your scan was scheduled last month, and work with them to get the test done as soon as possible, because we really don't want to be waiting any longer. I'm sorry. I will let you know today the outcome of the discussions'*

Exploring the Origin of the Anger

Do not assume the patient is angry for the reasons you might be in his circumstance. Allow them to explain their specific concerns, and address these individually and immediately. Three possibilities are below:

- Mr Gates may be well informed about his disease, knowing the possible treatments for each possible disease stage on CT scan. He may be frustrated knowing that that the delayed CT scan is necessary to start either curative or palliative treatment. Talking about the disease is not as relevant as focusing the discussion on practically arranging to get the scan done
- Mr Gates may be desperate to have the CT scan because he understands nothing about the disease, and associates the scan with finding out more information. In this case, counselling the patient about not just the CT scan, but also his disease may help relieve anger
- Mr Gates may have worsening symptoms, for example with worsening appetite, weight loss and tiredness. Anger may stem from feeling his disease is getting worse, yet appearing to be ignored by the system. Identifying and managing his symptoms, talking about the disease and arranging the scan all need emphasis here

The Complaints Procedure

- The patient is within their rights to complain, and this should normally be done within 12 months. The chief executive of the hospital will reply 'as soon as reasonably possible'
- It can be done through several channels, including the local complaints manager and the primary care trust complaints manager (many hospitals will have a Patient Advice Liaison Service and patients can be referred to this)
- They may also complain directly to a professional body (e.g. General Medical Council)
- In addition, help on practically filing a complaint can be obtained from organisations such as the citizens advice bureau

NOTE: if the patient does not calm down despite your efforts, put your own personal safety first, and get yourself out of harm's way. You probably will not be pushed this far in medical school OSCEs, but it is something to be aware of in post-graduate exams!

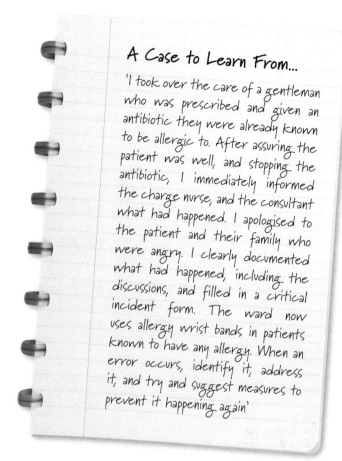

A Case to Learn From...

'I took over the care of a gentleman who was prescribed and given an antibiotic they were already known to be allergic to. After assuring the patient was well, and stopping the antibiotic, I immediately informed the charge nurse, and the consultant what had happened. I apologised to the patient and their family who were angry. I clearly documented what had happened, including the discussions, and filled in a critical incident form. The ward now uses allergy wrist bands in patients known to have any allergy. When an error occurs, identify it, address it, and try and suggest measures to prevent it happening again'

Station 10: BREAKING BAD NEWS

Mrs Gardner has come in to see you. You admitted her husband last week, who was suffering from a chest infection, on a long-term background of colorectal cancer. Despite antibiotic therapy, he is now rapidly deteriorating, and your consultant anticipates that Mr Gardner has days, if not hours, to live.

Breaking bad news is a difficult skill to master, especially within a short OSCE scenario. However, there are many different ways to do it successfully. Ensure that you are clear about the situation of the patient, who exactly you are talking to, and what you are trying to communicate.

*The **SPIKES** technique is an effective method to structure breaking bad news.*

Setting

- Ensure that you meet with the patient's relative in an appropriate setting, and that you have consent from the patient
- Turn to the examiner and say *'I have given my bleep to a colleague, found a private room, and drawn the curtains shut'*
- Tell the relative that you have all the time that they need to talk about the issue
- Ask them if they want anyone else to be present to make them feel more at ease. It is often useful to have a nurse present as well

Perception

- What does the relative know so far? What are their current expectations? Is Mrs Gardner aware of the reasons for the current admission, the management so far, and what her husband's response to treatment has been? This will help you assess the information you need to convey, and the language that is most appropriate. It will also highlight any initial misconception
- A simple question to ask is *'What do you know about his condition so far?'*
- Identify early in the consultation the concerns of the relative. These may not necessarily be the concerns you would have in a similar situation. For example, in this case, hypothetically Mrs Gardner may feel very guilty because she believes she gave her husband the chest infection. Until this guilt is addressed, it might be more difficult for her to focus on other discussions

Invitation

- Establish whether the relative would like to find out more information
- *'Would you like me to tell you more about what's going on?'*
- Set out a plan for what will happen in the consultation

Knowledge

- Warning shots are useful; for example phrases such as *'I have some difficult news'* or *'The chest X-ray does not look good'*
- Convey the important information
- In this example, explain that Mr Gardner has developed a chest infection, from which he is dying despite maximal treatment with antibiotics, and that he has days, if not hours, to live regardless of what treatment is given
- Emphasise that he will still be monitored closely, but that you believe the aim of all further management should be making sure he is as comfortable as possible (e.g. minimising pain)
- State that any further tests would not change his outlook, but might cause him unnecessary distress, and so you do not think doing any more tests are in his best interests
- State that he will be put in a room without other patients, so that he, and the family, have some privacy
- Depending on the scenario, it might be appropriate to introduce the concept of a 'Do Not Attempt CPR' form
- Deliver the information in small chunks and check that the relative understands it. Actively gauge their emotional response, and adapt the consultation to it

Empathy

- This is probably the most important part of the consultation, and involves specifically dealing with how the relative reacts
- If a relative becomes upset or angry, recognising this can be useful by using phrases such as *'I can see you are frustrated with what is going on'* or *'I know this isn't what you wanted to hear'*
- It is okay to allow a period of silence, and to offer to talk further when they have had time to think about the issues in more detail. Offer tissues if appropriate
- If the relative falls silent, it is tempting to fill the space with more reassurance but you should respect the silence for a while. If it goes on for long, you could say *'You seem to be finding it hard to talk about this and that is very understandable given the circumstances….'*

Issues involving the process of dying, pain and loss of independence may arise. Also wider issues with regard to family and money may be important. Acknowledging and allowing the relative to express such emotions is often beneficial.

Strategy and Summary

- Finally, the conversation should be closed
- Provide written information if appropriate, for example, about spiritual support or about bereavement
- A plan should be enacted incorporating the issues brought up in the discussion *'I'd like to decide, together with you, where to proceed from here'*
- It is useful to offer an opportunity to talk again
- Also, further empathy can be demonstrated by showing concern for the relative getting home after such a shock *'Do you have transport to get home? Do you want me to ring someone to help you?'*
- Lastly, offer some kind of hope. For example, *'we will make your husband as pain-free as possible'*

N.B. The above description can be used to break news directly to a patient by deleting relative and inserting 'patient' within the text.

5 Practical Skills

The best time to practice these skills is whilst on clinical attachments. This is when you have all the equipment available, and it gives you the time to develop a confident, seamless routine. Many universities offer dedicated clinical skills training sessions, and dedicated clinical skills revision sessions before exams. Utilise any learning opportunities that are presented to you.

Keep in mind that everyone makes mistakes, particularly with skills you may not have had the opportunity to practise as much. If you make a mistake in the OSCE, deal with it in the same manner you would in clinical practice: identify the problem, and address it appropriately, putting patient safety first.

Protocols for certain procedures vary with local guidelines. Follow those applicable to your NHS trust.

Study Action Plan

- The key to practical procedures is practice. A lot of these cannot be practised at home: e.g. urethral catheterisation. Therefore use the hospital as a learning resource
- Generally, you have the option of practicing on the wards (e.g. phlebotomy), practicing on friends (e.g. fundoscopy) or using the clinical skills laboratory (e.g. cannulation). Ask people to watch you whenever you do a procedure to ensure that you know how to improve for next time, and don't continue bad habits
- Try and practice some of the above skills in the context of a patient in front of you. This is very important in the context of, for example, interpreting ECGs: they form part of a clinical decision, and seeing investigations in the context of patients now will help ease the transition to being a junior doctor

This chapter contains the notes for the following skills:

Practical Skills

Station 1: INTERMEDIATE LIFE SUPPORT

You are on the medical wards and come across a patient collapsed on the floor. Approach the patient and perform resuscitation as necessary. Follow any instructions that are given by the examiners in this station.

PART 1

- A resuscitation manikin will be used to simulate a collapsed patient. Have a systematic approach. For example, follow the DR ABC mnemonic:

Danger

1) Ask, *'Is it safe to approach?'*

Response

1) Shake the dummy lightly and shout, *'Hello, can you hear me?'*
2) Call out for help. In the context of an OSCE, someone will be with you shortly

Airway

1) Check in the mouth for obstruction/foreign bodies
2) Perform head tilt, chin lift
3) If obstruction is present: a finger sweep under direct vision may be performed (and turn on side if necessary)

Breathing and Circulation

Simultaneously:

1) LOOK for chest movement
2) LISTEN for breath sounds
3) FEEL the carotid pulse for 10 seconds (count to 10)

Your help has now arrived: what do you do next?

1) Tell them to call the cardiac arrest team and say it is an adult cardiac arrest, specify your location, and ask them to come back with the crash trolley
2) Start chest compressions in the centre of the chest at the rate of 100/min and to one-third of the depth of the chest
3) After 30 compressions, give 2 breaths using a bag valve mask device. Make sure that you keep performing the head tilt and the chin lift, otherwise it will not work!
4) Continue compressions and breaths at the rate of 30:2

Once you have demonstrated that you can perform safe, effective basic life support, you will be asked to move to another dummy on a bed with the cardiac arrest trolley and defibrillator.

PART 2

1) Ask your helper to continue CPR: Rate of 100/min, 30:2, to one-third of the depth of the chest
2) Turn on the defibrillator and put on self-adhesive defibrillation/monitoring pads (ensure that you familiarise yourself with the defibrillators in local use)
3) One pad is placed below the right clavicle, the second is placed in the V6 position in the midaxillary line on the left
4) ENSURE that chest compressions continue while the pads are placed
5) Once the pads are connected, and once you are clear what actions you are going to take, ask your helper to stop CPR so that you can assess the rhythm
6) You will be particularly looking to see whether the rhythm is SHOCKABLE or NON-SHOCKABLE. If shockable, it may be either Pulseless Ventricular Tachycardia (VT) or Ventricular Fibrillation (VF). VT is a regular, broad complex tachycardia, and VF is irregular with varying amplitude and frequency

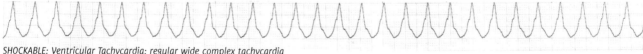

SHOCKABLE: Ventricular Tachycardia: regular wide complex tachycardia

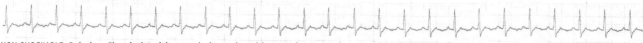

NON-SHOCKABLE: Pulseless Electrical Activity: regularly regular with normal p waves, but no pulse

7) Once you have identified the rhythm, say *'This is VT/VF; this is a shockable rhythm'*
8) IMMEDIATELY resume chest compressions
9) Turn the defibrillator up to 150J (biphasic) or 360 J (monophasic)
10) Tell all of the resuscitation team to *'stand clear'* EXCEPT the individual performing the chest compressions, who should continue with them. Remove any oxygen (at least one metre away from the defibrillator). Ensure that the only person touching the patient is the person continuing chest compressions
11) Press 'charge' (the yellow button) on the defibrillator, and say 'charging', ensuring that the chest compressions continue
12) Once the defibrillator is charged, tell the member of the team doing compressions to also stand clear
13) Double check the rhythm again. Whilst checking that everyone is clear, say *'Clear top, middle, bottom, me'*. Then deliver the shock, stating *'Shocking'* just before you do it
14) IMMEDIATELY resume CPR after the shock is delivered (for two minutes). Aim to minimise time 'off the chest' (i.e. the time that chest compression are not being performed), but be safe
15) During this time, say that you would ensure that someone is performing good quality chest compressions; check the electrode position; establish intravenous access; take venous gas for Hb, K+, and glucose; and perform an ABG (usually with a femoral stab)
16) You would ask for the patient's notes and consider the 8 reversible causes of cardiac arrest (4 H's and 4 T's)

The Four 'H's	The Four 'T's
Hypoxia	Toxins
Hypovolemia	Thromboembolism
Hypothermia	Tension Pneumothorax
Hypo/hyperkalaemia	Tamponade (cardiac)

17) At the end of 2 minutes, reassess the rhythm, and feel for a pulse. If pulseless, continue to follow the resuscitation protocol, as per the rhythm (shockable or non-shockable algorithms)
18) If a pulse is present, then you will want to give post-resuscitation care: oxygen, full set of observations, ECG, Chest X-ray, fluids, and inform HDU or ITU (if intubated)

Common Drugs Given In a Cardiac Arrest

Shockable Rhythm (VF, pulseless VT)

Deliver Immediate Shock

↓

CPR for 2 minutes and then reassess

↓

Deliver Second Shock

↓

CPR for 2 minutes and then reassess

↓

Deliver Third Shock

↓

Adrenaline 1 mg (with 20 ml saline flush) and Amiodarone 300mg (with 20 ml saline flush) both immediately AFTER the third shock

↓

Continue cycles of 2 minutes of CPR, followed by shock. Do not give any further amiodarone, but give adrenaline every 3-5 minutes (after every other shock)

Non-Shockable Rhythms (PEA, asystole)

Adrenaline 1 mg with 20ml saline flush immediately

↓

CPR for 2 minutes and then reassess

↓

Continue cycles of 2 minutes of CPR, followed by reassessment of the rhythm. Give adrenaline every 3-5 minutes (after every other shock)

Reversible Causes of Cardiac Arrest

Cause	Management
Hypoxia	You will be giving 100% O_2 by bag and mask. Once an anaesthetist arrives, they can intubate the patient to secure the airway and ensure optimal oxygenation
Hypovolaemia	Any fluid loss can be replaced intravenously. If the patient is septic and grossly vasodilated, then vasopressors can also be used
Hypothermia	Can be corrected by rewarming the patient at the same rate they were cooled down. Ways to rewarm include using a bear hugger, giving warmed fluids intravenously, catheterising and filling the bladder with warmed fluids, peritoneal lavage, and cardiopulmonary bypass
Hypo/Hyperkalaemia (and other metabolic disturbances)	This should be found on venous gas. If the potassium is elevated, give 10 ml of 10% calcium chloride (on the crash trolley) for cardiac protection. If the potassium is low, replace it intravenously
Toxins	Try to get any information from notes and staff. For example, give naloxone in the case of opiate overdose
Thrombosis (coronary or pulmonary)	If there is a history of ischaemic heart disease or DVT, or the patient had chest pain before they arrested, consider thromboembolism
Tension Pneumothorax	Look for asymmetrical chest movement, hyperresonance, and there may be resistance when using the bag and mask to ventilate the patient. Relieve with a large bore cannula in the second intercostal space, mid-clavicular line on the affected side
Cardiac Tamponade	Very difficult to diagnose in cardiac arrest. Suspect if there is history of trauma to the chest or recent cardiac surgery. Treat with pericardiocentesis

UK Resuscitation Council Guidelines

http://www.resus.org.uk/pages/als.pdf

Note: This station is based on the 2010 UK resuscitation guidelines

Station 2: PHLEBOTOMY

Mr Frederick is a 50-year-old man who is attending your clinic for an INR check, having recently been started on warfarin. Please explain to him what you are going to do, and then demonstrate how you would take blood on the mannequin provided.

- Introduce yourself, explain what you would like to do, and ask for permission. Wash your hands

'I would like to take a blood sample from you. This involves sticking a small needle into a vein near the surface of your skin. We will then analyse the blood, looking at its clotting tendency. This will guide us in adjusting your warfarin dose.'

- Ask about pain
- Check patient identification: 5 forms of identification e.g. name/age/DOB/address/postcode. Ask the patient, and check his bracelet
- Ask if they have had this done before: if not, explain what is involved
- Ask about needle phobia
- Ask if the patient has an arm preference
- Ask about allergies
- Ask about whether they have had a mastectomy or an AV fistula

'It is often easier to approach a vein at the junction where two veins join'

Zeshan Qureshi
Paediatric Trainee
London Deanery

Procedure Preparation

Gathering the Equipment: Checklist

a) Tray: either single-use, disposable sterilised tray, or a decontaminated plastic tray that is cleaned pre/post procedure
b) Vacutainer™
c) Venepuncture needle
d) Single use disposable apron
e) Disposable tourniquet
f) Non-sterile gloves (or sterile gloves if repalpation of venepuncture site after cleaning is anticipated)
g) Skin cleansing solution (2% chlorhexidine (CHG) and 70% isopropyl alcohol (IPA) (e.g. ChloraPrep®))
h) Blood bottles: put these in the order you need to take them
i) Sterile gauze
j) Sharps bin: sharps bin should always be taken to the point of care
k) Tape
l) Sterilised dressing

NOTE: Skin cleansing solutions and method will vary depending on local policy 'Scrub'. If taking blood cultures, blood culture bottle ports will need to be scrubbed for 15 seconds with ChloraPrep®, and allowed to fully dry

Preparing the Equipment

1. Clean hands (with soap and water or alcohol hand rub)
2. Clean tray according to local policy creating an aseptic field
3. Gather all equipment that may be needed
4. Assemble equipment using a non touch technique (attach needle to Vacutainer™)

Drawing Blood

1. Apply a single-use disposable apron
2. Apply a disposable tourniquet: explain to the patient that this is to 'bring up' the vein. Place the tourniquet 7-10 cm above the anterior cubital fossa
3. Select vein: ensure it is not thrombosed by palpating it. Loosen tourniquet
4. Clean hands, apply non-sterile gloves (use sterile gloves if re-palpation for the vein is likely or necessary), and retighten tourniquet
5. Clean site: say you would clean for 30 seconds with ChloraPrep® in an up-and-down, back-and-forth friction technique. Allow to fully dry
6. Puncture the vein using a non-touch technique (warning the patient of a 'sharp scratch') DO NOT REPALPATE the site (aseptic field), unless wearing sterile gloves
7. Draw blood, and invert bottles an appropriate number of times (see table). Inoculate blood to culture bottles using a non-touch technique (while attaching bottles, ask the patient how they feel)
8. Remove tourniquet
9. Remove needle and apply pressure with the gauze
10. Immediately dispose of sharps
11. Apply a sterilised dressing and secure with tape
12. Label the bottles at the bedside
13. Inform the patient to let a member of staff know if the site is painful, continues to bleed, or if they have any other concerns
14. Explain that they can remove dressing after a couple of hours

Finishing

1. Dispose of equipment
2. Clean the tray
3. Dispose of gloves and wash your hands

> 'Always fill the coagulation bottle right up to the line: it won't get processed otherwise!'
>
> **Zeshan Qureshi**
> *Paediatric Trainee*
> *London Deanery*

Blood Bottles (In Order of Draw, and colours may vary)

Tube	Tube Type	Example Tests	Inversion After Collection
Blood Cultures	Blue (aerobic) - 10ml followed by Pink (anaerobic) – 10ml	Blood culture and sensitivity	3-4 times
Light Blue	Sodium Citrate – 2.7 ml	Warfarin, Coagulation	3-4 times
Red	Plain – 10 ml	Hepatitis Status, Rubella Serology, Virology, CA125, Coeliac Screen	5-6 times
Gold	SST – 5 ml	Drug Level, TFTs, LFTs, Hormones, Lipids/Triglycerides, Cholesterol, U&Es , CK, Digoxin Levels, Paracetamol Level's, PSA	5-6 times
Green	Lithium Heparin – 6ml	Amino Acids, Cortisol, PTH	8-10 times
Lavender	EDTA – 3 ml	FBC, HBAl$_c$, HLAB27, Cyclosporine, ESR	8-10 times
Pink	EDTA – 6 ml	Group and Save, Cross Match, Blood Group	8-10 times
Grey	Fluoride Oxalate - 2 ml	Glucose	8-10 times
Royal Blue	EDTA – 5 ml	Trace Elements: Zinc, Copper, Selenium, Manganese, Lead	8-10 times

Station 3:
CANNULATION AND SETTING UP A GIVING SET

Mrs Jones has been diagnosed with small bowel obstruction. She requires intravenous fluids. Please obtain consent for this and then, on the mannequin provided, demonstrate how to insert an intravenous cannula.

- Introduce yourself, explain the process of inserting an intravenous cannula and obtain consent
- Decontaminate your hands before shaking/touching the patient's hands

'Mrs Jones - you are quite dehydrated and as we cannot let you drink for the time being, we would like to give you some fluid via a drip in your arm. For this, I will need to insert the drip, which involves a needle - a bit like having a blood test, but with a small plastic tube remaining in the vein. Would that be alright with you?'

- Identify the patient by asking them and by looking at their bracelet: name, date of birth, hospital number, address/postcode (5 points of identification check)
- Ask if they have had a drip before
- Explain the procedure, why they need it, and how long it will need to stay in
- Does the patient have any pain in the arm?
- Does the patient have an arm preference?
- Does the patient have any pre-disposing medical/surgical conditions that would not allow using a specific arm (stroke, renal fistula, cellulitis, mastectomy)?
- Does the patient have any allergies (chlorhexidine)?
- Position the patient comfortably. Lay the patient down if they have suffered vasovagal episodes with needles in the past
- **Talk to your patient throughout the procedure**

Procedure Preparation

Equipment checklist (remember to check expiry dates on all equipment) e.g. octopus

a) 1x 2% chlorhexidine in 70% alcohol (Chloraprep®) skin cleansing solution
b) 1x 2% chlorhexidine in 70% alcohol equipment wipes (Sani-cloth®)
c) 3x Draw up needle
d) 2x 5ml syringe
e) 2x 5ml saline ampoules (must be checked with examiner)
f) 1x Sterile adhesive dressing
g) 1x Cannula
h) 1x Disposable tourniquet
i) 1x Intravenous extension set e.g. octopus
j) 1x Sterile gauze
k) 2x Pairs of non sterile gloves (may require one pair of sterile gloves if repalpation of cannulation site after cleaning is anticipated)
l) 1x Cannula insertion record
m) 1x Tray (as with phlebotomy)
n) 1x Sharps bin

NOTE: Skin cleansing solutions and method with vary depending on local policy

Cannula Sizes

- Brown/Orange (14G): large infusion/emergency
- Grey (16G): rapid infusion/ obstetrics
- White/Green (18G): blood transfusion/fluid infusion/ certain medications e.g. amiodarone
- Pink (20G): fluids/bolus medications
- Blue (22G): fluids/bolus medications
- Yellow (24G): paediatrics
- Purple (26G): neonates/ paediatrics

'Patient comfort is very important in considering where to place the cannula, particularly in non emergency situations. Put it in the left arm if they are right handed, use a small cannula if that is all that might be needed, and remember that although the antecubital fossa is tempting, placing a cannula here makes moving the arm more difficult'

Zeshan Qureshi
Paediatric Trainee
London Deanery

Preparing Intravenous Extension Set

1x intravenous extension set, 1x draw up needle, 1x 5 ml syringe, 1x normal saline ampoule, 1x non sterile gloves

1. Decontaminate hands (with either soap and water or alcohol gel). Ask patient to wash their hands/arms if able
2. Clean tray according to local policy
3. Clean hands
4. Put on a non sterile pair of gloves
5. Gather equipment
6. Draw up saline using a draw-up needle and a 5 ml syringe using a non touch technique (NTT). Discard the needle into the sharps bin
7. Flush the intravenous extension set with saline (without attaching the intravenous extension set to the cannula), using NTT, and then close the line clamp. DO NOT REMOVE from the package the end of the intravenous extension set that is going to be attached to the cannula (maintain asepsis)

NOTE: Pre-filled syringes, with normal saline (depending on hospital) might be available. These save time, and reduce risk e.g. infection/ needlestick injury. If you are drawing up the normal saline from saline ampoules, before using them, some local policies suggest that you should decontaminate the top of each ampoule with a sterile 2% chlorhexidine in 70% alcohol equipment wipe (Sani-cloth®) for 30 seconds and leave to air dry

Preparing the Flush

2x draw up needle, 1x 5ml syringe, and 1x normal saline ampoule

1. Draw up a second saline syringe using a draw up needle and a 5-ml syringe using NTT
2. Discard the needle in the sharps bin, and attach the syringe to a second needle for storage (or if available, a sterilised cap for the syringe tip)
3. At this point, open the cannula packaging (check it is intact), cannula dressing, and sterile gauze, leaving the products in the packaging. This way they can be accessed later on without touching the outer packaging
4. Remove gloves and decontaminate your hands

DO NOT RESHEATH ANY NEEDLE

Performing the Procedure

Insert the Cannula

1x non-sterile gloves, 1x tourniquet, 1x Chloraprep®, 1x cannula, 1x sterile adhesive dressing, 1x pre-prepared intravenous extension set, 1x sterile gauze

1. Apply a single-use disposable apron
2. Position patient arm. Put on the tourniquet: explain to the patient that this is to bring up the vein: place the tourniquet approximately 7-10cm above the site of insertion
3. Select vein, then loosen tourniquet
4. Decontaminate your hands again, put on non sterile gloves (or use sterile gloves if it is anticipated you might need to repalpate the vein) and retighten tourniquet
5. Clean the site using Chloraprep®: say you would clean for 30 seconds and leave to air dry, and immediately dispose the chloroprep® in the sharps bin

6. Maintain traction on the vein that you have selected beneath the insertion site and insert the cannula at approximately 45 degrees using NTT (while warning the patient of a 'sharp scratch')
7. Advance the cannula until flashback is obtained. **Do not repalpate the aseptic area** of the skin at any time during the procedure (unless wearing sterile gloves)
8. Once the flashback has been obtained, advance the cannula (BUT NOT the needle) all the way into the vein. No part of the cannula tubing must be seen at the point of entry
9. Release the tourniquet
10. Occlude the vein and cannula with firm pressure, and then gently remove the needle
11. Dispose of the needle straight into the sharps bin
12. Attach the intravenous extension set to the cannula (remember to remove the cap/needle before attaching it to the end of the cannula)
13. Wipe away any blood that may have leaked around the cannula with sterile gauze
14. Apply sterile adhesive dressing
15. Write the date and time on the cannula dressing label (write this BEFORE you stick it onto the dressing)

> 'As a general rule, if you fail twice at putting a cannula in, ask a senior colleague to place it instead'
>
> **Zeshan Qureshi**
> *Paediatric Trainee*
> *London Deanery*

Flush the Cannula

1x pre-prepared flush, 1x Sani-cloth®

1. Decontaminate the end of the intravenous extension set that you are going to attach the flush to with a sterile 2% chlorhexidine in 70% alcohol equipment wipe (Sani-cloth®) for 30 seconds and leave to air dry
2. Attach the 5ml pre-filled syringe
3. Flush intravenous extension set, 1 ml at a time, ensuring that there is no subcutaneous fluid loss and checking with the patient if it is painful at all
4. Explain to the patient that they might feel coldness running up their arm as you are flushing the cannula
5. As the last ml of flush is being inserted, place the clip on the intravenous extension set across the line where it attaches onto the cannula (to maintain positive pressure, reduce the risk of complications and backtracking)
6. Remove the syringe

NOTE some local policies may suggest you decontaminate the end of the intravenous extension set after flushing the cannula (with a sterile 2% chlorhexidine in 70% alcohol equipment wipe (Sani-cloth®) for 30 seconds and leave to air dry)

Explain to the patient that if they have any pain or redness at or around the cannula site, or if they have any other concerns, they should speak to a member of staff

Finishing Off

1. Decontaminate tray as per local policy
2. Dispose of equipment in a clinical waste bin
3. Remove gloves
4. Decontaminate your hands

Complete a cannula insertion record, and place in notes

NOTE: A cannula SHOULD BE CHANGED every 72 hours unless it has been documented otherwise

> 'Take more than one cannula with you to the bedside: be prepared in case you miss!'
>
> ## Zeshan Qureshi
> *Paediatric Trainee*
> *London Deanery*

Setting Up a Giving Set

1. Decontaminate hands
2. Put on non sterile gloves
3. Check the bag of fluids with the examiner:
   - Is it the same fluid and quantity as what is prescribed on the fluid chart?
   - Are any additives required (e.g. potassium or magnesium)?
   - Is it in date?
   - Check that there is no sediment floating in the fluid bag
   - Check that the bag has not leaked into the packaging
   - Write down the batch number on the chart
4. Remove the bag of fluid from its outer casing
5. Remove the giving set from the bag (check expiry date and that it is the right giving set for the task) and close the tap. To maintain asepsis, do not remove the end of the giving set
6. Remove the cap from the fluid bag and attach it to the giving set: you may have to push it in hard, and make sure not to touch the sharp end as it should be aseptic
7. Place the bag on the stand
8. Squeeze the chamber at the top of the giving set until it is filled halfway with fluid
9. Then SLOWLY open the tap of the giving set so that fluid flows down the line; do this bit by bit until the line is full of fluid and there are no air bubbles seen; if the line is full of bubbles, the process needs to be started again with new sterile equipment
10. The line is now ready to be attached to the cannula (ensuring the port is cleaned first)
11. Remove gloves
12. Dispose of equipment in a clinical waste bin
13. Decontaminate your hands
14. Document the date and time of start of infusion on the fluid chart
15. Talk to your patient throughout the procedure

Practical Skills

Station 4: MALE URETHRAL CATHETERISATION

Mr Miller has lower abdominal pain and has been sent to the accident and emergency department by his GP. You diagnose acute urinary retention. Mr Miller requires a urethral catheter. Having already obtained his consent, demonstrate this procedure on the mannequin provided.

- Identify the patient by asking them and by looking at their bracelet: name, date of birth, hospital number/address
- Reconfirm that the patient understands what is going to happen
- Lay the patient on a trolley or bed and ask them to expose themselves from the belly button to the knees, covering the area with a blanket or towel
- Ask for a chaperone, and you will also require an assistant

Catheter Selection

- Size: Male generally 14Ch (may need 12Ch). Female generally 12Ch (may need 14Ch)
- Length: Male vs. Female. Do not use a female catheter for a male patient
- Material: Silicone (lasts up to 3 months), Coated Latex (lasts up to 2 weeks)
- If frank haematuria with clots, an irrigation catheter may be required

Get Out Equipment

a) 1x procedure trolley
b) 1x catheterisation pack (including disposable dish, plastic pots, cotton swabs and sterile drape)
c) 2x pairs sterile gloves
d) 2x sterile water sachets
e) 1x local anaesthetic/antiseptic gel syringe ('Instillagel®')
f) 1x catheter
g) 1x catheter bag
h) 1x disposable bag (for rubbish)
i) 1x draw up needle + 10ml syringe + sterile water vial (often pre-drawn up with catheter)
j) Disposable bag
k) Single use disposable apron
l) Leg bag (to be considered if patient mobile)

Prepare Procedure Trolley with Aseptic Field

1. Wash hands
2. Clean trolley according to local policy
3. Gather equipment, and wash hands again if contaminated whilst gathering equipment
4. Open the catheterisation pack using a non-touch technique on the centre of trolley
5. Using a non-touch technique, open the packaging and drop instillagel®, gloves and catheter onto the aseptic field
6. Open the packaging of the catheter bag (so that you can take it out later on)
7. If not pre-prepared, draw up sterile water using a draw up needle and a 10 ml syringe. Discard the draw up needle in the sharps bin

Prepare the Patient

1. Take your trolley to the bedside
2. Ensuring patient dignity (draw curtains, close the door or say that you would do this), expose the patient from umbilicus to knees with legs slightly apart and their arms by their sides
3. Wash your hands thoroughly, put on an single use disposable apron, and put on sterile gloves
4. Place a sterile drape with central hole over the patient, leaving his penis exposed

Causes of Urinary Retention

- Benign prostatic hypertrophy, usually in the context of another cause e.g. urinary infection or anticholinergic medication
- Prostatic or other pelvic malignancy
- Neurogenic bladder e.g. Cauda equina syndrome, Multiple Sclerosis or Parkinson's disease
- Urethral stricture, which may be traumatic or infective in origin e.g. due to Gonorrhoea or Chlamydia
- Infection, principally prostatitis
- Drugs e.g. Anticholinergics or psychoactive drugs such as amphetamines

Documentation of Catheter Insertion

In the medical notes, write the following (often a sticker from catheter pack is provided for this purpose):

- Date and time of insertion
- Size and material of catheter
- Ease with which catheter passed
- Colour of urine drained
- Volume of sterile water inserted into balloon
- Residual volume of urine (5-10 minutes after insertion)
- Sign and print your name under your entry

Asepsis and Anaesthesia

1. Ask an assistant to empty both sterile water sachets into plastic pot
2. Soak the cotton swabs in water
3. Hold the penis with the left (non-dominant) hand and retract the prepuce. This hand is contaminated and should now not touch the aseptic trolley
4. With the right hand, clean the penis in concentric circles beginning at the glans penis, and moving progressively outwards
5. Dispose of the swabs away from the aseptic field (a disposable bag is usually provided)
6. Explain to the patient that you are going to insert some anaesthetic gel to make the procedure more comfortable. Holding the glans, pull firmly upward, and insert the tip of the instillagel® syringe into the urethral meatus
7. Administer at least half the tube of instillagel®, allowing some to coat the glans
8. Leave the instillagel® for 2-3 minutes to take effect
9. Remove gloves and put on second pair of sterile gloves

Inserting the Catheter

1. Hold the base of the glans with the left hand. Apply gentle upward traction to the penis, while inserting the catheter with the right hand into the urethral meatus
2. Insert catheter using a non touch technique by touching only the packaging i.e. insert directly from sterilised packaging (without taking the catheter completely out of the packaging). Place the disposable dish between the patient's legs so that once the catheter is in, urine does not spill onto the bed sheets
3. Advance the catheter until resistance is felt. Now lower the penis and continue to advance the catheter until urine is seen to flow into disposable dish
4. Advance the catheter as far as the fork at the end, particularly if no urine is seen draining
5. Attach the sterile water syringe to the balloon port of the catheter. Insert 10ml slowly, (1ml first) asking the patient to tell you if there is any pain. STOP if there is pain or high resistance
6. Attach the catheter to the drainage bag. Remove the cap from the tubing and plug the plastic tube end into the catheter
7. If there is a leg-bag, attach it to the leg. Larger collection bags may be attached to the side of the patient's bed

8. REPLACE THE PREPUCE! If this is not done, a very painful paraphimosis may result, sometimes requiring surgery to repair
9. Clean the patient and ensure dignity by rearranging bed-clothes
10. Dispose of waste and gloves
11. Decontaminate hands
12. Clean trolley according to local policy
13. Decontaminate hands
14. Tell the patient to report any pain or other concerns to the nursing staff
15. Document insertion of catheter, including noting the residual volume of urine

What are the potential risks of urethral catheterisation?

- Inability to place a catheter
- Trauma
  - **Formation of a false passage:** if catheterization attempted against resistance. Necessitates urological input and possible suprapubic catheter
  - **Damage to urethral sphincters:** from balloon inflation within the urethra. Potentially leads to complete urinary incontinence
- **Infection:** commonly due to presence of foreign body, made more likely by poor aseptic technique. Not treated if asymptomatic, otherwise give a single dose of IV antibiotic (e.g. Gentamicin) and change the catheter
- **Paraphimosis:** caused by failure to replace the prepuce. Remedied by gentle bimanual pressure on the glans penis and traction to the ring of retracted prepuce skin (learn the technique from an expert: do not attempt this if you are untrained). May require surgery in extreme cases
- **Bladder spasm:** common due to presence of a catheter balloon. Treated by deflating the balloon by 5ml or giving an anticholinergic such as solifenacin

Station 5: URINALYSIS

Mrs Manpreet is a 35 year-old female who presents to your clinic with abdominal pain and vomiting. She has been going to the toilet more often than normal, and is concerned that her urine is foul-smelling. She has brought a urine sample with her. Please perform a urine dipstick and discuss the results with her.

Equipment

a) Non sterile gloves
b) Apron
c) Urine reagent strip
d) Sterile urine pot
e) Clinical waste bin

Obtaining the Urine Sample (if not provided)

- Give the patient the sterile urine pot
- Ask them to collect a mid stream urine
- (MSU) sample: Ask the patient, when they pass urine, to pass a small amount into the toilet first, and then without stopping the flow of urine, catch some into the bottle. They should immediately replace the cap of the pot. A MSU reduces the chance of contamination
- If the patient is unable to pass urine, a sample may be obtained from a catheter if clinically indicated. This is best obtained at the point of insertion. It carries a risk of introducing infection so should only be performed if absolutely necessary

Urine Dipstick

1) Wash your hands. Put on gloves and apron
2) Inspect the urine sample: does it look cloudy, dark yellow or red?
3) Remove the cap of the urine. Is it sweet smelling or foul smelling? Does it smell feculent?
4) Get the dipstick out of its container. Check the expiry date of the dipstick by looking at the container (make this obvious to the examiner)
5) Place the dipstick in the urine for 2-3 seconds. Make sure all of the reagents on the dipstick are immersed in the urine. Remove the dipstick
6) Place the dipstick horizontal to ensure that the chemicals do not mix. This can be achieved by placing the dipstick on top of the urine container. Leave it to dry for 1 minute before reading the result (although some tests are 30 or 45 seconds)
7) Look at each reagent on the dipstick in turn. With each reagent, look at the corresponding colour on the tub (the tub will have a colour code on its side so that you can interpret the results) and identify if the value is normal or high. If it is high, how high is it?

Causes of Haematuria

- **Kidney:** malignancy, calculi, trauma, glomerulonephritis, pyelonephritis, interstitial nephritis, infarction, polycystic kidney disease
- **Ureter:** malignancy, calculi, trauma
- **Bladder:** malignancy, calculi, trauma, infection
- **Urethra and prostate:** malignancy, stone, trauma, benign prostatic hypertrophy (BPH)
- **General:** anticoagulants e.g. warfarin, exercise, paroxysmal nocturnal haematuria
- **Not true haematuria:** May purely be vaginal bleeding. May not be blood at all (beetroot can give similar appearance, as can certain drugs e.g. rifampicin)

Interpretation

All of the results need to be interpreted in the context of the patient. A raised glucose on urinalysis does not necessarily mean that the patient has diabetes. For example, glycosuria can be transient in the context of pregnancy

Appearance	Smell
• Red indicates haematuria. What is the cause of the haematuria? • Cloudy urine can be due to an infection • Drugs can discolour the urine. For example, rifampicin or doxorubicin may turn it red. Desferrioxamine may turn urine a reddish-brown • Feculent and pneumaturia with bowel-bladder fistula	• Foul smelling with infection. Sweet smelling in diabetic ketoacidosis (DKA). Feculent with bowel-bladder fistulae

Blood

- A positive result can indicate either haematuria or, rarely, haemoglobinuria or myoglobinuria
- Bleeding can be from anywhere in the urinary tract. In a woman, ask if she is menstruating

Ketones

- Raised levels are seen in DKA and starvation
- The presence of raised glucose and metabolic acidosis, together with ketones in the urine, indicate DKA. The absence of ketones in the urine with a very high blood glucose suggests Hyperosmolar Non Ketotic State (HONK)
- Ask the patient if they are deliberately trying to lose weight and when they last ate

Nitrites and Leukocytes

- A positive test suggests a bacterial infection. However, leukocytes can be present in the urine non-specifically
- A urinary tract infection will only have a positive nitrite test if the bacteria can convert nitrates to nitrites (i.e. Gram negative bacteria). If they cannot, then the nitrite test will be negative even when infection is present

Protein

- This is raised in renovascular, glomerular or tubulo-interstitial renal disease. It is also raised in pre-eclampsia and hypertension. It may also be benign (exercise, postural)
- In nephrotic syndrome (low albumin, oedema, raised cholesterol, proteinuria), it is important to quantify the amount of protein loss by 24 hour collection

Glucose

- A raised glucose level is seen in diabetes, particularly if the patient is in DKA or HONK
- To further evaluate a new diagnosis of diabetes, further testing may be required, with a fasting or random glucose measurement
- Glucose may also be raised in pregnancy

Specific Gravity

- This represents the concentrating and diluting status of the kidney
- A high value occurs in dehydration, heart failure, liver failure, and syndrome of inappropriate ADH secretion (SIADH)
- A low value occurs in diabetes insipidus, and increased fluid intake

Urine pH

- Especially useful in the management of UTI and calculi (stones)
- If patients have symptoms of UTI, then alkaline urine can indicate an infection with a urea splitting organism (e.g. Proteus)
- Acidic urine is seen in calculi made of uric acid and cystine. Alkalinisation of the urine is an important part of the management of these patients (by giving potassium citrate)

Further Urine Investigations

- Pregnancy test is important in all fertile women presenting with lower abdominal pain
- If there is evidence of a urinary tract infection (leukocytes, nitrites, blood, protein) send the urine sample for microscopy, culture and sensitivity
- If there is a concern about myeloma (bone pain, anaemia, renal failure, elevated calcium, proteinuria) send the urine for protein electrophoresis
- Urine microscopy can reveal red-cell casts. These occur in the context of glomerulonephritis
- Urine can be tested for microalbuminuria in patients that have DM (newer dipsticks can measure this). This is a screening test for nephropathy

What methods are available for collecting urine samples in a baby?

- Clean-catch urine: Waiting for urination with a sterile pot after the nappy has been removed and the surrounding area has been cleaned (parents should be told to ask for a new sterile pot if it gets contaminated)
- Supra-pubic aspiration (ultra-sound guided)
- Catheter sample

'Don't throw away a urine sample after the dipstick is done: wait until a decision is made as to whether it needs to be sent for further tests'

Zeshan Qureshi
Paediatric Trainee
London Deanery

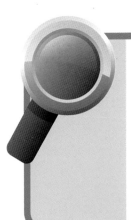

PRESENT YOUR FINDINGS...

'Mrs Manpreet is a 35 year-old lady who has presented with abdominal pain, vomiting and urinary frequency. On examination of her urine specimen, the urine appeared cloudy and foul smelling. Her urine dipstick was positive for nitrites++, leucocytes+ and blood+.

These results, in the context of her symptoms, suggest a urinary tract infection.

I would send her urine off for microscopy culture and sensitivity, and consider starting empirical antibiotic therapy according to local microbiology guidelines.'

Station 6: ECG INTERPRETATION

Mr Fredrickson has been having exertional chest pain. He is a smoker, and is known to suffer from diabetes. An ECG has been performed. Please assess the ECG, and present your findings.

The following information can be gained from an ECG:

Details	Derived Data
• Time and date of ECG • Patient details (name, date of birth) • Calibration • Paper speed: usually 25 mm/second [one small square = 40 msec]	• Heart rate • Heart rhythm • Cardiac axis • Morphology

Always put the ECG into context - how is the patient? Particularly, do they have chest pain? Are they haemodynamically stable?

General Points about the ECG Waveform

The P wave = atrial depolarisation

QRS complex = ventricular depolarisation

- Q wave = first negative deflection
- R wave = first positive deflection
- S wave = negative deflection after R wave
- Normally, the QRS complex is less than 3 small squares in duration (<120 ms). If it is prolonged, conduction through the ventricles is not occurring efficiently (and therefore is not occurring from the AV node through the bundle of His)

T wave = ventricular repolarisation

Heart Rate

This depends on if the heart rhythm is regular or irregular.

- If regular, count the number of large boxes between adjacent R waves
- Divide this number into 300

- For example, if there are **3 large boxes** between R waves, **300/3** = a heart rate of **100 beats per minute**
- If irregular, multiply the number of RR intervals in **10 seconds** by **6** (10 seconds is the standard rhythm strip on most ECGs which is typically the full strip for Lead II)
- For example, if there were **22** RR intervals on the **10 second** rhythm strip, the heart rate is **22 x 6 = 132 beats per minute** (alternatively dividing the number of large squares between 4 RR intervals into 900 is another way to calculate irregular rates)

When interpreting the heart rate: a heart rate over 100 bpm is described as 'tachycardia' and a heart rate under 60 bpm is described as 'bradycardia'. We will consider bradycardias and tachycardias separately

Bradycardia (HR<60)

- Are p waves present?
- Is each p wave followed by a QRS complex?
- What is the relationship between atrial depolarisation (p wave) and ventricular depolarisation (QRS complex)?
  - If there are p waves, is the PR interval the same for each QRS complex?
  - Is the PR interval the normal length (3-5 small squares (120-200 ms))?

Rhythm	P Waves Present?	Every P Wave Followed by QRS?	PR Interval
Sinus Bradycardia	Yes	Yes	Normal
1st degree heart block	Yes	Yes	Prolonged interval (regular)
2nd degree heart block (Mobitz 1, Wenckebach)	Yes	No	Lengthening each beat, until a QRS is 'dropped' from a non conducted P wave
2nd degree heart block (Mobitz 2)	Yes	No	PR interval is constant but occasionally the P wave is not conducted
3rd degree heart block (Complete)	Yes (unless in atrial fibrillation)	No	No relation between P and R wave

In second degree heart block, the degree of block is defined by the relationship between atrial and ventricular activity. If two p waves are present for each QRS, the block is 2:1.

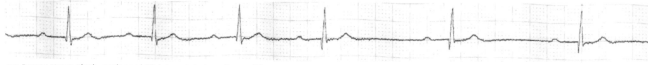

1st Degree Heart Block: prolonged PR interval, but no dropped beats

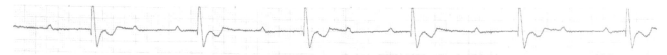

3rd Degree Heart Block: there is no relationship between atrial (p wave) and ventricular (QRS complexes) activity

Tachycardia (HR›100)

In tachycardias, is it useful to subclassify ECG patterns based on the heart rhythm.

Rhythm

First, ask: Is the rhythm originating in the atria or the ventricles?

- If QRS duration › 120 ms ('broad complex'), the focus of arrhythmia will usually be coming from within the ventricles e.g. ventricular tachycardia. The exception is if there is a bundle branch block or an aberrant conduction pathway (which results in inefficient ventricular depolarisation and a subsequent widened QRS complex)

- If QRS duration ‹ 120 ms ('narrow complex'), the focus of arrhythmia will always be supra-ventricular. This is because a narrow QRS complex implies efficient conduction through the ventricles (through the AV nodes and subsequently the bundle of His) which can only occur with a supra-ventricular focus

Second, ask: Is the rhythm regular or irregular?

- This can be done by checking the regularity of QRS complexes (RR interval should normally be the same between all complexes)

1. Irregular Atrial Tachycardia (QRS‹120ms)

Atrial Fibrillation	Sinus Rhythm with Ectopic Beats	Sinus Arrhythmia
• Irregularly irregular rhythm • QRS ‹120 ms • No p waves (baseline of ECG is chaotic: due to atrium fibrillating) • NOTE: heart rate may be normal, or even bradycardic, especially if already on treatment	• Background rhythm: Regular, normal P waves • QRS ‹120 ms • Occasional beats before expected (as predicted from the background regular sinus rhythm) • There is either an abnormal p wave followed by a QRS complex (atrial ectopic) or simply an isolated QRS complex with no p wave preceding it (ventricular ectopic)	• Regularly irregular rhythm (varying with breathing) • QRS ‹120 ms • Normal p waves

Atrial Fibrillation: irregularly irregular, with no visible p waves

2. Regular Atrial Tachycardia (QRS<120ms)

Atrial Flutter	Sinus Tachycardia
• Regular • QRS <120 ms • No p waves - Flutter waves are seen: 'saw toothed' appearance to baseline of ECG, typically at a rate of 300 bpm, with a 2:1 block (this is a physiological response of the AV node). Therefore, in this scenario, 150 bpm are conducted to the ventricle • NOTE: Atrial flutter is usually regular, but it can be irregular (if there is variable AV node block). Heart rate may be normal, or even bradycardic, especially if on treatment already	• Regular • QRS <120 ms • Normal p waves

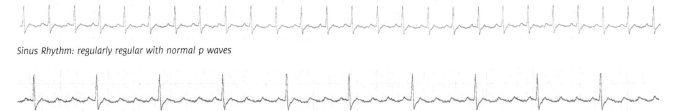

Sinus Rhythm: regularly regular with normal p waves

Atrial Flutter: 4:1 ratio of flutter waves to ventricular beats

3. Ventricular Tachycardia (QRS>120ms)

Ventricular Tachycardia	Ventricular Fibrillation
• Regular rhythm • QRS complex >120 ms • P waves may be present but no relationship with QRS complexes. There is no association between atrial and ventricular activity	• Irregular rhythm • QRS complex >120 ms • P waves absent

Ventricular Tachycardia: regular wide complex tachycardia

Fine Ventricular Fibrillation: irregular wide complex tachycardia: there will be no pulse/cardiac output!

Cardiac Axis

- The cardiac axis is the overall direction of the wave of ventricular depolarisation (measured in the vertical plane)
- This is measured from a zero reference point (from the same viewpoint as Lead I)
- An axis above this line is denoted by a negative number (of degrees) and an axis lying below this line is given a positive number (of degrees)

Left Axis Deviation	Normal Range	Right Axis Deviation
< -30° LEAD 1 POSITIVE LEAD 2 NEGATIVE	-30° to +90° LEAD 1 POSITIVE LEAD 2 POSITIVE	> +90° LEAD 1 NEGATIVE LEAD 2 POSITIVE

There are several ways to calculate the axis. Here is the simplest: A lead is 'positive' if there is a greater positive deflection in the QRS complex than the negative deflection (i.e. the R wave is taller than the S wave). A negative lead has a greater negative deflection. If leads I and II are +ve, the axis is normal; if lead I is +ve and lead II is –ve, this is left axis deviation; if lead I is –ve and lead II is +ve, this is right axis deviation

Wave Morphology

P Waves

- If all the p waves in the rhythm strip are of similar morphology, it is likely that they are arising from the same focus
- If tall: consider right atrium enlargement ('P pulmonale')
- If P waves are bifid: consider left atrium enlargement ('P mitrale')
- If flattened: consider hyperkalemia

QRS Complex

If widened, using the mnemonic 'WILLIAM MARROW' can be helpful:

- WiLLiaM (L for left bundle branch block: WM corresponds to V1 looking like 'W' and V6 looking like 'M')
- MaRRoW (R for right bundle branch block: MW corresponds to V1 looking like 'M' and V6 looking like 'W')

Causes of right bundle branch block	Causes of left bundle branch block
Normal variant	Myocardial infarction
Myocardial infarction	Hypertension
Pulmonary embolism	Conduction system fibrosis
Cor pulmonale	Cardiomyopathy
Congenital heart disease	
Cardiomyopathy	

ST Segments

The important changes to look for are either elevation or depression. The two important differentials for ST elevation are pericarditis and myocardial infarction (MI)

NOTE: in the presence of left bundle branch block, the ST segments cannot be accurately interpreted

	ST Elevation MI	Pericarditis
Site	ST elevation localised to ischemic territory	Widespread 'saddle-shaped' ST Elevation
ST Depression	Reciprocal ST depression e.g. ST depression in the anterior territory with an inferior infarct	No reciprocal change
PR Segment	Normal	PR depression

Other causes of ST elevation include left ventricular aneurysm. ST elevation may also be confused with early repolarisation

Causes of ST depression include:

- Myocardial ischaemia
- Digoxin ('reverse tick' appearance of ST segment)
- Left/right ventricular hypertrophy
- Bundle branch block
- Hypokalaemia

T Wave Changes

The two most important causes of T wave change are myocardial ischemia and hyperkalaemia

Ischemic T Wave changes:

- T wave inversion (can be normal in V1, III and aVR, especially if present in old ECGs)
- Flattened T waves
- Biphasic T waves
- Peaked T waves

If T wave inversion occurs across several leads, in the same myocardial territory, myocardial ischaemia becomes more likely

Hyperkalemia is associated will tall tented T waves

Q Wave Changes

- A pathological Q waves is one which is greater than 25% of the height of the R wave. This is suggestive of an old infarct
- In the context of an evolving infarct, if Q waves develop on serial ECGs, this is suggestive of a completed infarct

'It is very useful when seeing an ECG to compare it to a previous one (often located in the hospital notes). This way new changes (potentially associated with a new cardiac event) can be differentiated from known abnormalities.'

Zeshan Qureshi
Paediatric Trainee
London Deanery

Changes of ECG Seen in Myocardial Infarction

- ST segment elevation or depression
- T wave changes: peaked, flattened or inverted
- Poor R Wave progression (normally R waves get progressively larger from V1-6)
- Pathological Q waves

Anatomical Relations of ECG Leads

- II, III, aVF: inferior surface (right coronary artery or left circumflex)
- V1, V2, V3, V4: anterior surface (left anterior descending coronary artery)
- I, aVL, V5, V6: lateral surface (left coronary artery, circumflex)
- V5, V6: high lateral leads (left coronary artery, circumflex)
- Dominant R waves in lead V1-3, with significant ST depression: posterior surface (left circumflex or right coronary artery)

Finally, a note should be made about the ECG changes associated with hyperkalemia: flattened p waves, widened QRS complexes, tall tented T waves. ST segment depression and a prolonged PR interval may also be seen

Example ECGs (Illustration of how to 'present' follows at the end)

1. This is an ECG of Mr Fredrickson, a 65 year-old male, who is currently asymptomatic, and haemodynamically stable

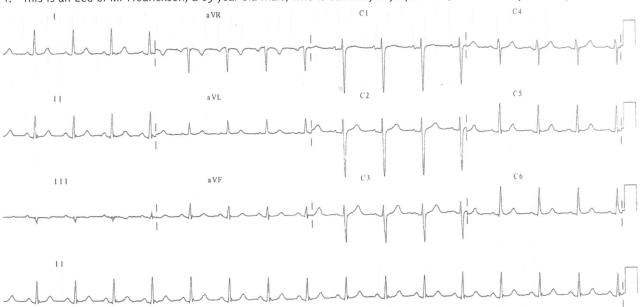

2. This is an ECG of Mr Fredrickson, a 65 year-old male, who is currently asymptomatic, and haemodynamically stable

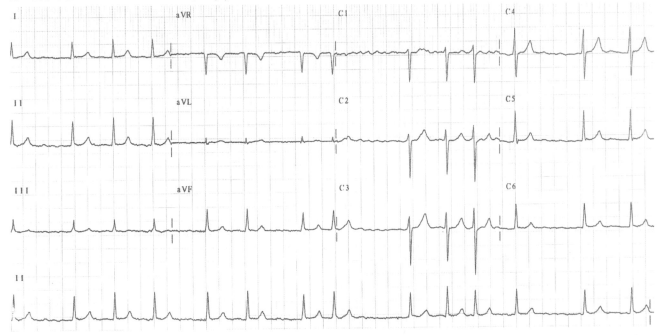

Practical Skills

3. This is an ECG of Mr Fredrickson, a 65 year-old male, who is currently asymptomatic, and haemodynamically stable

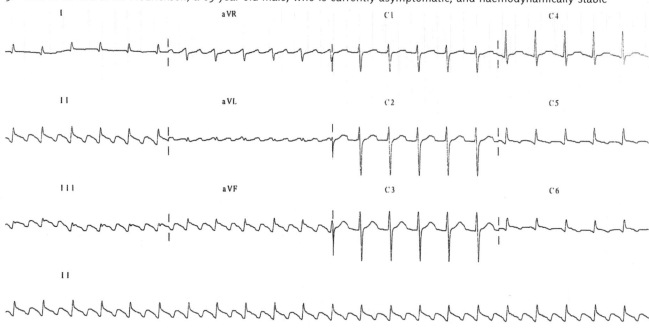

4. This is an ECG of Mr Fredrickson, a 65 year-old male, who presented with an episode of chest pain, and collapse. He is haemodynamically stable

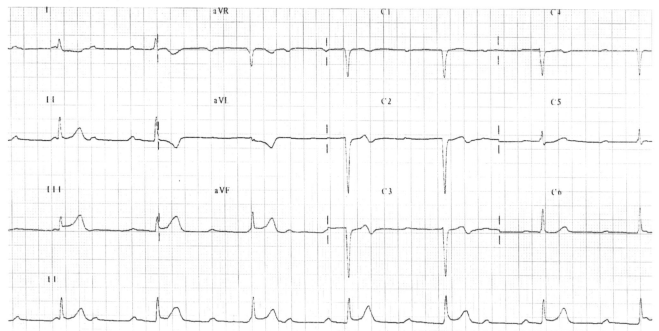

5. This is an ECG of Mr Fredrickson, a 65 year-old male, who is currently suffering from chest pain, but is haemodynamically stable

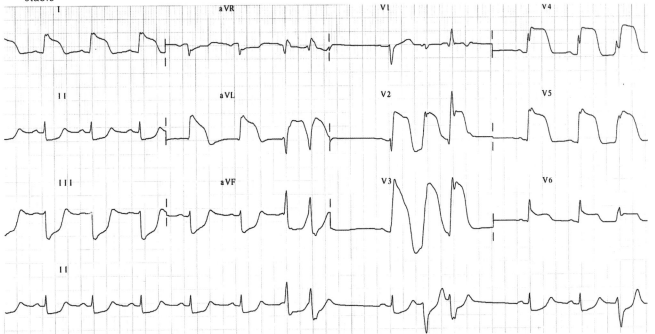

6. This is an ECG of Mr Fredrickson, a 65 year-old male, who is currently suffering from palpitations, has a peripheral pulse of 253, and a blood pressure of 92/60

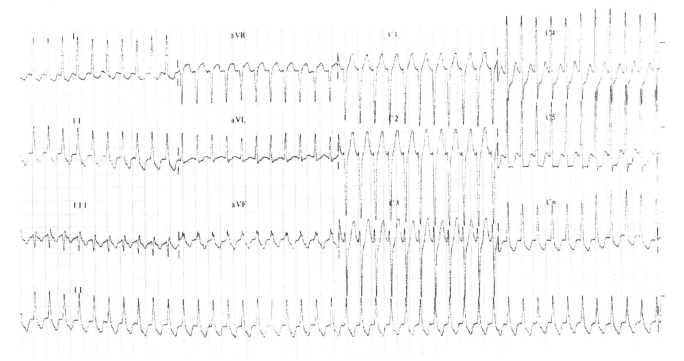

7. This is an ECG of Mr Fredrickson, a 65 year-old male, who has had a cardiac arrest

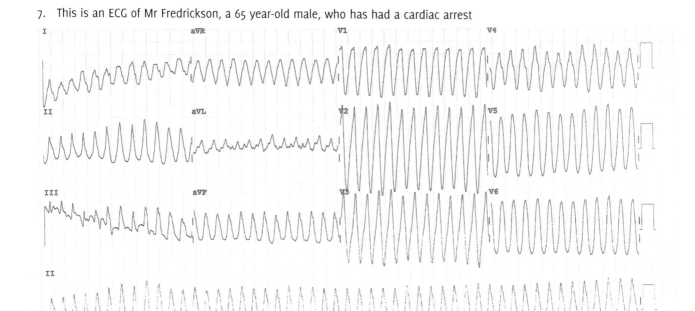

	Background	Rate, Rhythm, Axis	Morphology	Summary
1	This is an ECG of Mr Fredrickson, a 65 year-old male, who is currently asymptomatic, and haemodynamically stable	The heart rate is 94 bpm, the rhythm is regular. The axis is within normal limits	P waves are present, the PR interval is normal, QRS complexes are narrow, and there are no ST or T wave changes	In summary, this ECG is consistent with sinus rhythm
2	This is an ECG of Mr Fredrickson, a 65 year-old male, who is currently asymptomatic, and haemodynamically stable	The heart rate is 84 (14x6) bpm, the rhythm is irregularly irregular. The axis is within normal limits	No P waves are present. QRS complexes are narrow, and there are no ST or T wave changes	In summary, this ECG is consistent with atrial fibrillation
3	This is an ECG of Mr Fredrickson, a 65 year-old male, who is currently asymptomatic, and haemodynamically stable	The heart rate is 138 bpm, the rhythm is regular. The axis is within normal limits	P waves have a saw-toothed appearance, and there are two per QRS complex, which are narrow. There are no ST or T wave changes	In summary, this ECG is consistent with atrial flutter
4	This is an ECG of Mr Fredrickson, a 65 year-old male, who presented with an episode of chest pain, and collapse. He is haemodynamically stable	The heart rate is 42 bpm, the rhythm is regular. The axis is within normal limits	P waves are present, but there is no relationship with QRS complexes, which are narrow. There is 1mm ST elevation in leads II, III, and aVF, and 1mm of ST depression in aVL. There is T wave inversion in I, aVL, and aVR. There are biphasic T waves in V1-4	In summary, this ECG is consistent with complete heart block. The ST and T wave changes may represent a ventricular escape rhythm morphology OR an inferior MI causing SA node ischemia, and subsequent heart block
5	This is an ECG of Mr Fredrickson, a 65 year-old male, who is currently suffering from chest pain, but is haemodynamically stable	The heart rate is 82 bpm, the rhythm is regular. The axis is within normal limits	P waves are present, PR interval is normal, and QRS complexes are narrow. There is massive ST elevation, up to 16mm, in leads I, AVL, V2-6, and T wave inversion in lead aVL. There is ST depression in leads II, III and aVF. 4 ectopics are also present	In summary, this ECG is consistent with an anterolateral ST elevation myocardial infarction, with reciprocal inferior ST depression

Practical Skills

| 6 | This is an ECG of Mr Fredrickson, a 65 year-old male, who is currently suffering from palpitations, has a peripheral pulse of 253, and a blood pressure of 92/60 | The heart rate is 260 bpm, the rhythm is regular. The axis is within normal limits | P waves are not clearly visible (although if you look carefully, they can be seen buried in the T wave), and QRS complexes are narrow. There is ST depression (up to 5mm) in leads I, II, aVF, and V4-6 | In summary, this ECG is consistent with a supraventricular tachycardia, with probable rate related inferolateral ischemia |
| 7 | This is an ECG of Mr Fredrickson, a 65 year-old male, who has had a cardiac arrest | The heart rate is 300 bpm, the rhythm is regular. The axis is within normal limits | P waves are not clearly visible. QRS complexes are wide. ST segment and T wave changes cannot be seen | In summary, this ECG is consistent with a broad complex tachycardia (either ventricular tachycardia or supraventicular tachycardia with bundle branch block) |

Station 7: FUNDOSCOPY

Mr Wilson is a 55-year-old man with diabetes. Please examine his fundi. His pupils have already been dilated. Sketch your findings on the provided sheet.

- Introduce yourself, explain what you would like to do, and seek permission
- *'I'd like to examine the back of your eyes. To get a good view, I'll need to come quite close to your head. Keep looking straight ahead please' (pick something for patient to focus on e.g. light switch, so they keep their head still!)*
- In the exam, be prepared to examine a (pre-dilated) real patient or a model head

Positioning

- Sitting in a dark room
- For best results, dilate the pupil first e.g. using tropicamide drops
- To examine the right eye, use your right hand and right eye, and vice versa
- Keep your index finger on the dial at the side so you can adjust the focus whilst examining if needed: it may help to start on a low 'plus' setting, and ratchet anticlockwise towards minus until the image is clear (minus, anticlockwise, corrects for myopia)
- '0' is the equivalent of no refractive error, negative red numbers correct for myopia (short sighted) and positive green numbers correct for hypermetropia (long sighted)

Examination Sequence

Red reflex

- Before moving in to see the fundus, look for the red reflex from approximately 30cm, at approximately a 45 degree angle to the nose
- Incomplete/absent red reflex: think cataracts, corneal opacities or tumours

Optic disc

- Find a large vessel and trace it back to find the optic disc
- Assess the disc colour (pale e.g. optic atrophy); margin (blurred e.g. papilloedema); and cup (increased cup:disc ratio e.g. glaucoma)

Macula

- Look for abnormalities in this area haemorrhages or exudates (e.g. diabetes), pigmentation (e.g. macular degeneration)

Vessels

- Trace the 4 major vessel arcs out to the periphery
- Veins appear darker than arteries
- Look for **arteriovenous (AV) nipping** (at vessel crossing points) e.g. hypertension; look for **haemorrhages** or **vessel tortuosity** e.g. diabetes/hypertension; **microaneurysms** e.g. diabetes; and **silver wiring** e.g. hypertension

Thyroid Eye Disease

- Lid retraction (Dalrymple's sign)
- Lid lag on down gaze (von Graefe's sign)
- Exophthalmos (proptosis) due to oedema of extraocular muscles
- Restricted extraocular movements
- Chemosis (conjunctival oedema)

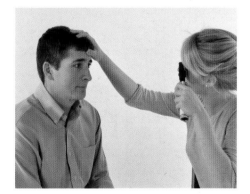

Fig 5.1: Assessing red reflex

Periphery

- Examine each quadrant, ensuring that the retina looks pink and healthy
- Due to the magnification of the ophthalmoscope, not much of the periphery is easily visible

Common Causes of Visual Loss

Acute	Gradual
Uveitis	Cataract
Keratitis e.g. due to corneal ulcer	Age-related macular degeneration
Optic neuritis	Optic neuropathy (including glaucoma)
Ischaemic optic neuropathy	
Retinal vein/artery occlusion	
Retinal detachment	
Vitreous haemorrhage	
Stroke	

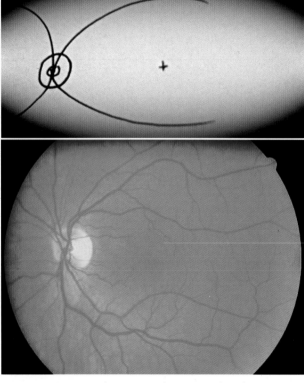

Fig 5.2: A healthy fundus (left eye, below) and sketch (above). Note the clear margins of the optic disc, the vessels branching away from it, and the macula (centre of the image, sketched as a plus sign)

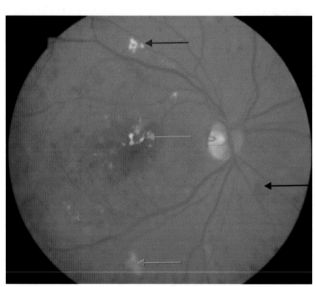

Fig 5.3: Severe non proliferative diabetic retinopathy with maculopathy (right eye)
'Multiple dot and blot haemorrhages (black arrow) are scattered throughout the retina. There are hard exudates in the superior field (blue arrow), and a cotton wool spot in the inferior field (grey arrow). The disc looks healthy, with no new vessels visible. These changes would be consistent with severe non-proliferative diabetic retinopathy. There are also hard exudates superior to the macula (green arrow), indicating diabetic maculopathy'

Diabetic Retinopathy

- The main risk factor is the duration of diabetes
- All patients with diabetes should be screened for retinopathy at least annually
- Incidence is lower with excellent glycaemic control (e.g. HbA1c of less than 7%)
- Below are listed the stages of diabetic retinopathy

Non-Proliferative Diabetic Retinopathy (NPDR)

- Microaneurysms (smaller, and more distinct that dot haemorrhage, but difficult to differentiate the two)
- 'Dot and blot' haemorrhages
- Hard exudates
- Cotton wool spots (due to local ischaemia)
- Normal visual acuity

- No treatment indicated, only regular follow-up

Severe Non- Proliferative Diabetic Retinopathy

- Venous beading/dilatation/tortuosity
- Larger and more widespread blot haemorrhages
- Intraretinal microvascular abnormality (IRMA)
- Closer follow-up

Proliferative Diabetic Retinopathy

- Neovascularisation (due to ischaemia): new vessels on the disc/elsewhere
- Risk of vitreous haemorrhage (new vessels are friable and prone to bleeding, particularly those close to the disc)
- Risk of tractional retinal detachment
- Severe loss of vision may occur secondary to these

Practical Skills

Diabetic Maculopathy

- Vessel leakage and/or ischemia at the macula
- Most common cause of visual loss in diabetes

Laser Treatment Scars

- Panretinal photocoagulation (PRP) for proliferative diabetic retinopathy
- Focal/grid laser photocoagulation for diabetic maculopathy

Hypertensive Retinopathy

- Arteriolar narrowing
- Arterio-venous nipping at crossing points
- Copper/silver wiring (increased central light reflex from arterioles)
- Cotton wool spots
- Hard exudates, which may surround the macula forming a partial or complete 'star'
- Blot or flame haemorrhages
- Usually asymptomatic if chronic

Accelerated Hypertension

- Disc swelling, indicating an optic neuropathy, as well as retinopathy changes above
- May have reduced visual acuity
- Usually severe hypertension (e.g. SBP >220mmHg) and evidence of other end-organ damage

Optic Disc Swelling

Papilloedema

- Bilateral disc swelling secondary to raised intracranial pressure
- Blurred disc margins ± disc pallor
- If long-standing, you may see dilated veins and hard exudates

Optic Neuritis

- Demyelination

Anterior Ischaemic Optic Neuropathy

- Infarction of the optic nerve head, usually secondary to giant cell arteritis or hypertension

Age-related Macular Degeneration (AMD)

- Commonest cause of blindness in the developed world for over 50s

Dry (atrophic) AMD

- Degeneration at and around the macula
- Atrophic (pale) +/- hyperpigmented areas
- Drusen (subretinal deposits of waste products)
- No treatment

Wet (neovascular) AMD

- Choroidal neovascularisation, which may leak, leading to oedema and haemorrhage
- More rapid loss of vision
- Anti-VEGF injections into the vitreous or sometimes laser treatment may be given

Management of Hypertension

- Aims of antihypertensive therapy are usually BP <140/90, or <130/80 if diabetic or target organ damage
- Look for evidence of target organ damage (renal, cardiovascular e.g. heart failure/PVD, cerebrovascular)

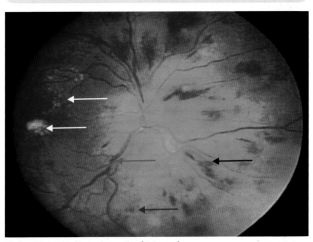

Fig 5.4: Hypertensive retinopathy (right eye)
'The most striking feature is the large number of blot (blue arrow) and flame-shaped haemorrhages (black arrow). The arterioles are narrowed in places and there is arterio-venous nipping (green arrow). There are hard exudates near the macula (white arrows)'

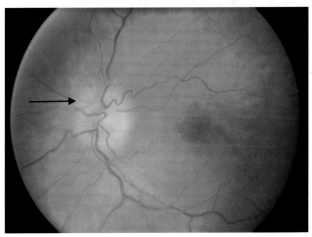

Fig 5.5: Papilloedema (left eye)
'The optic disc is pale with blurred margins (black arrow), indicating a swollen disc. If that patient has raised intracranial pressure this would be consistent with papilloedema. I would also consider other causes such as optic neuritis'

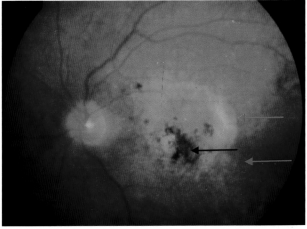

Fig 5.6: Dry AMD (left eye)
'There is a pale area around the macula (grey arrow), with some hyperpigmented areas (black arrow). There are some soft drusen (green arrow). I cannot see any areas of haemorrhage. This would be consistent with dry age-related macular degeneration'

Station 8: DEATH CERTIFICATION

You are called by the nursing staff to see a patient that has just passed away. You are asked to pronounce them dead and to write a death certificate.

Verification of Death

When certifying that someone is dead, the relatives may be present. If they opt to stay, you should explain what you need to do. For example, performing a sternal rub without prior explanation may cause further distress to the family.

- Patient unresponsive to painful stimuli (sternal rub)
- Absence of carotid pulse for over 1 minute
- Absence of breath sounds for over 1 minute
- Absence of heart sounds for over 1 minute
- Pupils dilated and unresponsive to light

NOTE: The use of adrenaline at a cardiac arrest can cause dilated pupils, so it is necessary to consider this detail

- When you have completed your examination, remember to leave your patient (mannequin) in a dignified manner. Cover the body up to the neck with sheet/bed linen
- Record date and time of death in the notes, and make arrangements for the family to be informed
  - The time of certification of death is recorded as the time of verification of death (not the time they were found by the nursing staff)

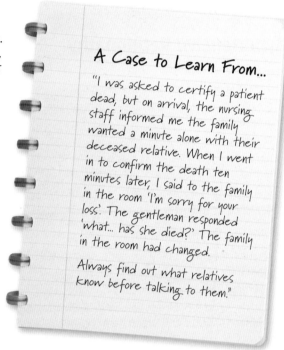

A Case to Learn From...

"I was asked to certify a patient dead, but on arrival, the nursing staff informed me the family wanted a minute alone with their deceased relative. When I went in to confirm the death ten minutes later, I said to the family in the room 'I'm sorry for your loss'. The gentleman responded 'what... has she died?' The family in the room had changed.

Always find out what relatives know before talking to them."

Writing a Death Certificate

- Only complete a death certificate if you know and understand the case. It is not necessary to have been present at the time of death or to have actually certified the death
- Understand the situations when a death should be referred to the Coroner or Procurator Fiscal (in Scotland) when it would be inappropriate to issue a certificate. If in doubt, seek senior advice
- Always write in block capitals and in black ink
- Avoid medical abbreviations
- Write the patient's full name and check the spelling carefully
- When writing the date of death, put the date in words
- State the place of death
- Remember to check the patient's employment history, as some industrial diseases attract financial compensation (e.g. exposure to asbestos)

You **must** circle either:

(1) The certified cause of death takes account of information obtained from post-mortem

(2) Information from post-mortem may be available later

(3) Post-mortem not being held

You **must** circle either:

(a) Seen after death by me

(b) Seen after death by another medical practitioner but not by me

(c) Not seen by a medical practitioner

'Understand local hospital policies relating to death certification – for example, some hospitals require the death certificate to be discussed with a consultant prior to being issued'

William Wallace
Consultant Pathologist
Edinburgh Royal Infirmary

Cause of Death

- Write the cause (e.g. myocardial infarction) rather than mode of death (coma, syncope, and cardiac arrest are modes of death)
- If you do not know the cause of death, you may not be able to issue the death certificate

Part I

- State the disease or condition directly leading to death on the first line [Part I (a)]
- Complete the sequence of diseases of conditions leading to death on subsequent lines for example, Part 1a: Intrapulmonary haemorrhage, Part 1b: Squamous cell carcinoma of the lung

Part II

- State significant conditions or diseases that contributed to the death, but which are not part of any sequence leading directly to death. For example, diabetes mellitus
- Duration of all conditions listed in Part 1 and Part 2 should be listed
- Print your name and bleep number clearly after your signature and add your medical qualification as registered with the GMC. If obtained in another country, state which university town it was obtained in and the year it was awarded
- Give the name of the Consultant responsible for the care of the patient

Copy what has been written on the death certificate into the medical notes, and in the death certificate booklet on the stub in the spaces provided. It is often useful to note which family members were present at the time of death, and whether the GP has been informed yet

> 'The certificate is usually given to the family. When doing this, explain what the certificate says and means. This is a legal document and therefore necessitates formal medical language that may be difficult for the family to understand — for example, the family may know what lung cancer is but not 'bronchial carcinoma'
>
> **William Wallace**
> Consultant Pathologist
> Edinburgh Royal Infirmary

Cremation Forms

- Do not complete the cremation form until you know that the case is not being investigated by the Coroner or Procurator Fiscal and a death certificate has been issued
- The first part can be filled in by any doctor, but they MUST have seen the patient alive and seen and examined the body after death
- The presence of pacemakers or any type of radioactive implant must be recorded as these may preclude cremation unless they are removed
- All parts of the form must be completed in full and then signed
- After filling out the first part of the form, a second doctor (who has been fully registered for more than 5 years) must fill out the second part
- The form should not be given to the relatives but will be passed to the undertakers, usually via the mortuary staff or bereavement officers

Give some examples of when a death might be reported to a coroner (or procurator fiscal)

1. Any uncertified death (i.e. for which the clinician is unable or unwilling to issue a death certificate)
2. Any death that is sudden and unexpected, or that is due to any violent, suspicious or unexplained cause
3. Any death resulting from an accident at work or arising out of the use of a vehicle, or involving burns or scalds, or a fire or an explosion, or of any other similar cause

This includes deaths occurring as a late result of trauma i.e. months afterwards

4. Any death due to poisoning, including drug overdose (even as a late result)
5. Any death resulting from an industrial disease
6. Any death where the circumstances indicate that suicide is a possibility
7. Any death where there are indications that it occurred as a result of medical mishap

8. Any death following an abortion or attempted abortion
9. Any death where the circumstances seem to indicate fault or neglect on the part of another person or organisation including hospitals
10. Any death occurring while the deceased was in legal custody
11. Any death occurring as a result of food poisoning or a notifiable infectious disease
12. Any death of a foster child

Station 9: INSTRUMENTS

On this table are a number of instruments. Please take one and tell me what you know about it.

Instruments

- If you are given a choice, take your time and pick something simple that you are familiar with. This will help you to gain confidence and momentum before you approach more difficult items
- Take the item and hold it delicately but with familiarity. Turn to the examiner and try not to look back at your hands. Remember to stop talking, as it is easy to ramble on. The following structure can be applied to almost any instrument and will give you a framework for your answers:

1) Name and type of instrument
2) Indications for use or real scenario of where you have seen it used
3) How it is used
4) Complications of using said instrument

What can you tell me about this object?

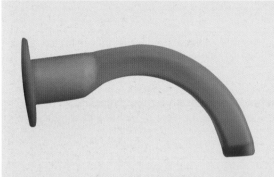

1) *'This is an oropharyngeal (Guedel) airway; it is an example of a non-definitive airway adjunct.'*
2) *'I have seen this being used in a patient with an impaired conscious level, and an unprotected airway presenting to accident and emergency.'*
3) *'It is sized by measuring the distance from the incisors to the angle of the jaw. It is then introduced to the oral cavity, with the spout pointing superiorly and rotated 180° as it descends passed the hard palate, entering the oropharynx. This approach reduces the risk of pushing the tongue backwards.'*
4) *'Complications include trauma to the oropharynx, upper airway obstruction and stimulation of vomiting.'*

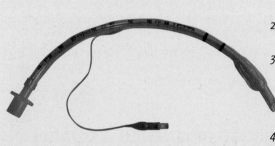

1) *'This is a cuffed endotracheal tube, it is an example of a definitive airway.'*
2) *'I have seen this being used in intensive care for the ventilation of an unconscious patient.'*
3) *'It is inserted by a trained health professional in a controlled environment. I have seen it inserted using direct laryngoscopy to identify the glottis. After insertion, a balloon cuff is inflated to secure it in place and to reduce the risk of aspirate entering the respiratory tract.'*
4) *'Complications include those associated with the tube (subglottic stenosis, vocal cord paralysis) and those associated with the intubation procedure (misplacement, dental trauma, intubation of oesophagus, pulmonary aspiration).'*

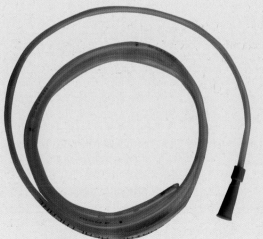

1) *'This is a Ryles nasogastric tube, of which there are two types: fine and wide-bore.'*
2) *'I have seen fine-bore tubes being used to provide enteric feeding and witnessed wide-bore tubes used to provide gastric decompression in bowel obstruction.'*
3) *'The lower 10cm is lubricated. It is then inserted into the patent nostril of an upright patient. It is advanced in a horizontal plane along the base of the nasal cavity. When it reaches the posterior pharynx, the patient is asked to swallow water through a straw, thereby introducing the tip into the oesophagus. The nasogastric tube is inserted to the 40cm mark and correct positioning is confirmed with pH aspirate (pH<4) and chest X-ray.'*
4) *'Complications include damage to the nasal turbinates and oesophageal perforation. Care should be taken not to place the tube in the trachea.'*

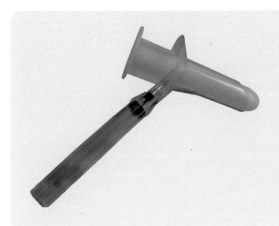

1) 'This is a disposable proctoscope.'

2) 'I have seen this being used in an outpatient clinic to visualise and treat haemorrhoids.'

3) 'The patient is positioned in the left lateral position with their buttocks to the edge of the examination couch. The anus and perineum is inspected for evidence of fissures, fistula, prolapsed haemorrhoids or skin tags. A digital rectal examination is then performed. The proctoscope is connected to a non-disposable light source and then lubricated before being inserted slowly under direct vision. The obturator is removed and rectum visualised for diagnostic and therapeutic intervention.'

4) 'Complications include pain, perforation of the rectum, bleeding and damage to the anal sphincter.'

Other objects to think about:

Fluids

Crystalloids:
Hartmann's Solution
Normal Saline
Dextrose Saline

Colloids:
Gelofusin
Albumin
Blood products

Airways

Laryngeal Mask Airway
Tracheostomy
Nasopharyngeal Airway

Lines

Central Venous Line
Hickman Line
Swan Ganz Catheter

Colorectal

Rigid Sigmoidoscope
Flexible Sigmoidoscope
Gabriel Syringe
Laparoscopic Ports

Orthopaedic

Knee Prostheses
Hip Prostheses
External Fixation
Dynamic Hip Screw
Intramedullary Nail

Station 10: SUTURING

Mr Harrison, 27, has presented to A and E with a simple laceration to his forearm. Please suture the wound together using a simple technique.

Always mention that you would assess the wound in order to see if you need to refer it on to a senior surgical colleague (hand, plastic, vascular). Most simple lacerations can be sutured by junior doctors, however always get a senior opinion on lacerations that involve tendons, nerves, or large vessels (remember to check the neurovascular supply). Order an X-ray where there may be retained or deep foreign bodies.

Always bear in mind that wound suturing restores function and form; therefore, a plastic surgery referral is essential for complex facial lacerations, especially those involving the vermilion line (the border between the lips and skin).

Equipment Needed

a) **Wound cleaning equipment:** Sterile pack with gloves, povidone Iodine solution +/- sterile water, gauze/swabs to clean the wound

b) **Suturing pack (often disposable):** Needle holder, toothed forceps, scissors

c) **Suture(s):** e.g. 4/0 synthetic, non-absorbable monofilament with a curved needle

d) **Local Anaesthetic (LA) equipment:** LA e.g. Lignocaine with 1/200 000 adrenaline (to minimise bleeding), 5 ml syringe, 21G needle (to draw up LA), 25G needle to administer LA

e) +/- Tetanus Injection

f) Sharps bin

g) An assistant (not essential, but very helpful)

In the examination, examiners often simply want to see you suturing; however it is important to know how to prepare a wound and administer local anaesthetic, as they will often test this through questioning.

Wound Preparation

1) Use an aseptic technique to put on your gloves. Assemble the suturing equipment on a sterile field

2) Remove visible debris from the wound using the forceps

3) Use a gauze soaked in sterile water to clean the wound. Administer the LA at this point (see below) as cleaning the wound with the betadine soaked gauze will sting a great deal

4) Dry the wound with a clean gauze

Local Anaesthetic Administration

Remember that LA containing adrenaline causes vasoconstriction, this is advantageous on one hand as it aids in haemostasis; however, it can also cause avascular tissue necrosis. Therefore, never use LA containing adrenaline on high-risk sites such as the fingers, nose, toes, ears or penis.

1) Draw up 5ml of LA using the 21G needle. LA date and dose needs to be double checked with a second person

2) Detach the needle without re-sheathing, and discard it in a sharps bin

3) Attach a 25G needle and inject the LA into the skin and soft tissues around the wound

4) Draw back on the syringe before injecting in order to ensure you are not inadvertently in a vessel; administering LA intravenously can cause convulsions, CNS depression, arrhythmias or acute heart failure

5) LA can take 5-10 minutes to reach full effect; therefore, always check with forceps that the patient cannot feel anything

Suturing (basic interrupted suturing technique)

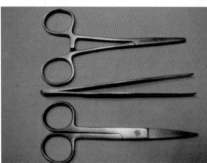
Fig 5.7: Equipment

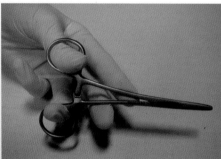
Fig 5.8: Holding the needle-holder

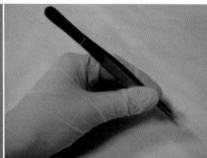
Fig 5.9: Holding the forceps

1) Hold the needle holder in your dominant hand with your thumb and fourth finger (Fig. 5.8)
2) Hold the toothed forceps in your other hand like you would hold a pen (Fig. 5.9)

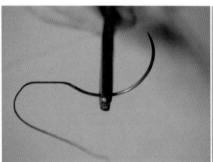
Fig 5.10: Holding the needle

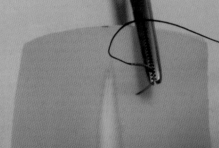
Fig 5.11: Inserting the needle

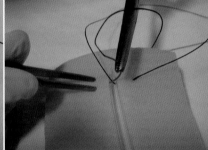
Fig 5.12: Exiting the wound

3) Remove the needle and suture from the packaging with the needle holder. Reposition the needle in the holder using the forceps (never handle the needle with your fingers). You should be holding the needle 1/3 away from the end where the suture is attached, and it should be at 90 degrees to the needle holder (Fig. 5.10)

4) With the forceps, gently manipulate the wound's edge. Being rough with the tissues will increase the chance of necrosis and wound infection

5) Insert the needle perpendicular to the skin's surface and about 5mm from the wound edge (Fig. 5.11). In one smooth and curved movement (supinating at your wrist), advance the needle, aiming to exit in the middle of the wound (Fig 5.12)

6) Re-insert the needle from within the wound and aim to exit about 5mm from the wound edge

7) Release the needle from the needle holder, re-grasp the tip of the needle and pull the suture through, leaving about 4cm of suture length

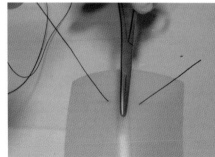
Fig 5.13: The first "V"

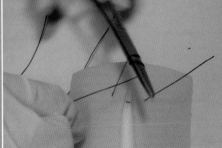
Fig 5.14: Looping the suture

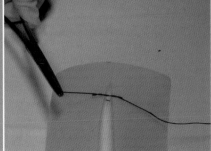
Fig 5.15: The first knot

8) The two bits of suture sticking up and out of the skin now form a V-shape. Reposition your needle holder (now not holding the needle) in the middle of this 'V' (Fig. 5.13)

9) Wind the long end (the end with the needle attached) around the needle holder 3 times (Fig. 5.14). Keep hold of this long end of the suture

10) With your needle holder, grasp the very tip of the short end of the suture. At right angles to the wound, pull the two ends of sutures in opposite directions. This is your first knot (Fig. 5.15)

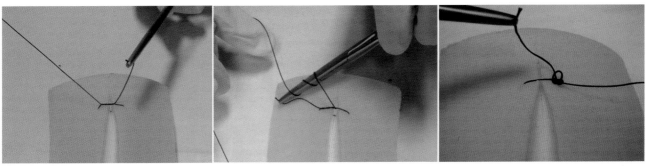

Fig 5.16: The second "V"   Fig 5.17: The second knot   Fig 5.18: Correct positioning of the knot

11) This knot, with some imagination, will also resemble a 'V' (Fig. 5.16)

12) Repeat the process of knot tying, but alternate the direction you pull each suture end in (Fig 5.17). This enables you to lay down knots in opposite directions in order to prevent the suture from unraveling

13) Reposition your knots so that they are not lying over the line of the wound (Fig. 5.18); this helps improve scar formation

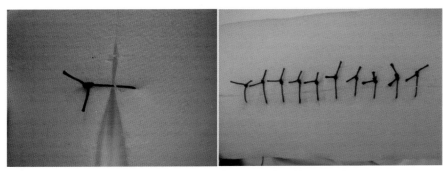

Fig 5.19: An interrupted suture   Fig 5.20: A series of interrupted sutures

14) When you have laid down at least 3 knots, cut the ends of the suture, leaving about 5mm each end (Fig. 5.19)

15) Repeat the process 5-10mm along from your first suture if a second suture is required (Fig 5.20)

16) Ensure that all the wound edges are successfully brought together

Wound Aftercare

- If necessary, apply a dressing over the wound
- ALWAYS administer a tetanus booster if the patient has not had one in the past 10 years, or if the wound is contaminated
- Advise the patient to keep the wound dry whilst showering/washing
- Educate the patient on signs of wound infection (e.g. red, sore, discharging) and advise them to seek medical help if this occurs
- Sutures will normally be removed in 7-14 days (4-5 days if it is the face); this can usually be done with the agreement of their GP or district nurse

6 X-Ray Interpretation

Presented below are systematic ways to approach chest, abdominal, and orthopaedic X-rays, including examples of commonly seen abnormalities that junior doctors will be expected to recognise.

Remember, junior doctors will often be expected to act on the results of the X-rays before the formal report is issued. On the other hand many possible subtleties can exist on X-rays, which only radiologists will pick up. Therefore X-rays may need to be discussed with specialists. If they are formally reported, (as they will be in most departments) always check the formal report, regardless of how confident you are in your initial interpretation.

- At each station, you will have a brief patient history to read before viewing the X-ray. Read this carefully, as it should be fairly obvious which major abnormality you should be looking for. For example, if any mention is made of smoking, as well as changes associated with COPD, make sure you have a good look for lung cancer and its complications on a CXR. A young asthmatic becoming acutely short of breath should make you focus on the periphery of the film, looking for a pneumothorax
- Do not touch any of the X-rays, and do your best to provide a verbal description of what you see and its location, rather than pointing at it. Keeping your hands behind your back is a good strategy to avoid touching or pointing at the film

There are 5 main densities on X-rays:

- **Black** for gas
- **Dark grey** for fat
- **Grey** representing soft tissue
- **White** for bone and other calcified structures
- **Intense bright white** for metal (other manmade structures are also usually white)

This chapter contains the following scenarios:

Study Action Plan

- X-ray interpretation is all about pattern recognition, so the key to becoming competent and confident is practice. If possible, go down to the radiology department and sit in with a radiologist reporting X-rays: you will see more X-rays, and often higher quality images on their screens
- Try looking at the X-rays of patients you are involved with and come up with your own report before checking the formal report
- Practice presenting X-rays to doctors on the ward in a systematic way

X-rays

Station 1: CHEST X-RAY

Mr Jones is a 68-year-old smoker who has had a cough for the last two months, and is becoming increasingly breathless. Tell the radiologist what films you would like to request, and then describe the findings of the film that is shown.

1. Projection AP/ PA

- Somewhere on the film you should see something that indicates whether it is Anteroposterior (AP) or Posteroanterior (PA)
- If not, assume it is a PA film and say so
- AP films are more difficult to interpret and are usually only performed for haemodynamically compromised (all patients are usually "sick"!) patients. If you cannot remember which one is the standard view, remember AP is 'crAP', so PA is standard
- If you are asked to justify why a film is PA, remember that the arms are raised up during PA films, so the scapulae are pulled almost fully out of the lung fields. In AP films, the patient is unwell so you can see a humerus down either side of the film and scapulae in the lung fields

2. Patient Details

- These will be on the film (unless anonymised for the exam)
- Say the name, age/date of birth, and when the film was taken

3. Technical Quality

- Check you can see both lung apices, both lateral sides of the ribcage, and both costophrenic angles on the film
- It is unlikely that they will give you a film in the exam that does not show the entire lungs, but some parts are occasionally missed in practice

RIP – Rotation, Inspiration, Penetration

- **Rotation:** heads of the clavicles (medial ends) should be equidistant from the spinous processes of the vertebral bodies
- **Inspiration:** PA films are taken in held deep inspiration. Count the ribs to assess inspiratory effort. The last rib to count is the one going through the diaphragm. Six anterior ribs or 10 posterior ribs indicate adequate inspiratory effort. More ribs, particularly with flattened diaphragms, indicate airway obstruction, such as chronic obstructive airway disease (COPD), and fewer ribs indicate poor inspiration
- **Penetration:** assume adequate penetration when you can just see the vertebral bodies behind the heart. Underpenetrated means you cannot see behind the heart and over penetrated means that you will be able to see the vertebral bodies very clearly
- Rotated, under inspired or under/over penetrated films hinder accurate assessment

Suggested Approach

1. Projection (AP/PA)
2. Patient details
3. Technical quality
4. Obvious abnormalities
5. Systemic review of the film
6. Summary

4. Obvious Abnormalities

If you can see obvious abnormalities, say so and describe them:

- **Which lung?**
- **Which zone (upper, middle or lower)?** If possible, suggest which lobe it is most likely to be. Remember: this is not always obvious without a CT
- **Size**
- **Shape:** well or poorly demarcated?
- **Density/texture:** uniform, patchy, dense, cotton wool-like. If there is anything else in the abnormality, such as air bronchograms or fluid levels, then mention these as well

5. Systematic Review of the Film

- Initially assess from about four feet away to see difference in lung shadowing/obvious masses, then reassess close up
- It doesn't matter what system you have, as long as you stick to one and don't miss any areas. A useful system is ABCDD (Airway, Breathing, Circulation, Diaphragm/ Delicates)
- Also comment on manmade abnormalities e.g. lines, pacemakers, a nasogastric tube

A – Airway

- Is the trachea central?

B – Breathing

- Start in the apices and work down to the costophrenic angles, comparing both lungs to look for differences
- Ensure that you inspect the apices, hila, mediastinum, and costophrenic angles
- The left hilum should never be lower than the right (except in dextracardia), and they should both be the same density
- Look around the edge of the lung fields, assessing for pneumothoraces

C – Cardio

- **Cardiomegaly:** defined as the heart shadow being more than half the width of the chest cavity on a PA film
- **Heart borders:** if the left and right heart borders are not clearly visible, consolidation or collapse should be considered
- **Cardiophrenic angles:** should be clear – masses or pericardial cysts can obliterate this space
- **Behind the heart:** look for any abnormalities: e.g. lung masses

D – Diaphragm

- Both hemi-diaphragms should be visible and not flattened
- **Costophrenic angles:** are they clearly demarcated? If not, does it contain any fluid?
- **Right hemi-diaphragm:** is normally slightly higher than left (due to the liver)
- Look for air under the diaphragm (a gastric air bubble on the left is normal)

D – Delicates

- **Bones:** look for fractures and any rib space narrowing suggesting collapse
- Look for gas in the soft tissues (black areas) – surgical emphysema

Important Findings on CXR

Pneumonia

- Dense or patchy consolidation, usually one-sided
- May contain air bronchograms
- In the lower zones, it may be difficult to distinguish from effusions, so both should be on your differential list
- It is important to know which lobes touch the heart and diaphragmatic borders since loss of clarity of the borders indicates the affected lobe (silhouette sign)
  - **Diaphragms:** left and right lower lobes
  - **Right heart border:** right middle lobe

Review Areas

Double-check the following areas at the end, since they are easy to miss on initial viewing:

- Apices
- Hila
- Behind the heart
- Costophrenic angles
- Around the pleura/edge of the lung fields assessing for pneumothoraces and pleural thickening
- Under the diaphragm

6. Summary

Summarise your findings and give a differential list. Think about the history as well as the findings when making your differentials.

> 'Remember you are looking at a **CHEST** X-ray not a **LUNG** X-ray! Ensure you assess all of the X-ray, including the soft tissues, bones, such as the clavicles, scapulae and upper humeri, and the upper abdomen'
>
> **Mark Rodrigues**
> *Radiology Trainee*
> *Edinburgh Royal Infirmary*

- **Left heart border:** lingula
- If in doubt about the lobe, describe it as 'upper, middle or lower zone'

Pleural Effusions

- Look for loss of the costophrenic angles, a homogenous opacification, and fluid level (manifests as a meniscus)
- Bilateral effusions are more likely to be transudates; unilateral effusions are more likely to be exudates
- Pleural aspiration helps identify the cause of the effusion

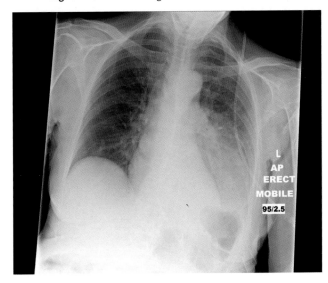

Fig 6.1: Left lower lobe consolidation. Note the left hemi-diaphragm is obscured but the left heart border is well defined. Therefore the consolidation must be in the lower lobe

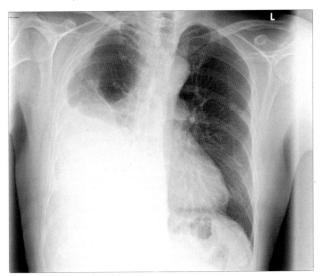

Fig 6.2: Large right pleural effusion. Note the homogenous pattern of the opacity obscuring the right hemi diaphragm and heart border, and the crisp upper border of the effusion. An effusion of this size will be approximately 3-4 litres in volume

Causes of a Pleural Effusion

Exudates (>30g/l protein)	Transudates (<30g/l protein)
Infection – pneumonia, TB	Heart failure
Pulmonary embolism	Liver failure/cirrhosis
Malignancy – metastases, bronchial, mesothelioma	Protein loss – nephrotic syndrome, protein-losing enteropathy
Rheumatoid arthritis, systemic lupus erythematosus	Reduced protein intake – malnutrition
Pancreatitis	Iatrogenic – peritoneal dialysis
Trauma/surgery (blood)	Meigs syndrome (triad of ovarian fibroma, ascites and right pleural effusion)
	Hypothyroidism

The amount of protein (above or below 30g/l) can be used as a rough guide to determine whether the effusion is a transudate or exudate but is not always accurate; therefore Light's Criteria should be used. The effusion is an exudate if:

Pleural fluid protein to serum protein ratio > 0.5 (more than twice as much protein in pleural fluid than in blood)

OR

Pleural fluid LDH to serum LDH ratio > 0.6

OR

Pleural fluid LDH is greater than 2/3rds the upper limit of normal serum LDH

To assess if heart failure is the cause, remember **ABCDEF:**

A: **A**lveolar (interstitial) shadowing

B: Kerley **B** lines (little white horizontal dashes usually in the lateral lower edges)

C: **C**ardiomegaly (**C**ardiothoracic ratio of greater than 50% on a PA film)

D: Upper lobe blood **D**iversion (prominent upper lobe vasculature)

E: **E**ffusions

F: **F**luid in the horizontal fissure

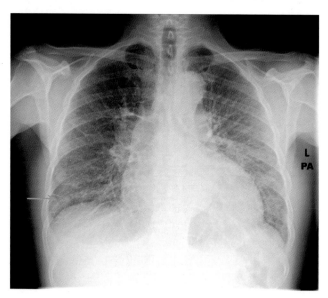

Fig 6.3: Heart failure. Note the cardiomegaly, upper lobe venous diversion and Kerley B lines (arrowed)

Pneumothorax

- Loss of lung markings in the peripheral lung field
- You may also identify a discrete lung edge
- If under tension, there may be tracheal/mediastinal deviation away from the pneumothorax and flattening of the ipsilateral dome of the diaphragm. A tension pneumothorax should never be diagnosed by a CXR! It is a medical emergency, is diagnosed clinically and treated immediately with needle thoracocentesis

Causes of a Pneumothorax

- **Spontaneous**
- **Iatrogenic/ trauma:** pleural tap, transbronchial biopsy, central venous line insertion, mechanical ventilation
- **Obstructive lung disease:** asthma, COPD
- **Infection:** pneumonia, tuberculosis, cystic fibrosis
- **Connective tissue diseases:** Marfan's, Ehlers-Danlos

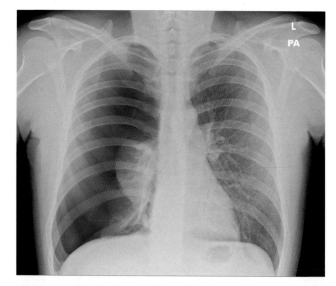

Fig 6.4: Large right simple pneumothorax. Note: in contrast to a tension pneumothorax, the trachea is central and the heart and mediastinum is not deviated. The right hemi diaphragm is not flattened

Lobar Collapse

- Look for loss of volume
  - Narrowing of the space between the ribs compared to the opposite side
  - A raised hemidiaphragm ipsilaterally
  - There may be tracheal and mediastinal shift towards the collapsed side
- **Left Upper Lobe:** Veil sign – the whole lung field looks like it's covered by a veil
- **Left Lower Lobe:** Sail sign – sharp line like the edge of a sail at the same angle as the left heart border
- **Right Upper Lobe:** hazy RUL, with raised horizontal fissure, and the abnormality well demarcated by the fissure

> *'Inverting the image (if viewing on a digital viewer) can make pneumothoraces more obvious'*
>
> **Mark Rodrigues**
> *Radiology Trainee*
> *Edinburgh Royal Infirmary*

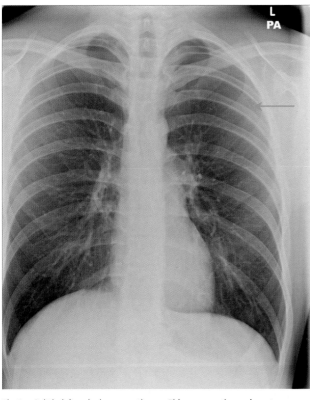

Fig 6.5: Subtle left apical pneumothorax. This pneumothorax is not easy to see at first glance but note the visible lung margin in the left apex (arrowed) and the loss of lung markers beyond this

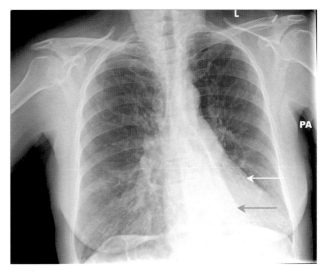

Fig 6.6: Left lower lobe collapse with evidence of the sail sign (pink arrow). Left heart border shown (white arrow)

- **Right Middle Lobe:** loss of the right heart border (can be difficult to differentiate from consolidation)
- **Right Lower Lobe:** hardest to differentiate from effusion. Normally, complete loss of diaphragmatic border due to haziness while the right heart border is normally clear

Demarcated Lesions (single or multiple)

- Large differential diagnosis
- Tumour, TB, abscess, localised pneumonia and rheumatoid nodules should be the top differentials, unless the history suggests otherwise

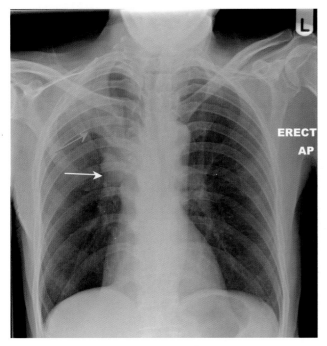

Fig 6.7: Right upper lobe collapse (pink arrow) with a right hilar mass (white arrow)

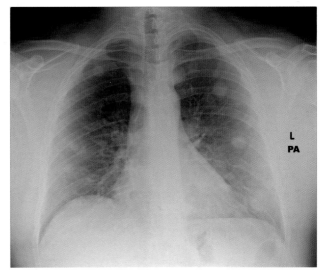

Fig 6.8: Multiple round opacities in keeping with metastatic deposits

Causes of a Single Coin Lesion

- **Malignant tumour:** bronchial, single pulmonary metastasis
- **Infection:** pneumonia, abscess, TB, hydatid cyst
- **Benign tumour:** hamartoma, schwannoma
- **Infarction**
- **Rheumatoid nodule**

Causes of Cavitating Lung Lesions

- **Abscess** *(Staph or Klebsiella)*
- **Neoplasm** (usually squamous cell)
- **Cavitation** around a pneumonia, TB
- **Infarct**
- **Rheumatoid nodule** (rare cause)

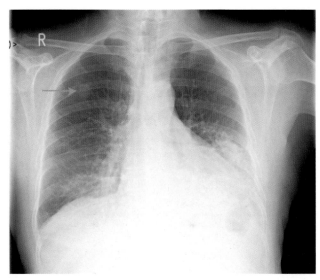

Fig 6.9: *There is loss of the left hemi diaphragm and a heterogenous opacification in the left lower zone signifying left lower lobe consolidation. Also note the single coin lesion in the right upper zone (arrowed). A CT of the chest and biopsy will help diagnose the cause of the coin lesion*

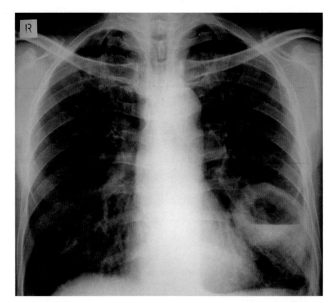

Fig 6.10: *Circular lucent area in left lower zone with surrounding "wall" and air fluid level. Common causes are infection (abscess or pneumonia) and neoplasia*

Causes of Numerous Calcified Nodules

- **Infection:** TB, histoplasmosis, chickenpox
- **Inhalation:** silicosis
- **Chronic renal failure**
- **Lymphoma** following radiotherapy
- **Chronic pulmonary venous hypertension**

Causes of Hilar Lymphadenopathy

- **Neoplastic:** spread from bronchial carcinoma, lymphoma
- **Infective:** TB
- **Sarcoidosis** (rarely unilateral)

Causes of Bilateral Hilar Enlargement

- **Sarcoid, berylliosis**
- **Tumours:** lymphoma, bronchial carcinoma, metastases
- **Infection:** TB, recurrent chest infections, AIDS

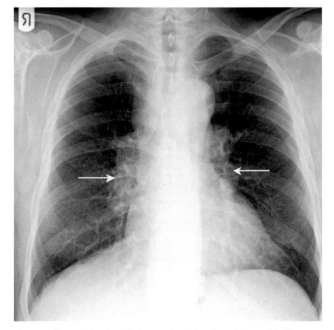

Fig 6.11: *Bilateral hilar lymphadenopathy in keeping with sarcoidosis*

Causes of Bronchiectasis

- **Structural:** Kartagener's syndrome, obstruction (carcinoma, foreign body)
- **Infection:** childhood pertussis/measles, TB, pneumonia
- **Immune:** hypogammaglobinaemia, allergic bronchopulmonary aspergillosus
- **Metabolic:** Cystic Fibrosis
- **Idiopathic:** 2° to stasis

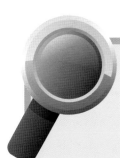

PRESENT YOUR FINDINGS...

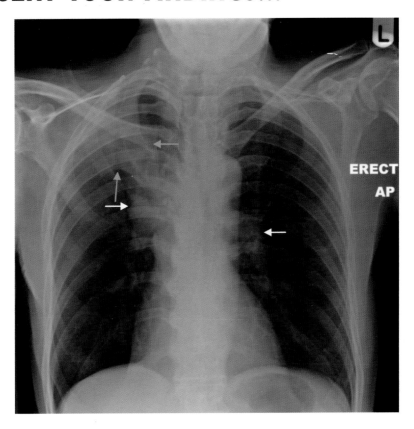

'This is an AP chest radiograph. There are no identifying markings. I would like to ensure that it is the correct patient and to check the date that it was taken.

It is a technically adequate film: it is not rotated, has adequate penetration, and good inspiratory effort. There are no important areas cut off at the edges of the film.

The most striking abnormality is a well-demarcated area of increased opacification in the right upper zone (pink arrows). The right hilum is increased in size, with a round opacity, and higher than the left (white arrows), suggesting loss of volume.

Reviewing the rest of the film, the trachea is not deviated. Comparing the left and right lungs, I can see no other obvious abnormalities in the lung fields. The heart is not enlarged (noting that this is an AP film), heart borders are clear, as are the cardiophrenic angles. There is no abnormality visible behind the heart. The diaphragms look normal, the costophrenic angles are clear, and there is no air under the diaphragm. There is no evidence of fractures.

In summary, this chest radiograph shows right upper lobe collapse with associated right hilar enlargement.

The most likely differential diagnosis is neoplasia, although hilar lymphadenopathy may also be due to infection or sarcoidosis.'

Station 2: ABDOMINAL X-RAY

Mr Pai is a 68-year-old gentlemen who has presented with vomiting, abdominal pain, and a distended abdomen. He has not opened his bowels in one week, and has previously had bowel surgery. Tell the radiologist what films you would like to request, and then describe the findings of the film that is shown.

1. Projection

- The standard abdominal radiograph (AXR) is taken AP (anterior-posterior) in the supine projection, so assume this is the case unless told otherwise

2. Patient Details

- These will be listed on the film
- State the name, age (or date of birth), and the date on which the film was taken

3. Technical Adequacy

- Make sure the entire abdomen is present on the film
- Ideally, the region from the diaphragm down to past the pubis should be visible

4. Obvious Abnormalities

- Abnormalities are not always obvious on initial viewing but if, for example, there is a dilated loop of large bowel measuring 12cm in diameter, comment on this before conducting your systemic review of the film

5. Systematic Review of the Film

Foreign Bodies

- Mention clips from previous surgery and any indwelling lines

Assess the Bowel

When looking at the bowel it is important to identify:

- Large or small bowel
- Size of bowel
- Cause of abnormalities
- Extraluminal and intraluminal content (Note – air is black; faeces are mottled grey)

Large Bowel

- The large bowel is normally the easiest to identify as it classically runs around the outside of the abdomen, so start by looking for the large bowel
- Apart from its position, the large bowel can also be identified by haustra (horizontal lines that only partially cross the width of the large bowel)

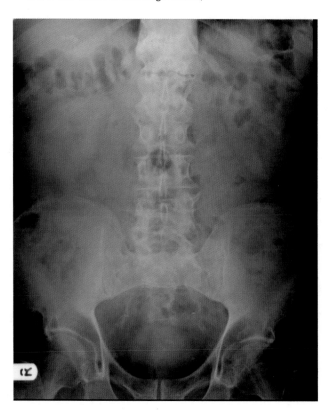

Approach
1. Projection
2. Patient details
3. Technical adequacy
4. Obvious abnormalities
5. Systematic review of the film
6. Summary

- The large bowel should be no wider than **5 cm**, except the caecum, which can be up to **8 cm**
  - Identify the rectum, it usually contains air
  - Follow this around to the left edge to the sigmoid colon, and up the descending colon to the splenic flexure
  - Follow the transverse colon (often, this hangs down through the middle of the film before rising again to the hepatic flexure)
  - Follow the ascending colon from the hepatic flexure down to the caecum

If you can follow the entire large bowel around, then identifying the small bowel is easy as it is the remaining part of the intestine.

Small Bowel

- The small bowel normally lies more centrally and should be no more than 3 cm in diameter
- The small bowel can also be identified by the valvulae conniventes, which are lines that traverse the full width of the small bowel

Remember: in a "normal" abdominal X-ray the large and small bowel can often be difficult to see clearly. Instead a "nonspecific bowel gas pattern" is usually seen. The small and large bowel become much easier to recognise when there is bowel dilatation from mechanical obstruction or an ileus.

The most common finding in an exam AXR is bowel obstruction. The first thing to do is identify which part of the bowel is obstructed.

Fig 6.12: Normal abdominal X-ray showing a nonspecific bowel gas pattern. It is difficult to make out with confidence the small or large bowel

If it is the large bowel:

- The level of obstruction is normally clear

- Malignancy commonly causes large bowel obstruction; this requires further imaging for identification

- The other cause not to be missed on the AXR is a caecal or sigmoid volvulus; these usually twist inwards so they appear like balloons in the middle of the film

- If the small bowel is also enlarged, then the ileo-caecal valve is incompetent (in the short term, this is a good thing, since it reduces the risk of perforation of the large bowel)

If the small bowel is dilated alone:

- The cause is most likely either adhesions or a hernia

- Evidence of previous surgery, such as surgical clips, may suggest adhesions

- Looking at the inguinal hernia orifices is essential for identifying inguinal hernias

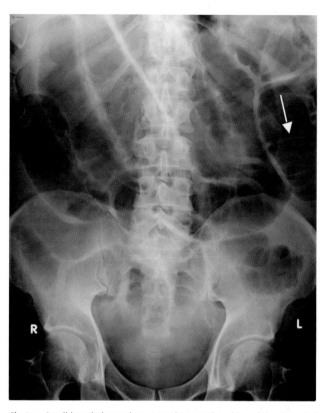

Fig 6.14: Small bowel obstruction – note the central position of the distended bowel loops and the valvulae conniventes (arrowed)

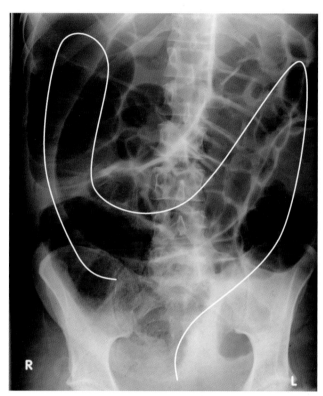

Fig 6.13: Large bowel obstruction with associated small bowel dilatation. The white line outlines the position of the rectum, descending, transverse and ascending colon

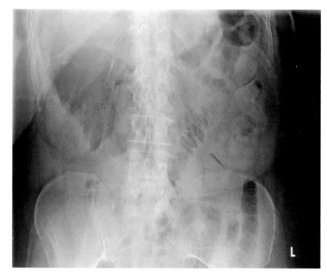

Fig 6.15: Pneumoperitoneum demonstrating Rigler's sign

Extraluminal Gas (Pneumoperitoneum)

- The best evidence of perforation is free air under the diaphragm (a gastric air bubble under the left diaphragm normal) – always ask for an erect CXR to assess for this

- On the AXR, air under the diaphragm may be visible, so comment on this if you see it

- **Rigler's sign**: where you can clearly see both sides of the bowel wall. Normally only the inner wall of the bowel is visible. This is due to the contrast of the inner wall against air present inside of the bowel. Therefore, when air is also outside the bowel, you can see the outside of the bowel wall as well

- **Football sign**: a round area of air, usually towards the top of the film, mainly found in neonates

Always look for perforation, even without bowel obstruction; perforation can occur in gallstone disease, inflammatory conditions such as Crohn's disease, appendicitis or trauma.

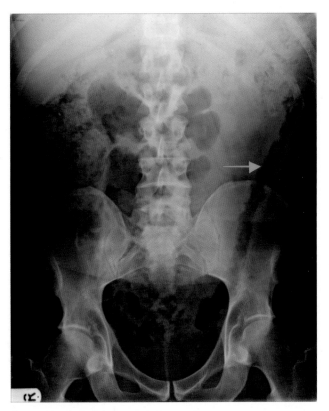

Fig 6.16: Thumbprinting

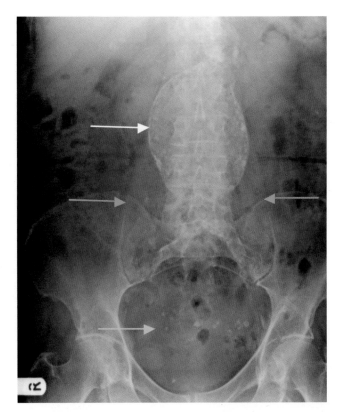

Fig 6.17: Non-specific bowel gas pattern. Large calcified abdominal aorta (white). Psoas shadows are visible (pink). Incidental phleboliths (grey).

Oedema of the Bowel Wall

- Thumb printing is thickening of the bowel wall caused by oedema, which is so named because it looks like someone has pushed their thumb into it in several places; this gives a wavy pattern and occurs in inflammatory bowel disease and ischaemic colitis

- If you see a massively enlarged colon, always question if this is inflammatory bowel disease-related (particularly Ulcerative Colitis) toxic megacolon

Liver, Spleen and Gall bladder

- Look at the size of the liver and spleen

- Look for gallstones within the gallbladder

- Remember that the majority of gallstones are radiolucent and will not be seen on X-ray

Abdominal Aorta

- Always look for the aorta and iliac vessels

- Often the aorta is calcified, so the 2 edges can be seen and measured; an aorta less than 3 cm is normal but if it is larger than 3 cm, then this suggests an aneurysm and requires further investigation and possible surgery

- If you are suspecting dissection, look closely at the psoas muscle shadows that are normally present on AXR films

- If they are absent, this suggests blood in the retroperitoneal cavity

Kidney Stones

- Look for calcification along the renal tract; with practice, the kidneys can be visualised on most AXRs (T12-L2)

- Stones classically obstruct the renal pelvis, pelvo-ureteric junction (PUJ) and vesico-ureteric junction

- There may be stones within the bladder itself

- Beware of phleboliths (calcified pelvic vessels), which are common. If you do not look at their position carefully, you may mistake them for renal or bladder stones

Bones

- Look for pelvic and hip fractures

- Look at the spine – often, osteoporotic fractures can be seen, as well as scoliosis and metastatic deposits

6. Summary

State your key findings (either as a diagnosis or a description), and put forward a management plan and a differential diagnosis.

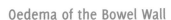

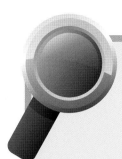

PRESENT YOUR FINDINGS...

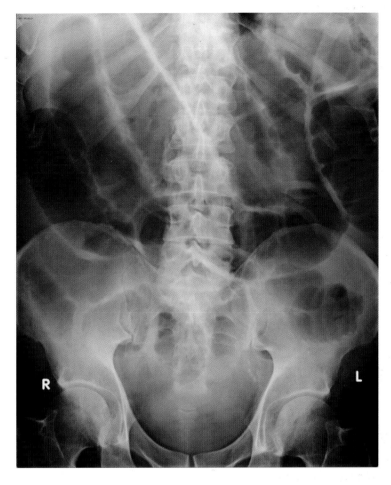

'This is an AP supine abdominal radiograph. There are no identifying markings. I would like to ensure that it is the correct patient and check the date it was taken. The upper abdomen and the lateral extremes of the patient are not included in this film.

There are multiple loops of small bowel dilatation. It is small bowel due to its predominantly central distribution and the presence of valvulae conniventes.

There is no evidence of hernia and no evidence of previous surgery. There is no evidence of extra-luminal air. The abdominal aorta is not visible and the bladder appears normal in size. There are no apparent bony abnormalities.

In summary, this is an abdominal radiograph showing small bowel obstruction with no evidence of perforation. I would like to arrange an erect CXR specifically to look for free air under the diaphragm.

Differential diagnosis of the cause of small bowel obstruction includes adhesions, neoplasia, incarcerated hernia and strictures.'

How would you manage this patient?

In the context of small bowel obstruction, management may include:

- Place patient nil by mouth
- Intravenous access with intravenous fluids and a naso-gastric tube ('drip and suck')
- Bloods – FBC, U&E, LFT, CRP, clotting, group and save to prepare for theatre if appropriate and an arterial blood gas
- Erect CXR
- Urgent surgical review regarding the need for further imaging (CT Scan) or surgical intervention

Station 3: ORTHOPAEDIC X-RAY

Mrs Jones is a 68-year-old lady who has recently fallen. Her leg is shortened and externally rotated. Tell the radiologist what films you would like to request, and then describe the findings of the film that is shown.

General points to cover in all Orthopaedic X-Rays

- Type of films
    - At least two views – 'one view is one too few!'
    - Normally antero-posterior (AP) and lateral views
    - For some sites, such as the scaphoid, where fractures are difficult to detect, it is routine procedure to obtain more than two views
    - For some patients in whom the clinical suspicion of a fracture is high but is not evident on the usual two views, additional views may be requested, such as internal rotation views of the hip
    - If the shaft of a long bone is fractured, it is imperative to X-ray the joint above and below because of the potential for fracture or dislocation at these sites
- **Patient demographics:** name, date of birth/age, when the film was taken
- **Technical Adequacy:** the film needs to show all of the joints in question from at least 2 different angles and it needs to be correctly exposed so that bone and soft tissues can be seen and differentiated
- Review the bone for fractures, subluxations and dislocations
- Review for inflammatory/chronic changes (particularly in the hands)

If no fractures are obvious, look around the edges of all the bones for fractures (new fractures appear as black lines through the cortex and old fractures may have callous around the bone). If a fracture results in bone fragments that overlap, the result is an area of increased X-ray absorption and thus a whiter area on the X-ray.

There are also some specific extra bits to look at in each joint (see individual joints).

Features Used to Describe Fractures

Being able to provide an accurate description of a fracture is vital for conveying the correct information to other members of the team (e.g. the on-call consultant who is at home during the night).

- **Which bone is involved**

- **Which part of the bone is fractured**
    - Proximal third
    - Middle third
    - Distal third
    - Intra-articular

- **Fracture pattern**
    - Simple (skin is intact) or open (skin not intact)
    - Comminuted (more than 2 fragments of bone)
    - Impacted (when bone fragments are driven into each other)

- **Type**
    - Transverse (i.e. perpendicular to the long axis of the bone)
    - Oblique (i.e. angled less than 90º to the long axis of the bone)
    - Spiral (i.e. curving around the bone)
    - Greenstick (occurs in children, a break in one cortex with the other cortex remaining intact, often associated with angulation)

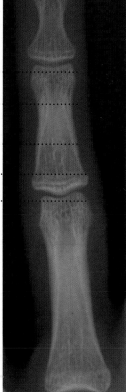

Distal third

Middle third

Proximal third

Intra-articular

Fig 6.18: Describing the part of a bone fractured

X-rays

- Displacement
  - Relationship of the distal fragment to the proximal fragment
  - Non-displaced or anterior, posterior, medial, lateral displacement
  - It is essential to use both films to assess this
- Angulation
  - The movement of the distal fragment relative to the proximal bone in degrees
- Rotation
  - Measured along the longitudinal axis of the bone
  - Generally detected on clinical examination but may be diagnosed on X rays
  - Requires knowledge of normal anatomical alignment
  - Either internal or external rotation
  - Important to assess all long bone fractures for rotation
- Shortening
- Joint space: may be smaller than it should be, asymmetrical, or foreign bodies may be present
- Joint cartilage: look for outline symmetry and any fractures on the surface of the bones
- Bone lucency
  - If most of the bone is radiolucent (dark), this suggests osteoporosis
  - Radiolucency just around the joint suggests an inflammatory/infected joint
  - Radio-opaque (bright) areas are rare (Paget's, osteochondritis, sclerotic bone metastases)

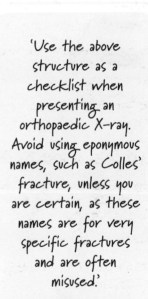

Fig 6.19: Ulnar subluxation of the distal phalanx of the fifth digit. The dotted pink line highlights the contact that remained between the articular surfaces

Subluxation versus Dislocation

The difference between these two terms may not appear obvious in the first instance:

- Subluxation
  - The normal anatomy of the joint is disrupted but some contact remains between the articular surfaces of the joint
- Dislocation
  - Complete disruption of the joint with no contact between the joint surfaces (Fig 6.20)

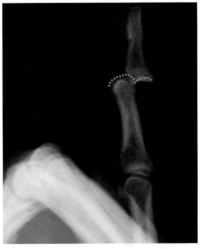

Fig 6.20: Posterior dislocation of the distal phalanx of the fifth digit. The dotted lines highlight the two articular surfaces, which are not in contact

'Use the above structure as a checklist when presenting an orthopaedic X-ray. Avoid using eponymous names, such as Colles' fracture, unless you are certain, as these names are for very specific fractures and are often misused.'

Mark Rodrigues
Radiology Trainee
Edinburgh Royal Infirmary

Cervical Spine Film

- Adequacy
  - At least 3 views:
    1. Lateral, which must show all 7 cervical vertebrae and the top of the 1st thoracic vertebra
    2. AP
    3. Open mouth AP/Peg view, to view C1 and C2
- Normal anatomy – Lateral view
  - Vertebral alignment (arcuate lines)
    - Anterior spinal line: goes along the anterior margins of vertebral bodies
    - Posterior spinal line: goes along the posterior margins of vertebral bodies
    - Spinolaminar line: joins the bases of the spinous processes

} These curves should be smooth and unbroken

X-rays

- Vertebral bodies
  - From the third cervical vertebrae downwards, the vertebral bodies should have a regular rectangular shape
  - There should be no wedging (i.e. the height of the anterior and posterior aspects of the vertebral bodies should be equal)
  - The intervertebral discs should be the same size
- Prevertebral soft tissues
  - The distance between the anterior spinal line and the edge of the prevertebral soft tissues should be <7mm between C1-C4 and <22mm between C5-C7
  - An increase in these distances suggests the presence of a haematoma and thus an important injury
- Normal anatomy: AP view
  - Alignment
    - The spinous processes should follow a straight line
    - Alignment may look abnormal with asymmetric bifid spinous processes
- Spacing
  - The spinous processes should be roughly equidistant
  - The intervertebral disc spaces should be a uniform height
- Normal anatomy – Peg View
  - Alignment
    - The lateral masses of C1 and C2 should line up
  - Spacing
    - The peg should be equidistant from the lateral masses of C2
- Fractures
  - Look for deformity in the lines of the vertebra on both AP and lateral views. Any sign that a vertebra has 'stepped out' could be a fracture and requires further imaging
  - Roughly 10% of patients with a c-spine fracture have a second non-contiguous vertebral column fracture

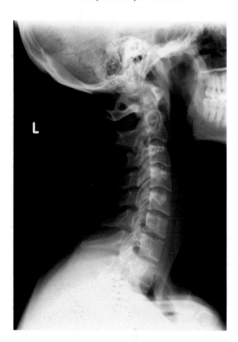

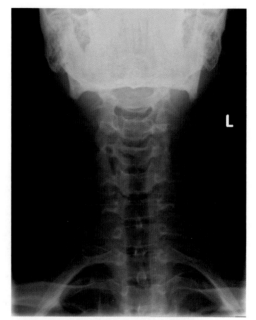

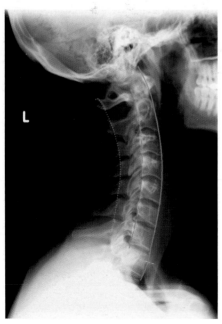

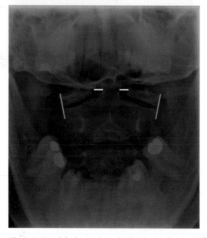

Fig 6.21: Top left: lateral cervical spine radiograph (normal)
Top right: AP cervical spine radiograph (normal)
Below left: lateral cervical spine radiograph showing anterior spinal [solid line], posterior spinal [dashed line], spinolaminar [dotted line]
Below right: PEG view showing the odontoid peg equidistant from the lateral masses of C1 (white lines), and normal alignment of C1/2 (pink lines)

'1. Always ask an experienced observer to review c-spine films — it's important not to miss an abnormality!
2. Normal X-rays do not exclude significant injury; if there is clinical concern and a normal film, further imaging should be considered'

Mark Rodrigues
Radiology Trainee
Edinburgh Royal Infirmary

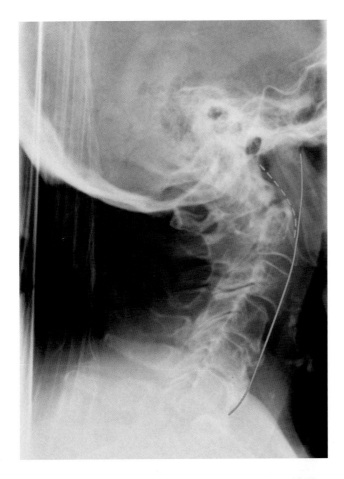

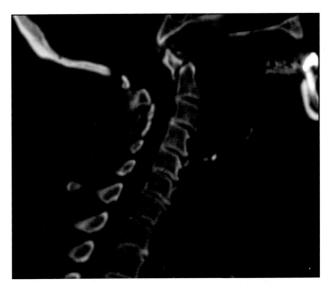

Fig 6.22: Left: Lateral X-ray showing disruption to the arcuate lines (Solid and dotted line) due to a fracture through the odontoid peg. Degenerative changes of the lower cervical spine. Note: this lateral view is inadequate as the C7/T1 junction cannot be visualized. The patient proceeded to CT. Above: Sagittal view showing the fracture through the odontoid peg. The odontoid peg is displaced posteriorly relative to the body of C2

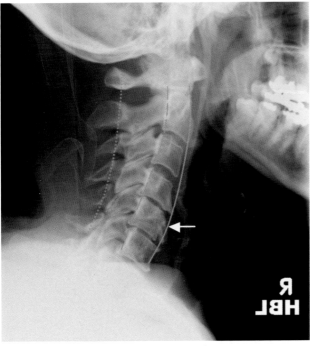

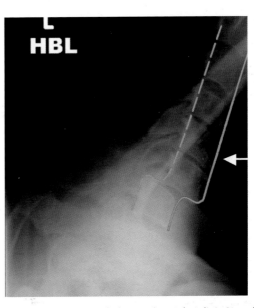

Fig 6.23: The importance of adequate views. Left: Only C1-C6 can be seen on this lateral view. There is a possible fracture through the C5 vertebral body (arrowed). Above: Swimmer's view shows C7 and the T1 junction. The C5 fracture can be clearly seen (arrowed) but disruption of the arcuate lines is also now evident due to anterior subluxation of C6 on C7

Thoracic and Lumbar Spinal Radiographs

- The three columns of the spine should be assessed:
  - Anterior
    - Anterior longitudinal ligament and the anterior 2/3 of the vertebral body and the anterior part of the annulus fibrosus
  - Middle
    - Posterior 1/3 of the vertebral body, the posterior part of the annulus fibrosus and the posterior longitudinal ligament
  - Posterior
    - Posterior ligaments and bone arch

Instability is present if two of the three columns are disrupted (breaks, steps or kinks)

Normal anatomy – Lateral view:

Alignment:

- Smooth, unbroken contour to the lumbar spine
- No breaks, steps or kinks in any of the three columns

Vertebral bodies:

- Anterior and posterior margins should be equal in height
- Posterior margin is normally slightly concave

Normal anatomy – AP view:

Alignment:

- The spinous processes should follow a straight line

Pedicle:

- The pedicles from L1 to L5 become slightly wider apart

- **Fractures:** Look at the height of the vertebral bodies, comparing each side and comparing above and below, as crush/osteoporotic wedge fractures are common
- Most fractures will be evident on the lateral film
- **Stability:** If a fracture is present, comment on whether the abnormality is stable or unstable (by assessing the columns of the spine as above)
- Joint space narrowing is common in the spine and may cause nerve root compression
- Comment on:
  - Kyphosis (anterior convexity i.e. outward curvature of the spine. Normally there is a thoracic and sacral kyphosis)
  - Lordosis (anterior concavity i.e. inward curvature of the spine. Normally there is a cervical and lumbar lordosis)
  - Scoliosis (side to side curvature of the spine)
- Osteoporosis is also common in the spine

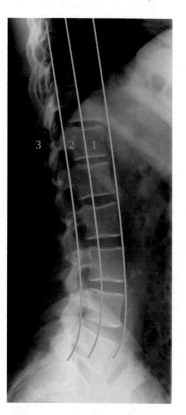

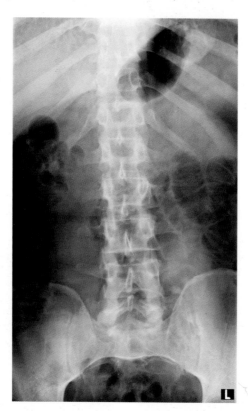

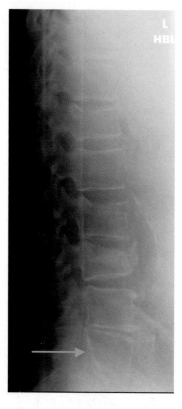

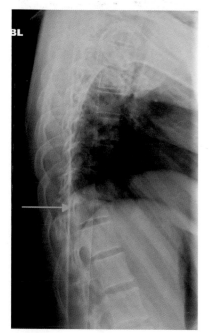

Fig 6.24: The top left (lateral) and the centre (AP) radiographs are normal lumbar spine films. The anterior (1), middle (2) and posterior (3) columns are shown on the lateral film

The top right radiograph shows multiple compression fractures (T12, L2 and L3). To identify which vertebrae are involved, count up from the L5 vertebra (arrowed pink)

The bottom left radiograph shows a vertebral compression fracture at T11 with anterior wedging (arrowed pink). There is also evidence of subluxation of T10 on T11 of approximately 25%

Hip Film

- Probably the most likely orthopaedic film you will be shown
- Most neck of femur fractures are displaced and easy to detect
- Characterise the site of the fracture as this affects management and prognosis:
  - Draw a line between the greater and lesser trochanters

- A fracture proximal to this line is intracapsular
- A fracture distal to this line is extracapsular (roughly speaking)
- Intracapsular (subcapital, transcervical). There is risk of disruption to the blood supply to the head of the femur. This fracture type usually requires some form of arthroplasty (total or hemiarthroplasty, depending on premorbid mobility), unless there is minimal displacement, in which case cannulated screws can be considered

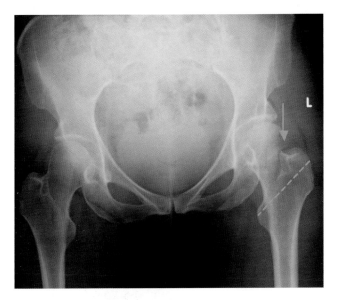

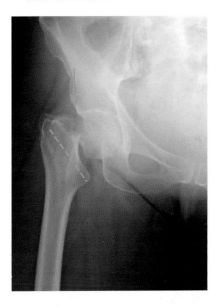

Fig 6.25: Intracapsular neck of femur fractures (the dotted line signifies the boundary between intra and extracapsular fractures). The left image shows a minimally displaced fracture, which can be fixed with cannulated screws, whereas the right image shows the more commonly encountered displaced fracture, which needs hemi-arthroplasty fixation

- Extracapsular (intertrochanteric, subtrochanteric). No risk of avascular necrosis. These fractures are typically treated with internal fixation (a dynamic hip screw for intertrochanteric and a gamma nail for subtrochanteric)

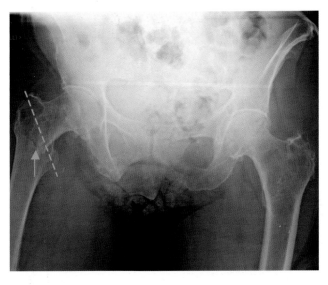

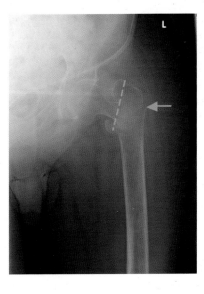

Fig 6.26: Extracapsular neck of femur fractures (the dotted line signifies the boundary between intra and extracapsular fractures). The left film shows a right intertrochanteric fracture; the right a left subtrochantreric fracture

- If you cannot identify a fracture, look closely for:
  - Disruption to the cortex – look for a step, buckle or gap
  - Interrupted trabecular pattern
  - A transverse region of sclerosis (caused by impacted fracture)
  - Shenton's line (normally a smooth curve drawn along the inferior edge of the superior pubic rami and the medial side of the femur and femoral neck); if Shenton's line shows a sudden sharp angle, the fracture is nearby
  - Changes on the lateral view (more easily missed than on the AP view)
- Look for acetabular and pubic rami fractures, which can present with similar symptoms to neck of femur fractures
- Acetabular and pubic rami fractures – if the pelvis is broken in one place, it must actually be broken in another place as well (same as Polo mints!)
- Look for any signs of osteoarthritis
- Observe the pelvis and vertebrae for fractures and osteoporosis

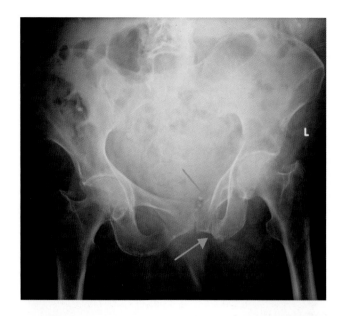

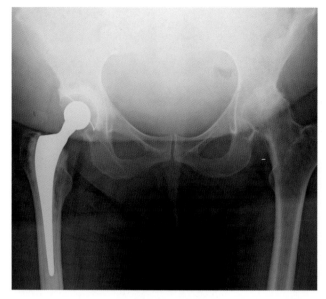

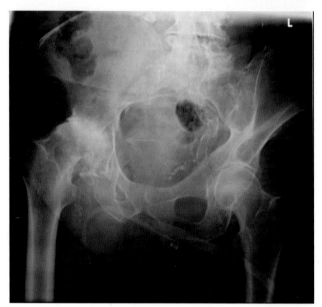

Fig 6.27: All of these patients presented with hip pain following a fall. None of the films show a neck of femur fracture, however they each show alternate causes for the patient's symptoms.

The radiograph in the top left shows superior and inferior left sided pubic rami fractures (pink arrows)

The top right X-ray shows severe osteoarthritis of the left hip, with loss of joint space, sub-chondral sclerosis, cysts and osteophytes. There is also a right total hip replacement

The bottom left X-ray also shows severe osteoarthritic change, this time affecting the right hip but in addition there is a right-sided acetabular fracture (arrowed)

Knee Film

- Fractures
  - Most are easily seen
  - A fat-fluid level, detectable on a horizontal beam lateral X-ray, signifies a lipohaemarthrosis and may be the only sign of an intra-articular fracture
  - The majority of tibial plateau fractures affect the lateral plateau
    - Look for an area of depression/ increased density
- Soft tissue injuries
  - Injury to the ligaments or menisci usually cause no abnormality on X-ray
  - Effusions can be seen as a soft tissue density deep to the quadriceps tendon
- Carefully look for signs of osteoarthritis
  - Joint space narrowing
  - Osteophyte formation
  - Sub-chondral sclerosis
  - Bony cyst formation

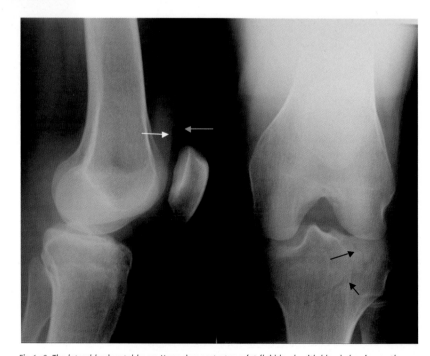

Fig 6.28: The lateral horizontal beam X-ray demonstrates a fat-fluid level, with blood showing as the denser fluid (white arrow) and fat adjacent to this (pink arrow). The AP X-ray demonstrates a fracture of the proximal tibia with intra-articular involvement (black arrows)

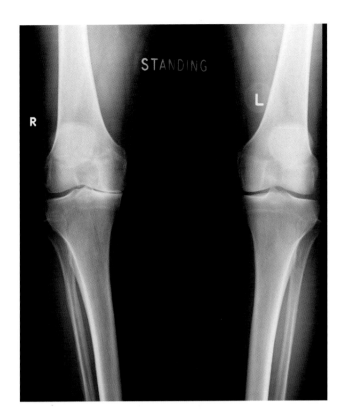

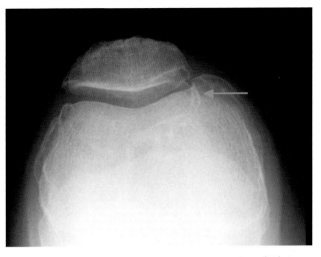

Fig 6.29: These X-rays show osteoarthritis of the right knee. The AP (left) shows loss of joint space and sub-chondral sclerosis. The skyline patella view (above) shows degenerative change with marginal osteophyte formation (arrowed) on the femoral surface of the patella and distal femur. The joint space is reasonably preserved

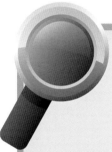

PRESENT YOUR FINDINGS...

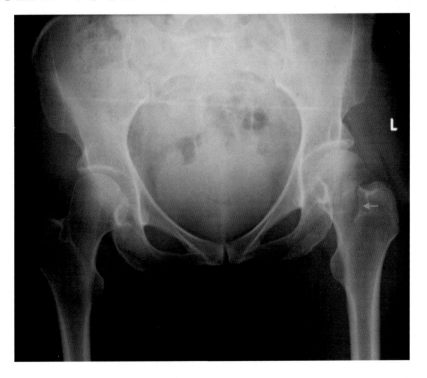

'This is an AP Pelvis radiograph. There are no identifying markings. I would like to ensure that this is the correct patient and check the date that it was taken. The film is not rotated and there are no important areas cut off at the edges of the film.

There is an oblique intracapsular fracture involving the left femoral neck (pink arrow). It is a simple fracture with minimal displacement. There is no angulation, rotation or shortening. There is no intra-articular involvement. Bone lucency is normal.

There are no other abnormalities on the radiograph.

A lateral x ray is needed to complete the radiological assessment of the fracture.'

7 Obstetrics and Gynaecology

As well as gaining the appropriate Obstetrics and Gynaecology experience, the O&G attachment, if planned well, is an excellent opportunity to brush up on some of your weaker clinical skills. Clerking anxious obstetric patients will refine your communication skills, and you should find opportunities to watch and learn from experienced clinicians delivering bad news. With the high turnover of patients, the pro-active student will be able to practice examination technique for most systems and commonly elicit clinical signs (such as anaemia, flow murmurs, clonus and hyper-reflexia). Sessions in theatre can be used to brush up on anatomy, and there is always an anaesthetist in theatre and another covering the delivery suite who can assist with physiology revision.

Study Action Plan

- When on the delivery suite, make sure you introduce yourself to the senior midwives, as they co-ordinate the unit and will get you involved in the normal deliveries. Do not fall into the classic trap for medical students of leaving the unit when it is quiet with the intention of returning later, as invariably you will miss opportunities. Instead, have reading materials with you and stay as long as you can

- Attend 'Family Planning' clinics to learn about contraception, and how best to counsel patients. Similarly, colposcopy clinics are excellent for learning about cervical smear counselling and further management of abnormal results

- Becoming proficient at the obstetric examination will take practice, but remember that midwives carry out the examination as well as the doctors, so ask them to watch you examine patients and then check your findings

- If you are scheduled time in theatre, meet with the consultant beforehand, and ask if the patients can be consented before the procedure for you to undertake a vaginal and speculum examination whilst they are under general anaesthetic

This chapter contains notes on the following scenarios:

O and G

Ms Jones is a 26 year-old lady who is 20 weeks pregnant in her first pregnancy. Her routine abnormality ultrasound scan demonstrates placenta praevia. Her husband works overseas and she has come to clinic to discuss the result of her scan. Please explain the scan result to her, including a discussion of the risks associated with this condition and how this may be managed.

Introduction

- *'Do you know why you had the scan?'*
- *'Your scan shows that you have a condition called placenta praevia. Do you know what that means?'*

Description of Placenta Praevia

- *'The placenta is the organ that allows your blood to reach your baby so that the baby receives the oxygen and nutrients it needs'*
- *'Usually, the placenta grows near the top of your womb (a picture here can demonstrate this more clearly)'*
- *'In your case, the placenta has grown near the bottom of the womb (draw another picture to explain this), so it is covering the entrance to the womb'*
- *'Sometimes, the placenta moves up as the pregnancy progresses, which can allow for a normal vaginal delivery, but in 1/200 women the placenta remains at the bottom of the womb, at which point caesarean section is often the safest delivery method'*

Impact on Pregnancy

- *'You may not have any symptoms at all'*
- *'However, since the placenta is covering the entrance to your womb at the moment, sometimes it might start to bleed'*
- *'We advise abstinence from sex since sex can increase the risk of bleeding for women with placentas covering the entrance to their womb'*
- *'You would notice this as blood from your vagina, like when you have a period. This might be a small amount of blood but it is also possible that you could bleed more heavily'*
- *'If you were to bleed, you should come into hospital for assessment urgently because if you lost a significant amount of blood it could cause problems for both yourself and your baby'*
- *'If the bleeding settles, you may be able to go back home'*
- *'If the bleed was significant or recurred, we would advise staying in hospital for the duration of your pregnancy, especially since your husband works and there may not be someone with you all the time at home'*

Classification of Placenta Praevia

Minor: the placenta is in the lower segment, near to (or touching) the os. There is a potential for vaginal delivery (depending on the distance of the lower edge of placenta from the internal os)

Major: the placenta is completely or partially covering the os. Caesarean section is required (vaginal delivery not possible)

Delivery Options

- *'As your womb grows more, the placenta might move away from the opening of your womb. If it does this, it is less likely to cause you any problems and you may be able to deliver your baby vaginally'*
- *'However, if the placenta continues to stay low down in the womb, it will block the passage for your baby to be delivered vaginally. If this happens, we would recommend you have a planned Caesarean section at 39 weeks to deliver your baby, as this would be the safest option for both you and your baby'*
- *'If before your planned Caesarean, a bleed occurred that was threatening to cause harm to yourself or your baby, the Caesarean may be brought forward as an emergency'*

Management Plan

- *'We will arrange another ultrasound scan around 36 weeks to assess whether or not the placenta has moved away from the opening of the womb'*
- *'In the meantime, if you have any vaginal bleeding, please come to hospital for assessment'*

Confirm rhesus status, as rhesus negative mothers will need anti D given if they bleed.

> *'Remember information sheets may be useful if giving important information or choices'*
>
> **Colin Duncan**
> *Consultant Obstetrician and Gynaecologist Royal Infirmary of Edinburgh*

O and G

Mrs Rae is 37 weeks pregnant and has been diagnosed as having a frank breech presentation of her first pregnancy. Please explain the diagnosis. Then discuss the possibility of external cephalic version (ECV) to put the baby into a normal position, and delivery options if ECV is unsuccessful.

What is a Breech Presentation?

- *'We have done an ultrasound scan to see how your baby is positioned in the womb. We have found that your baby is in 'breech presentation'*
- *'3-4% of term pregnancies are breech presentation'*
- *'In your case, this means that your baby's bottom is at the exit of your womb (whereas usually the baby's head is at the exit of the womb). This means that if you were to give birth vaginally, your baby would come out bottom first, which could potentially place them at higher risk of complications than if they were born head first'*

Conditions Increasing Risk of Breech Presentation

Twins
Polyhydramnios
Oligohydramnios
Uterine fibroids
Placenta praevia
Pelvic tumour
Pelvic deformities

What has Caused Breech Presentation?

- *'No cause is identified in most cases'*
- *'It may be associated with certain conditions (which prevent engagement of the foetal head)'*

How do we Manage Breech Presentation?

- *'A procedure called 'External Cephalic Version' (ECV) at 36 weeks (or 37 weeks if it is second or subsequent pregnancy) may put the baby into a normal position'*
- *'This involves an obstetrician attempting to rotate the baby in your womb, by putting their hands on your tummy. We will give you some medication to relax your womb for this to help facilitate the procedure'*
- *'This procedure decreases the need for Caesarean Section. The immediate success rate is around 50%, but in around 10% of these cases, the baby subsequently reverts back to the 'breech' position'*

Contraindications for ECV

Previous Caesarean Section
Foetal compromise
Twins
Ruptured membranes
Antepartum haemorrhage

- *'There are some risks associated with this manoeuvre, which include a small risk of umbilical cord entanglement, placental abruption (premature separation of the placenta from the womb) or induction of labour. Although the risks are small, this procedure is done where there is access to an operating theatre to make sure any problems can be managed'*
- *'Given that the risks of ECV are lower than that of a Caesarean, we would advise an attempt at ECV first, if you are in agreement'*
- *'If ECV is unsuccessful or if there is a good reason not to do it, then we would advice an elective Caesarean section'* (although a vaginal delivery may still be attempted)

Vaginal Breech Delivery

Problems Associated with Vaginal Delivery of a Breech Presentation

- *'Labour is potentially more hazardous'* (cord prolapse, foetal hypoxia following obstruction of head, intracranial injury, spinal cord transsection, damage to internal organs)

Indication

'Each case can be judged individually. In some circumstances, it may still be reasonable to go ahead with a vaginal delivery, providing certain criteria are met (detailed below)'

- Skilled attendant
- Anaesthetic and neonatal personnel available
- Patient selection
    - Not footling breech (foot is presenting part)
    - Estimated foetal weight on ultrasound <4.0kg
    - Head not hyperextended
    - No maternal or foetal complications
    - No pre-eclampsia
    - Willing mother who is aware of potential complications
    - Access to operating theatre
- Intrapartum care
    - Adequate progress
    - Continuous monitoring
    - No foetal distress

O and G

Mrs Taylor is pregnant at term with her first child. Her foetus has a breech presentation. Delivery options have been discussed and she is considering an elective Caesarean Section. Please explain the risks and benefits of this procedure to her.

Explain

Why is it Being Done?

- *'If your baby were to be born as a vaginal delivery, due to its position, rather than the head coming out first, the bottom or the legs would be coming out first. This makes the baby technically more difficult to deliver vaginally, which results in an increased risk to the baby's health. A Caesarean section is a safer option for the baby, but does come with its own risks, which we can discuss'*

How will it be Done?

- *'It is a surgical procedure that involves making a cut in your bikini line and bringing the baby out through that cut. Then we sew everything back together'*
- *'We will use a spinal or epidural anaesthesia, which will numb the lower half of your body. You should not feel any pain, just some pushing and pulling'*
- *'Before we start the operation, we will also need to empty your bladder with a catheter'*
- *'You will be awake during the operation and we will put up a screen so you cannot see the actual operation'*
- *'Once your baby is born, there will be a paediatrician contactable in case there are any problems. After the baby has been checked over, it may be possible for you to hold your baby while the rest of the operation is finished'*
- *'There will be many people in the theatre – an anaesthetist, obstetricians, midwives, and theatre staff. Your partner can also be in the theatre by your side'*
- *'Once the baby is born, we will give you a drug to contract your womb and reduce bleeding, as well as antibiotics to reduce the risk of infection'*

Risks to the Mother

During The Operation

- Bleeding
    - *'Everyone will lose blood to some extent during the procedure; depending on the degree of bleeding we could give you iron tablets or a 'top up' blood transfusion. There are also surgical techniques to stop bleeding, but in some cases (5:1000), these measures are not enough and removing the womb may be the only way to definitively stop bleeding – this would only be done as a last resort'*
- Damage to surrounding organs (1:1000) – bladder, ureters, bowel
    - *'If damage occurs, this can usually be fixed at the time by an appropriate surgeon'*

After The Operation

- Blood clot (Deep Vein Thrombosis/Pulmonary Embolism) (1:1000)
    - *'To reduce the risk, blood thinning medication (5 days of subcutaneous heparin injections) is given, early mobilisation is encouraged, and special stockings, Thromboembolic Deterrent Stockings (TEDS), are worn'*
- Infection (wound or chest) (5:100)
    - *'Antibiotics are given routinely to reduce this risk'*
- Ileus
    - *'Your bowels might not work properly for a while'*
- Post operative pain

Future Pregnancies

- *'In subsequent pregnancies, 50-60% of women who have had a caesarean are able to give birth vaginally'* (referred to as VBAC – vaginal birth after caesarean)
- *'There is an increased risk of a tear in the womb, stillbirths and placenta acreta (all around 4:1000).' 'Placenta acreta is where the placenta sticks to the uterine wall for a longer time than normal after delivery of the baby'*

Risks to the Baby

- Cuts to the baby's skin (1:100)
- Breathing difficulties can occur, but these are usually minor and get better on their own (contextualise the risk by saying that paediatricians will be in theatre to help if there are any problems)

O and G

Station 4: ANTEPARTUM HAEMORRHAGE

Mrs Patel is 30 weeks pregnant. She has noticed blood passing from her vagina and is very concerned. Please take a history from her and establish a differential diagnosis.

- First resuscitate using an ABCDE approach (antepartum haemorrhage at 30 weeks can be associated with major haemorrhage which may be concealed)

Presenting Complaint

- How much? Quantify e.g. number of sanitary towels, egg cups
- Clots? Signifies large amounts of bleeding or an old bleed
- Precipitating factors? Trauma, local or systemic infection, intercourse
- Associated pain?
- Are there foetal movements? IF NOT, when did the patient last feel her baby move?
- Has there been a previous caesarean section or myomectomy?

History of Present Pregnancy

- **Ultrasound Scan:** dating of pregnancy, placental position, foetal abnormalities
- **Complications:** hospital admissions, previous bleeding
- **Rhesus Status**

Past Obstetric History

- **Past deliveries:** year, gestation, mode of delivery, birth weight, complications (hypertension, pre-eclampsia, haemorrhage, infection)
- **Past pregnancy losses:** miscarriages, terminations, still births
- **Parity (births beyond 24 weeks) + others:** for example, if this patient had one previous normal delivery and a termination you would record Para 1+1

Ensure that you also ask about past medical and surgical history, drug history (including allergies) and social history (particularly exploring current support at home)

Investigations and Management of Antepartum Haemorrhage

- **Resuscitate:** using an ABCDE approach (before taking a detailed history)
- **Intravenous access:** if a significant bleed is suspected, insert two large-bore intravenous cannulae in the largest veins you can find
- **Bloods tests:** FBC, U&E's, coagulation screen, group and save or cross-match (depending on the size of the antepartum haemorrhage)

> 'Remember when you see an obstetric case that there are two patients and ask about the baby, for example, foetal movements'
>
> **Colin Duncan**
> *Consultant Obstetrician and Gynaecologist*
> *Royal Infirmary of Edinburgh*

If clinically stable:

- **Cardiotocography (CTG):** assess foetal well-being
- **Ultrasound:** low lying placenta, intra uterine growth restriction (IUGR)
- **Anti-D:** administered to Rhesus-negative women
- **Consider steroids:** (if <34 weeks gestation)
- **Speculum:** (**only** if ultrasound confirms no placenta praevia) – 'no PV if PP'

If clinically unstable or becomes unstable:

- **Further resuscitation:** (IV fluids/blood and urethral catheterisation aiming for urine output of more than 0.5ml/kg/hour)
- **Urgent senior obstetric and anaesthetic assistance**
- **Consider emergency delivery:** the risk to the mother's life takes precedent over that of baby

Causes of Antepartum Haemorrhage

Common	Rare
Obstetric	**Obstetric**
• Placenta praevia (painless)	• Ruptured vasa praevia
• Placenta abruption (painful)	• Uterine rupture
• Bloody show	
Non- Obstetric	**Non Obstetric**
• Benign gynaecology - vaginal lacerations, ectropium (often after intercourse)	• Sinister gynaecology - cervical cancer, polyps
• Undetermined origin (diagnosis of exclusion)	• Coagulopathy

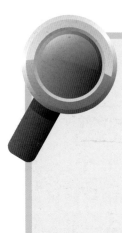

PRESENT YOUR FINDINGS...

'Mrs Patel is a 30 year-old lady presenting with vaginal bleeding. She is Para 0+0 and is currently 30 weeks pregnant. Her pregnancy has been uneventful so far, and she is rhesus positive. She is normally fit and well.

Mrs Patel has passed around 500ml of fresh blood from her vagina over the last 24 hours, associated with severe lower abdominal pain. She has not felt any foetal movements in the last day. She lives at home on her own, having recently separated from her partner.

This is consistent with a diagnosis of placental abruption with associated foetal compromise.

This lady requires urgent hospital admission. I would like to establish intravenous access, fluid resuscitate the patient, check her haemoglobin and request a cross-match for 4 units of red cells. A cardiotocogram should be performed, and I would seek an urgent obstetric review for ongoing management, and the potential need for delivery.'

Station 5: OBSTETRIC EXAMINATION

Mrs Pfannenstiel is 32 weeks pregnant. Please perform an obstetric examination and present your findings.

Volunteer to assist the lady on to the examining couch

General Inspection

- Get the patient to lie comfortably at 45° and expose them from xiphisternum to pubic symphysis
- General appearance, weight, height, oedema
- Blood pressure and pulse
- Eye (conjunctival pallor of anaemia)

Inspect Abdomen

- Size, scars (e.g. Pfannenstiel scar from a previous Caesarean Section), linea nigra, striae gravidarum

Palpation

CHECK THAT THE PATIENT DOES NOT HAVE ANY PAIN

- Measure fundal height
- Feel for the fundus (starting from xiphisternum with your right hand if examining from the right side)
- Measure the distance from the fundus to the superior edge of the pubic symphysis with a tape measure – turned over so the numbers are hidden

- Assess foetal lie
- Feel for the foetal spine (the long hard part of the foetus, often the easiest foetal part to identify) – this will either be longitudinal, oblique or transverse
- Assess foetal presentation and engagement

- Warn the patient that this may be uncomfortable for a few seconds
- Using either one hand (using thumb, index and middle fingers) or two hands depending on your preferred technique, firmly palpate the presenting part to assess whether presentation is breech or cephalic. If unsure, try to assess what the non-presenting end is
- If you can palpate inferiorly to the presenting part (i.e. between baby and the pelvis), then the presenting part is non-engaged and is five-fifths palpable. If you cannot palpate inferiorly, then estimate how many fifths are palpable. For example, if the head is the presenting part, and you can only palpate one finger width of 'head' above the pelvis, it is one-fifth palpable; two fingers is two-fifths and so on
- Assess liquor volume
- This is clinically difficult to assess (hence the importance of ultrasound scanning), but a very low liquor volume is suggested by very easy palpation of the arms and legs of the baby. Conversely, if there is a very large liquor volume it becomes difficult to palpate the baby

Auscultate

- Doppler (or Pinard stethoscope) over anterior shoulder of the foetus
- Normal rate 110-160 bpm
- Remember to use ultrasound gel and have a tissue ready to wipe the gel off afterwards
- If you cannot find the foetal heart, try the other end of the foetus as you may have misinterpreted the foetal presentation

- Thank the patient and cover them up. Depending on the clinical presentation, you may also examine or offer to examine:
  - Reflexes, clonus (pre-eclampsia)
  - The calves (deep vein thrombosis)
  - Chest (pulmonary embolism)
  - Vaginal/speculum examination (but never in suspected placenta praevia)

Tell the examiner that, to complete the examination, you would like to look at an observation chart, a cardiotocogram tracing and perform urinalysis and fundoscopy. Also offer to assist the lady in alighting from the examining couch

Definitions

Lie: the relationship between the head-to-tailbone axis of the foetus and the head-to-tailbone axis of the mother. If the two are parallel, then the foetus is said to be in a longitudinal lie, if perpendicular, the foetus is said to be in a transverse lie

Presentation: the part of the foetus that lies closest to or has entered the true pelvis of the mother. Can be:

- 'Cephalic' (vertex, brow, face, chin)
- 'Breech' (buttocks or feet)
- 'Shoulder'
- 'Compound' (entry of more than one part e.g. head and hand)

Engagement: fixation of the presenting part of the foetus in the maternal true pelvis (past the level of an artificial line drawn between the ischial spines). Measured in fifths of presenting part i.e. a free head abdominally would be 5 fifths palpable

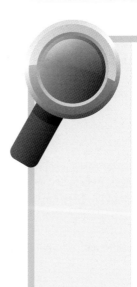

PRESENT YOUR FINDINGS...

'Mrs Pfannenstiel is a 28 year-old primigravida lady of 32 weeks gestation whose symphysis-fundal height is 32cm. She has linea nigra and striae gravidarum. The foetal lie is longitudinal with a cephalic presentation. The foetal head is not engaged, with five-fifths palpable.'

Station 6: ANXIOUS PREGNANT WOMAN

Mrs Brown is a 44 year-old primigravida who has presented to your GP practice after having had a positive home pregnancy test. She is very anxious about her pregnancy. Please explore her anxieties and establish whether her pregnancy is high or low risk

There are two aspects to this station: dealing with an anxious patient and identifying problems in pregnancy

- What has made them come into to see you? What is she anxious about? The Ideas, Concerns, Expectations (ICE) structure can be helpful in dealing with this

Ideas

- *'So how can I help you today?' 'I understand you might be pregnant?'*

Concerns

- Does she have any particular worries or issues she would like to discuss? Has she or anyone close to her had problems during previous pregnancies? Has she read about problems with pregnancy in the media? Does she have a poor support network? Does she want to continue the pregnancy?
- There may be concerns about symptoms such as urinary frequency, tiredness, breast tenderness or constipation that might purely be a consequence of the pregnancy

Expectations

- What does the patient expect will happen during the pregnancy?
- Ensure that they are aware of what they can expect from healthcare services during their pregnancy. Multiple professionals are available to help, including midwives, GPs and obstetricians. The first 'Booking visit' is usually between weeks 8 and 12 of pregnancy

Next, find out more details about the pregnancy itself, which have not been covered in the above discussion.

- Age
- Was the pregnancy planned? When was the last menstrual period?
- Have there been any problems in the pregnancy so far?

Obstetric History

- Ask about previous pregnancies - any complications, termination of pregnancies or miscarriages, type of delivery
- Ask about any problems with other children, particularly congenital problems such as Spina Bifida and chromosomal problems such as Down syndrome
- Pre-conception folic acid (decreases the risk of neural tube defects)

> 'If bad news is of complex information, ask if there is someone that the patient would like to be present"
>
> **Colin Duncan**
> *Consultant Obstetrician and Gynaecologist
> Royal Infirmary of Edinburgh*

Social History

- Social support - partner, family, domestic violence
- Smoking, alcohol and substance misuse
- Diet
- Ethnic origin of parents may be important in determining risk of certain inherited diseases e.g. thalassemia, sickle cell disease

Other History

- Past medical and surgical history
- Systematic enquiry
- Current medication and allergies

> 'Don't ignore non verbal clues. If someone seems upset, angry or anxious, then acknowledge it'
>
> **Colin Duncan**
> *Consultant Obstetrician and Gynaecologist
> Royal Infirmary of Edinburgh*

Is this a High-Risk Pregnancy?

Maternal Factors	Foetal Factors
• Age - younger than 15 or over 35 • Previous obstetric complications - still birth, preterm labour, pre-eclampsia, foetal loss • More than five previous pregnancies • Medical co-morbidities - hypertension, diabetes, heart disease (particularly valvular)	• Exposure to infection e.g. herpes simplex • Exposure to toxic medication e.g. phenytoin • Exposure to addictive substances e.g. smoking • Identified physical abnormality during screening e.g. congenital cardiac disease

The risk of the pregnancy is important in determining the management of the patient. High risk pregnancies require more regular input from obstetricians and may require further specialist input depending on the underlying reason for being high risk.

How do you calculate Estimated Date of Delivery?

Gestational age and calculation of Estimated Date of Delivery by Last Menstrual Period (LMP) is calculated according to Naegele's rule:

LMP + 7 days + 9 months

However this should be corrected for the length of the menstrual cycle. The above calculation is based on a 28 day cycle. An extra day should be added on to the calculation for each day over 28, and subtracted for each day below 28
E.g. for a 33 day cycle, the calculation is **LMP + 7 days + 9 months + 5 days**

What Screening Tests Are Available to Pregnant Mothers?

At the booking visit, parents can opt for screening tests (see NICE Antenatal Care Guidance for further details):

Blood Tests
- Red cells: blood group, rhesus D status and screening for haemoglobinopathies, anaemia, red-cell alloantibodies
- Infection: hepatitis B virus, HIV, rubella susceptibility and syphilis

Urine Tests
- Check for proteinuria, glycosuria and screen for asymptomatic bacteriuria

Ultrasound Scan
- **12 week dating scan (between 10+0 to 13+6 weeks)** - used to confirm foetal number, gestational age using crown-rump measurements (or head circumference if the crown-rump measurement is > 84mm); nuchal translucency is also measured to calculate an estimated risk of trisomy 21 (in conjunction with maternal age, serum markers (free BhCG and PAPP-A), smoking status and previous obstetric history)
- **20 week detailed anomaly scan (between 18+0 to 20+6)** - used to look in more detail for structural anomalies

Down Syndrome
- See section 9.8 'Down Syndrome'

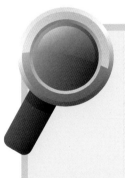

PRESENT YOUR FINDINGS...

'Mrs Brown is a 44 year-old lady with aortic regurgitation and type 1 diabetes mellitus who presents following a positive home pregnancy test, with a planned pregnancy. She is currently well and is keen to continue the pregnancy. She is Para 0+1, with a previous miscarriage in 2008 at 10 weeks and has a family history of congenital heart disease. Mrs Brown is a non-smoker, is married and has very supportive parents living close by.

This is a high risk pregnancy, and I would address Mrs Brown's concerns and refer her to secondary care for more intensive antenatal care.'

Station 7:
COMBINED ORAL CONTRACEPTIVE PILL (COCP)

Miss Williams is a 36 year-old lady in a long-term relationship. She is looking to start using the combined oral contraceptive pill as her partner no longer wishes to use condoms – she worries about the risk of future pregnancy. Please counsel her as to what this would mean for her and establish whether she is suitable for this form of contraception.

Background

- Discuss all methods of contraception available
- Gynaecological history
  1. Menstrual cycle – length, regularity, pain and bleeding
  2. Contraceptive history
  3. Sexual health history
  4. Smear history
- Past medical history
- Drug history (interactions)
- Allergies
- Family history (particularly breast carcinoma and thromboembolic disease)
- Social history (smoking – this is a good opportunity for health promotion)
- Body mass index

Explain how the COCP Works

- Stops the ovary from releasing an egg
- Affects the lining of the womb and the cervical mucus to make pregnancy less likely
- It is suitable for many women, including older women with no risk factors

Benefits and Side Effects of Taking the Pill

Benefits	Side Effects
• 99% effective (if used properly) – reliable, reversible, easy to take • Lightens the period, reduces dysmenorrhoea and pre-menstrual changes • Reduces the risk of ovarian and endometrial cancer, ovarian cysts and benign breast disease	• Weight gain • Dizziness • Nausea • Breast tenderness • Mood swings

Taking the Pill

- The pill comes in a pack of 21 tablets; each day is marked
- Women should be advised to start taking this pill on the first day of their next period, (between now and then alternative contraception is necessary). Protection also begins immediately if the pill is started on the 2nd, 3rd, 4th or 5th day of their period
- Alternatively, they can start the pill on any day of the menstrual cycle but will require barrier contraception for 7 days in addition
- After completion of the packet (i.e. 21 pills) there is a 7 day break from taking the pill; during this time, they will have a withdrawal bleed. The period will likely be lighter and less painful than usual
- The pill should ideally be taken at around the same time each day

Contraindications to Taking the Pill

Contraindications

- Age over 50 years
- BMI >35
- Venous thrombosis or arterial disease
- Breast cancer history
- Severe migraine, or migraine with associated focal aura/neurology
- Cardiovascular risk factors:
  1. Hypertension (>160 systolic, >95 diastolic)
  2. Diabetes mellitus (with associated complications)
- Undiagnosed vaginal bleeding
- Pro-thrombotic blood disorders
- Taking liver enzyme inducing drugs (e.g. carbamazapine, rifampicin), antibiotics
- Hepatic impairment
- Gallstones

Cautions
(contraindicated if more than one present)

- Age over 35 years
- BMI > 30
- Family history of venous thrombosis, arterial disease, or breast cancer
- Migraines without focal aura
- Cardiovascular risk factors:
  1. Hypertension (but <160 systolic, <95 diastolic)
  2. Diabetes mellitus (uncomplicated)
  3. Smoking
- Long-term immobility

Any enzyme-inducing medication decreases the pills efficacy by increasing the rate of pill metabolism. There is a long list of medications to consider, so when prescribing always check for interactions using the British National Formulary. Common enzyme-inducing medication categories (although not all drugs within a category have the same pharmacokinetics) are anti-depressants, anti-psychotics, anti-epileptics and antibiotics.

Development of Complications Whilst on the Pill

The patient must be made aware of symptoms associated with potential complications whilst using the pill and advised to seek medical help urgently if symptoms develop

- **Blood clots:** discuss calf pain, leg swelling, chest pain and shortness of breath
- **Migraines:** any increase in headache frequency should be reported to the GP and any development of focal neurological signs (either as an aura with a migraine or signs alone) also require discontinuation of the pill
- **Hypertension:** advise the patient that they will need regular blood pressure checks with the practice nurse

Advice for Missed Pills

- *'A pill is late if less than 24 hours have elapsed since it was meant to be taken: in this case, take the pill anyway and continue as usual'*
- *'A pill is missed if more than 24 hours have elapsed since the time it should have been taken'*
- *'If one pill is missed, take the last missed pill when remembered (even if that involves taking two pills at once). Continue taking the rest of the pack as usual;*

take the normal seven day break. There is no need for additional contraception. Emergency contraception is not usually required, but it should be considered if pills have been missed earlier in the packet, or in the last week of the previous packet'

- *'If two or more pills are missed, (more than 48 hours without taking the pill), take the last pill missed when remembered (even if that involves taking two pills in one day). Leave any earlier missed pills. Use additional contraception for the next 7 days. If the pack is due to end in these seven days, run the packs together without the normal 7 day break. Consider emergency contraception (particularly if the pills are missed in the first week of taking the pill after a 7 day break)'*

Other Things to Discuss:

- Antibiotics alter the gut flora and reduce the enterohepatic circulation of oestrogen - therefore, alternative methods of contraception should be used for the duration of the course of antibiotics and for 7 days after (4 weeks in the case of rifampicin)
- Similarly, any episodes of diarrhoea and vomiting require the same advice for an additional method of contraception
- Immobility i.e. long-haul flights - encourage hydration, mobilising
- Contraceptive pills do not protect against sexually transmitted infections – therefore also use barrier method
- There are different formulations of contraceptive pills to ensure that one will suit the individual
- There are other contraceptives agents available, for example, long-acting reversible contraception such as the Implanon and Mirena intra-uterine system

O and G

Sarah is a 16 year-old female who had unprotected intercourse last night, and is worried she may be pregnant. Please advise her as to what her options are with regard to emergency contraception and explain the risks and benefits of different methods.

History of Presenting Complaint

- When was the last episode of unprotected intercourse?
- Brief past medical history (including last menstrual period, previous pelvic inflammatory disease - Chlamydia specifically), previous pregnancies, drug history and social history

Levonelle

- 'Morning-after' pill
- It can be used within 3 days of unprotected sexual intercourse but the earlier the better

Explain what it is (including effectiveness) and how to take it

- Tablets contain levonorgestrel (a progestogen)
- Stops ovulation or stops implantation
- Levonelle – one pill (1.5mg)
- Success rate depends on the gap between unprotected sex and taking the pill: 95% success rate if Levonelle used within 24 hours, 85% within 48 hours, and around 60% effectiveness at 72 hours
- If the patient vomits within 3 hours, they need a replacement dose (consider an anti-emetic if the patient is persistently nauseated)

Contraindications

- Allergic (have they had this pill before?)
- Severe liver disease
- Malabsorption
- Acute intermittent porphyria

Note: If the patient is taking enzyme-inducing drugs (e.g. rifampicin), they require a higher dose of Levonelle

Side Effects

- Nausea
- Spotting/irregular bleeding after taking the pill until the next period
- Minor headaches, breast tenderness
- Next period may be early or late

They must return to the clinic if:

- No period after 3 weeks (do a pregnancy test on first urine specimen upon waking up in the morning) – although advise the lady that her next period may be lighter or shorter than normal
- They have any concerns – although these can also be addressed by the GP as well as Genitourinary Medicine (GUM) or Family Planning clinics

Intrauterine Contraceptive Device (IUD)/Emergency Coil

- The IUD is 99% effective up to 5 days after intercourse
- Can be fitted up to 5 days after unprotected sexual intercourse
- Absolute contraindications to its use are **pelvic infections** (current or in the past 3 months), **pregnancy, unexplained genital bleeding, severely distorted uterine cavity, pelvic cancer**
- IUDs are easier to insert if the patient has previously given birth
- Provide ongoing contraception afterwards
- Can be removed after first period
- Risks of these devices include prolapse, perforation, ectopic pregnancy and infection

Essential Advice to Deliver

- The patient needs to use condoms until her next period
- STIs – discuss need for screening. The best time to screen is from 2 weeks after exposure
- Give contraceptive advice for the future – *'I'd like to see you again to discuss contraception for the future, or if you'd rather, I could refer you to the family planning clinic'*

Ethical and Legal Note

For females under the age of 16, contraceptive treatment and advice can be given without parental consent providing the criteria of the 'Fraser Guidelines' are met:

- They understand the professional's advice
- They cannot be persuaded to inform their parents
- They are likely to continue or begin having sexual intercourse with or without contraception
- Unless they receive contraceptive treatment, they are likely to suffer physically and/or mentally
- It is in their best interests to receive contraceptive treatment with or without parental consent

If there are any child protection concerns (e.g. the male partner is significantly older), then confidentiality can and should be broken with the appropriate safeguarding steps taken (see section 9.5)

Station 9: CERVICAL SMEAR COUNSELLING

Mrs Smith has arrived at your clinic after having a routine cervical smear. The result states she has moderate dyskaryosis. Please counsel her as to what this means and what options are available for management.

- Screening is done to pick up early changes in the cells of the cervix – 'early warning cells' - abnormal cells that are not cancerous, but have the potential to become malignant
- Abnormal smears are a common finding (1 in 12 smears – commonest cause is HPV, acquired from sexual intercourse)
- Detecting abnormal cells potentially allows the early treatment and prevention of cancer development

Smear Results and Management

Mild dyskaryosis	Moderate dyskaryosis	Severe dyskaryosis
- Mild changes often return to normal - No need for immediate action - Follow up repeat smear in 6 months - if still abnormal, then refer for colposcopy	- Reassure the patient that there is no evidence of cancer, but you need to assess her further and treat her if there are cells present that could become cancerous - Requires colposcopy	- Explain that the smear suggests there are abnormal cells and that further investigation is required to reduce the risk of cancer transformation - Requires urgent colposcopy

Colposcopy

- *'Colposcopy is a short procedure – it is done in a colposcopy clinic in hospital; and lasts 10-15 minutes'*
- *'Colposcopy involves passing a speculum (similar to a smear) into the vagina, but also involves using a microscope to be able to see the cervix in more detail'*
- Performed if the cervical smear shows signs of moderate or severe changes, or persistent mild
- Aims to detect the presence and grade of cervical intraepithelial neoplasia (CIN)
- *'The cervix is 'stained' to look for any abnormal regions'*
- *'A biopsy may be taken of any abnormal region and will subsequently be analysed in a laboratory'*
- *'If there is just a small abnormal region, no procedure would be done until the results of the biopsy come back. However, if there is quite a bit of abnormality, then it is better to perform a treatment straight away, and remove that part of the cervix (by doing a Large Loop Excision of the Transformation Zone (LLETZ)). Some local anaesthetic is injected into the cervix if a treatment is needed'*
- Abnormal appearances include acetowhite (hyperkeratosis), 'iodine negative', neovascularisation and mosaicism
- If the biopsy appearance is consistent with:
  - CIN I – either observed (60% return to normal), or LLETZ
  - CIN II or III – LLETZ (large loop excision of the transformation zone) and histological examination (may require further treatments)

After Colposcopy

- Repeat colposcopy 4-6 months later if any treatment is performed
- Avoid sex, swimming and tampons for 2 weeks after biopsy/LLETZ (bleeding risk)
- Follow-up smears will be more frequent if CIN II or III diagnosed, often every 6 months to a year, for a number of years, before returning to the normal 3-year programme

Potential Concerns to Discuss

- Human papillomavirus (HPV) as the cause of cervical carcinoma
- Cigarette smoking - patient may be concerned about the link between this and cervical cancer. Note smoking also (because it suppresses immunity) increases the likelihood of persistent abnormal cells despite treatment
- Sex will not make abnormal cells worse and cellular changes are not passed on to the partner
- Abnormal cell changes will not affect fertility, but treatment can; for example, LLETZ increases the risk of pre-term labour and premature rupture of membranes
- An abnormal smear is nothing to be embarrassed or ashamed about
- *'By having a smear test, you've taken positive action to protect your health and reduce the risk of cancer'*

8 Psychiatry

Psychiatry is often perceived to be a daunting, or even difficult, attachment. To some extent, it involves a different skill set than other specialities; for instance, like being able to assess the content of a patient's thoughts. However, developing these types of skills is what the placement is for! Even for those who do not want to pursue it as a career, psychiatry offers excellent training in generic skills that a doctor needs, such as the ability to communicate in sensitive circumstances like taking a history from 'the depressed patient'.

Study Action Plan

- Speak to the staff on your ward to determine the most suitable patients for you regarding obtaining histories and performing mental state examinations
- Discuss your findings with ward staff afterwards to consolidate your learning
- Interviewing a patient in pairs is often a helpful experience, especially when starting your rotation in Psychiatry – provide feedback to each other on your performances
- Practice the routine for a Mini Mental State Exam (MMSE) on friends to ensure that you are familiar with it: this is a common OSCE station
- Sharing the experiences of psychiatry patients can often be quite a difficult emotional task, often more so than with other medical patients. This is common. If you think it might help, speak to psychiatry doctors to 'debrief' from such experiences

This chapter contains notes on the following systems:

Psychiatry

Mr Chang is a 58-year-old man who has recently lost his job and has gone through a difficult divorce. Recent routine blood tests revealed an elevated GGT, and you are worried that this may be secondary to an alcohol problem. Please take a detailed alcohol history from him

CAGE

This is a widely used screening method for alcohol abuse or dependence.

C: *'Have you ever felt that you should **CUT** down on your drinking?'*

A: *'Have other people **ANNOYED** you by criticising the amount you drink?'*

G: *'Have you ever felt **GUILTY** about your drinking?'*

E: *'Do you ever need a drink first thing in the morning – an **EYE-OPENER?'***

The recommended cut-off for CAGE is ≥2 to screen for alcohol abuse or dependence.

Alcohol Intake

- *'How much do you drink in a typical week?'* (maximum weekly intake is 14 units for women and 21 units for men; with a maximum daily intake 3 units for women and 4 units for men)
- *'How often do you drink?'*
- *'Binges or steady drinking?'*
- *'What time do you start drinking?'*
- *'What makes you start drinking?'* e.g. stress, alcohol availability
- *'Where do you drink? Is it alone or with company?'*
- *'What do you drink – beer, wine or spirits?'*
- *'Describe how much you'd drink on a typical day'*

> 'Poor nutrition is common in the alcohol dependent and the consequences of thiamine deficiency can be catastrophic. Doctors should have a low threshold for the administration of parenteral thiamine'
>
> **Killian Welch**
> *Specialist Registrar Psychiatry*
> *Royal Edinburgh Hospital*

> 'CAGE is reasonably sensitive for moderate to severe alcohol dependence, but its sensitivity for less advanced problem drinking is poorer. Positive screens should always be followed by a full alcohol history.'
>
> **Killian Welch**
> *Specialist Registrar Psychiatry*
> *Royal Edinburgh Hospital*

Past Alcohol History

- *'At what age did you start drinking?'*
- Longest period of abstinence
- *'Is there a family history of alcoholism?'*

Physical Complications of Alcohol Abuse

'Have you experienced any health problems associated with alcohol?'

Health problems related to alcohol abuse include:
- Anaemia
- Liver damage: cirrhosis
- Pancreatitis
- Gastro-oesophageal reflux, peptic ulcer disease
- Neurological: epilepsy, ataxia, peripheral neuropathy, amnesia
- Psychiatric: depression (assess mood), hallucinations, Wernicke's encephalopathy, Korsakoff's syndrome (assess cognition)
- Cardiovascular: ischaemic heart disease, cardiomyopathy, hypertension

It is also important to ask about the presence of symptoms of the alcohol dependence syndrome. Furthermore, the complications of poorly managed alcohol withdrawal can be life threatening. These include seizures, Wernicke's encephalopathy/Korsakoff's syndrome and delirium tremens.

Social Complications of Alcohol Abuse

- Absenteeism, loss of job, divorce, driving convictions
- Reduced job productivity
- *'Any problems in getting along with people close to you?'*
- *'Have you ever been in trouble with the police?'*

Previous Treatments (And Outcomes)

- Ask what previous help has been sought e.g.
  - Detoxification programs
  - Counselling e.g. Alcoholics Anonymous (AA)

Enquire about Maintaining Factors

- Access to alcohol
- Motivation to drink: social isolation, avoidance of withdrawal symptoms

Assess Motivation to Change

- Has the patient expressed a desire to change now?

N.B. Success in changing drinking behaviour depends on the individual's preparedness to change. This can be illustrated by the "Stages of Change" model (Prochaska and DiClemente, 1984). An individual progresses through all 5 stages before successfully achieving a new behaviour such as becoming sober. This does not necessarily occur in a strictly linear manner, and the patient may return to earlier stages on the path to achieving abstinence.

PRECONTEMPLATION: No intention to take action in the next six months

⇕

CONTEMPLATION: Intends to take action in the next six months

⇕

PREPARATION: Intends to take action in the next 30 days: has taken some steps in the direction

⇕

ACTION: Has changed behaviour for less than 6 months

⇕

MAINTENANCE: Has changed behaviour for greater than 6 months

What are the features of alcohol dependence syndrome?

According to ICD-10, three of the six criteria below must be met (over a 12 month period) to diagnose dependence:

- Strong desire or sense of compulsion to take the substance
- Difficulties controlling intake of the substance (either its onset, termination or levels of use)
- Physiological withdrawal state or the use of the same (or similar) substance to prevent such a withdrawal state – *'What happens when you stop drinking?'*
- Tolerance (increasing amounts required to achieved desired effects) – *'Are you finding yourself drinking more to get drunk?'*
- Lack of other activities and interests
- Ongoing substance misuse despite clear evidence of harmful consequences

With regard to the management of alcohol withdrawal, standard benzodiazepine reducing regimes (20mg chlordiazepoxide qds, decreasing gradually over 6 days) are there for guidance. Administration of benzodiazepines should be titrated according to need on the basis of objective symptoms (BP, pulse, tremor etc). The severely alcohol dependent generally require doses of benzodiazepines that are substantially greater than those outlined in a standard protocol.

'The experience of withdrawal is not a prerequisite for the diagnosis of dependence — an individual can be dependent on a substance even if they do not experience a clear withdrawal syndrome on ceasing use'

Killian Welch

Specialist Registrar Psychiatry
Royal Edinburgh Hospital

Psychiatry

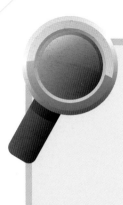

PRESENT YOUR FINDINGS...

'Mr Chang is a 58-year-old man who has recently divorced and lost his job. Before this he claims to have been a 'social drinker'. He now consumes 50 units of alcohol a week, mainly beer, often drinking alone and at the expense of missing meals. He is increasingly tolerant to the effects of alcohol and experienced withdrawal symptoms on previous attempts to stop drinking.

He has no other health problems. He has good insight, acknowledging his drinking excess, and the effect it has on his relationships. He is actively seeking help, although he has been unsuccessful in the past at giving up.

In conclusion, Mr Chang has features of alcohol dependence syndrome and is preparing to abstain from alcohol in the future.'

Station 2: DEPRESSION

Mr Wood is a 50 year-old man who recently separated from his wife. His mood has been low and he has stopped caring about life. He has now lost his job. Please take a history from him and elicit any features of depression.

Core Depressive Symptoms

- **LOW MOOD:** *'How do you feel in your spirits?', 'Does it vary throughout the day?'*
- **LOSS OF INTEREST [ANHEDONIA]:** *'Do you still enjoy things that you used to?'*
- **LACK OF ENERGY:** *'Do you find that you tire more easily?'*

Biological Symptoms

- **Sleep Disturbance:** *'How is your sleep?', 'When do you go to sleep?', 'How long does it take you to fall asleep?', 'Do you wake up in the night?', 'When do you wake in the morning?', 'How do you feel on waking?', 'Do you sleep much during the day?'*
- **Reduced Appetite:** *'How has your appetite been?'*
- **Weight Loss:** *'Have you noticed any change in your weight?'*
- **Constipation:** *'Have you noticed any change in your bowel movements?'*
- **Loss of Libido:** *'Any change in your interest in sexual things?'*

Cognitive Symptoms

- **Worthlessness:** *'How do you see yourself compared to other people?', 'How do you think other people see you?'*
- **Self-esteem:** *'How do you feel about yourself?' 'How confident a person are you?'*
- **Poor Memory:** *'Has your memory changed over time?'*
- **Poor Concentration:** *'Has your ability to concentrate changed; for example, can you watch a television programme all the way through or read a book?'*
- **Guilt:** *'Do you feel guilty about anything?'*
- **Tearfulness:** *'Is there anything that makes you cry?', 'Have you been more tearful recently?'*
- **Agitation:** *'Is there anything that makes you angry?'*

Mnemonic for some of the symptoms of depression:
SAW EMAIL

- **S**leep disturbance
- **A**ppetite reduced
- **W**eight loss
- **E**nergy low
- **M**ood low
- **A**nhedonia
- **I**rritability
- **L**ibido loss

Differential Diagnosis

- *Physical illness e.g. hypothyroidism, Cushing's syndrome, cancer*
- *Drugs e.g. alcohol/ withdrawal from stimulants, oral contraceptives, some anti-hypertensive drugs*
- *Bereavement*
- *Bipolar affective disorder*
- *Psychotic depression*

Differential Diagnosis

- **Psychotic depression:** *'Have you ever heard things said when there is no one about and nothing to explain it?' 'Do you ever feel as if people are against you or may wish to do you harm? Do you seem to have special powers? Do things ever look changed or different – and if so, do they look as if they are dying or rotting?'*
- **Bipolar affective disorder:** *'Do you ever have episodes where your mood is very elated or you do things which you later regret?'*
- **Physical causes:** *'Are you taking any drugs – prescription or recreational?', 'Do you have any health problems?'* e.g. hypothyroidism, Parkinson's disease, malignancy (hypercalcaemia)

General Questions

- **Pre-morbid personality:** *'How would you describe yourself before all of this?'*, *'How would others describe you?'*
- **Psychiatric illness:** *'Have you ever had any issues relating to your mental health?'*, *'Have any family members had issues with their mental wellbeing?'*
- **Insight:** *'Do you think that there has been a change in your behaviour?'*, *'Would you say that this might be depression?'*, *'Do you think you might benefit from help?'*
- **Social history:** *'Where do you live?'*, *'Who do you live with?'*, *'Who could you go to for help?'*
- **Substance use:** Particularly enquire about alcohol

Suicide Risk

It may not be possible to take a full suicide history in a depression station. However, it is an important area to cover. Tell the examiner that you would go on to ask about it, if you run out of time. Ask questions such as:

- *'How do you feel about life at the moment?'*
- *'How do you feel about the future?'*
- *'Have you ever felt that life is not worth living?'*
- *'Do you ever wish it would end?'*
- *'Have you ever thought about ending it?'*
- *'Have you ever thought how you would do this?'*
- *'Have you ever attempted to end your life before?'*

Other suicide risk factors should be assessed such as unemployment, relationship status, chronic pain or disability, previous family history of deliberate self harm or completed suicide.

Atypical Depression

- *Reactive affect*
- *Weight gain*
- *Increased appetite*
- *Hypersomnia*
- *Leaden paralysis (heavy, leaden feelings in arms or legs)*

What are the most alarming features of depression one should look out for?

- *Psychotic features e.g. nihilistic/persecutory delusions, auditory hallucinations*
- *Self-neglect e.g. reduced appetite may result in significant weight loss*
- *Potential for harm to self or others*
- *Suicide risk*

Aetiological Factors

Predisposing	Precipitating	Perpetuating
Long-term adversity: employment/marital difficulties	Acute stressful life events	Inability to solve precipitating or predisposing adversity
Poor support network: Lack of close-confiding relationships	Poor compliance with medication	Poor insight
Female gender		Alcohol/ substance misuse

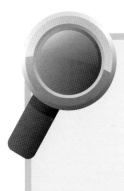

PRESENT YOUR FINDINGS...

'Mr Wood is a 50-year-old gentleman with a 2 month history of low mood following separation from his wife. He has anhedonia, poor energy and poor appetite associated with 5kg weight loss. He sleeps poorly with early morning wakening. Mr Wood describes feelings of worthlessness and guilt about his relationship. His pre-morbid state is described as cheerful and active.

He displays no evidence of psychosis or mania and denies thoughts of self-harm or suicide. He has no relevant psychiatric or medical history and is not on any medication.

This history is consistent with a diagnosis of depression, perhaps reactive in nature, with evidence of self-neglect.'

Psychiatry

Mr Jones is worried about his wife. He reports that she has been acting out of sorts and has been on huge shopping sprees resulting in considerable debt. She often does not return home until the early hours of the morning. She has previously suffered from depression. Please take a history from her.

Elicit Symptoms Suggestive of a Manic Episode

- **Mood:** 'How would you describe your mood?', 'Have you found yourself more excitable than normal?', 'Do you find others irritate you more than they used to?', 'Do you ever have periods of feeling low?'
- **Increased activity:** 'How would you describe your energy levels?', 'Do you find yourself taking on a lot more than you used to?', 'How would you spend a typical day?'
- **Sleep:** 'How is your sleep?', 'When do you go to sleep?', 'Would you say you need a lot of sleep?'
- **Increased libido:** 'Has your interest in sex changed?'
- **Disinhibition:** 'Would you describe yourself as impulsive?', 'Have you been on any shopping sprees?', 'Do you feel you've been taking a lot more risks than you used to?', 'Have you got into any trouble lately or broken the law?', 'Have you done anything which you later regretted?'
- **Self-worth:** 'How do you see yourself compared to other people?', 'How would you describe yourself as a person?'
- **Concentration:** 'Do you have any difficulties concentrating on things, e.g. reading a book or watching TV?'

General Questions

- **Pre-morbid personality:** 'How would others describe you?', 'Do you feel you've changed at all?'
- **Psychiatric illness:** 'Have you ever had any issues with your mental health?', 'Have any family members ever suffered from depression or any other aspect of their mental health?'
- **Insight:** 'Do you think everything is okay right now?', 'What do you think is causing your change in behaviour?' 'Do you feel you need any help?'

Symptoms (mnemonic for features of a manic episode – MANIC)

- **M**ood: *elated, excited, enthusiastic*
- **A**ctivity increased
- **N**aughty: *spending sprees, use of alcohol and drugs, increased sexual activity*
- **I**nsomnia
- **C**onfidence increased

Differential Diagnosis

- **Physical causes:** 'Are you on any drugs – prescription or recreational?', 'Do you have any health problems? (e.g. frontal lobe disease)'
- **Psychosis:** 'Do you have any special powers?', 'Do you ever hear anything unusual which cannot be explained?'

Get a collateral history if possible.

Define a manic episode and describe features necessary for its diagnosis

A manic episode is a distinct period of persistently elevated, expansive and irritable mood. It must last for <u>at least one week</u> and features include:

- Inflated self esteem or grandiosity
- Decreased need for sleep
- Talkative – more than usual
- Flight of ideas/racing thoughts
- Distractibility
- Increased goal-directed activity and psychomotor agitation
- Excessive involvement in pleasurable activities

What is the difference between mania and hypomania?

Although many of the same symptoms are experienced in hypomania as in mania (see above), these are usually less severe.

Hypomanic periods must last for several days and should not necessitate hospitalisation or have psychotic features.

With hypomania an individual's ability to function in everyday life is not significantly impaired.

Psychiatry

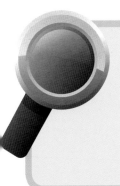

PRESENT YOUR FINDINGS...

'Mrs Jones has a 2-week history of unusual behaviour. Her mood has been unusually elevated. She has had more energy than usual, she has been getting little to no sleep, and she has been spending excessively. She has a history of depression but has otherwise been fit and well. She reports no thoughts of self-harm or harm to others and displays no features of psychosis.

This history is consistent with a manic episode. Given the history of depression, the mostly likely diagnosis is Bipolar Affective Disorder.'

Station 4: POSTNATAL DEPRESSION (PND)

Mrs Roberts is a 24-year-old lady who has recently given birth to her first child. Her husband is concerned because Mrs Roberts doesn't appear to be coping well. Her mood has been persistently low and she has been very tearful. Please take a history from her.

- Approximately 1 in 10 mothers suffer postnatal depression (PND) in the year after birth
- This is usually gradual in onset
- 50% onset by 6 months
- Non-psychotic depression – no loss of contact with reality

Clinical Features

Features of PND are similar to those of depression (low mood, tearfulness, anhedonia, self harm etc), but suicidal thoughts are less common and anxiety is particularly marked. Patients tend to have feelings of:

- Guilt or inadequacy towards the baby
- Inability to cope, overwhelmed
- Getting anxious/worried for no apparent reason
- **Thoughts of harming the baby** (rarely act on thoughts)

Other forms of low mood post-partum:

- **'Baby blues':** more than 50% of mothers will experience this type of low mood within the first week after childbirth – this generally resolves and requires reassurance as management
- **Puerperal psychosis:** the most severe form of depression following childbirth. It occurs in approximately 1-2 per 1,000 mothers and is characterised by depression with psychotic features, often associated with thoughts of harming their baby. Hospitalisation is invariably required in a Mother and Baby Unit

Assess those at risk of PND

- Personal or family history of PND/depression
- Poor social support/marital discord
- Difficulties with breastfeeding
- Unplanned/unwanted pregnancy
- Recent adverse life events e.g. family death, loss of income

> *'Keep postnatal depression in your mind when seeing mothers: it can present up to two years after birth. Even as a paediatrician seeing their child, symptoms in the mother may become apparent when taking the history'*
>
> **Zeshan Qureshi**
> *Paediatric Trainee*
> *London Deanery*

Advice for the Mother

- PND is common
- It will usually improve with treatment. Psychological interventions (cognitive behavioural therapy or interpersonal therapy) and anti-depressants can play a role. It is important to discuss the risks and benefits of anti-depressants in a breast feeding mother as some psychotropic drugs are secreted in breast milk. However, it is thought that low dose amitriptyline will not harm the baby. At higher doses, one may advise against breast feeding
- Tell the mother that it is helpful to discuss any concerns and her feelings

Psychiatry

Management

- The use of the Edinburgh PND scale can be a useful screening tool. It is a self-reported 10-item questionnaire that can be completed at 6-8 weeks post partum
- In cases of mild PND, anti-depressants should be avoided. At this stage, guided self-help, exercise or watchful waiting should be attempted
- However, if severity warrants it, offer referral to psychiatry and offer anti-depressants

Adequately assess and monitor safety of the mother and child:

- Increase visits by health visitors and regularly see the mother yourself
- If serious concerns arise regarding child and/or mother safety, urgent assessment by Mother and Baby Psychiatry is required
- It may be advisable to admit the patient to a Mother and Baby Unit to allow treatment (generally with the baby being present in the unit)
- Child protection issues may arise and need to be addressed

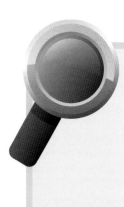

PRESENT YOUR FINDINGS...

'Mrs Roberts is a 24-year-old married lady who is 5 days post-delivery of her first child. She is tearful and feels 'down in the dumps'. She has no previous background of psychiatric illness. She has no thoughts of harm to herself or others (including her baby). She describes finding it difficult coping being a mother.

This is consistent with a diagnosis of 'baby blues.'

Reassurance and support should be provided in the community, with involvement of the health visitor/GP.'

Station 5: SUICIDE RISK

James Smith is a 45-year-old recently separated gentleman who has attempted to hang himself. However, the rope gave way. He is now medically fit for psychiatric assessment and you are asked to see him. Take a history from him to establish his suicide risk.

There is a lot of information to be obtained in a psychiatric history. Conduct your questioning in a structured manner, whilst simultaneously showing sensitivity by being flexible and exploring what the patient wants to talk about in greater detail.

A good approach to assessing suicide risk is to invite the patient to take you through an autobiographical timeline (starting at least 24 hours before the act of self-harm). Further assessment of risk can then be determined by:

- Taking into consideration the patient's risk factors
- The nature of the self-harm attempt

The Suicide Attempt

- What was the method?
- If a medication overdose, what was taken? Was it taken with alcohol?
- How long had they been planning to do this?
- Was an effort made to avoid detection? Did the patient think the dose/act would be lethal?
- How was the patient found? Did they seek help or were they 'discovered'?
- Was there a suicide note? Did they make a will?
- How does the patient feel about the suicide attempt?

Risk Factors (mnemonic for suicide risk factors – SAD PERSONS)

- **S**ex – *male*
- **A**ge – *over 40, or under 19*
- **D**epression
- **P**revious attempts/Plans to re-try
- **E**thanol or drug abuse
- **R**ational thinking loss *(e.g. psychosis)*
- **S**ocial isolation *(e.g. single, separated, widowed)*
- **O**rganised plan *(e.g. leaving a suicide note, getting affairs in order)*
- **N**o hobbies
- **S**ickness *(e.g. chronic pain)*

Also unemployment, recent change in life circumstances

Relevant History

- Have they attempted suicide before? Do they self-harm? Have they sought medical attention previously?
- Did anything happen to make them want to try to end their life?
- Do they suffer from any major illnesses? Depression: ask about mood, energy and enjoyment of life (mnemonic for some of the symptoms of depression – *SAW EMAIL* (**S**leep disturbance, **A**ppetite reduced, **W**eight loss, **E**nergy low, **M**ood low, Anhedonia, Irritability, Libido loss))

Future Risk

- Thoughts, intentions or plans for self-harm in the future
- *'How do you feel about the future?'*
- **Support network:** *'Where do you live?'*, *'Who do you live with?'*, *'Is there someone you can you talk to?'*
- **Insight:** Do they understand that they may require help to deal with this?

How may the patient be helped?

Any underlying disease could be treated, including depression. The patient could be counselled to deal with underlying emotions.

- Specialist groups such as 'Relate' could more specifically deal with relationship problems

- Methods to reduce work stresses (reducing hours and reducing tight deadlines) and financial problems could also be explored

- Beliefs could be challenged using Cognitive Behavioural Therapy

'If a patient has written a 'suicide note' you should read it, as it may provide insight into their motivation. A note that reads like an emotionally charged rant suggests a writer who desperately wants to be heard — the self harm may be a 'cry for help', whereas a note that reads like the instructions someone with a terminal illness would leave for surviving relatives is highly suggestive of suicidal intent — the writer expected to die'

Robby Steele
Consultant Liaison Psychiatrist
Royal Infirmary of Edinburgh

Psychiatry

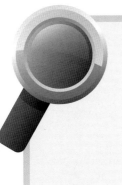

PRESENT YOUR FINDINGS...

'This patient has a high risk of successfully completing suicide. He has multiple significant risk factors for completed suicide (sex, age, social isolation). He believed and intended the suicide attempt to take his life, and made efforts to avoid detection. The attempt was pre-planned, and the stresses that led to it are still present.

The patient has evidence of untreated depression, and has a poor support network to help with adaptation to life stressors. I would encourage the patient to stay in hospital for further psychiatric assessment, ideally on an informal basis.'

Please take a history from this 19 year-old student, whose parents are worried is acting 'strange'. He has recently been hearing voices and believes his friends are out to get him.

Delusions

- *'Is there anything you're worried about?'*
- **Persecutory:** *'Do you feel like anyone's out to get you?', 'Do you feel safe?', 'Has anyone tried to harm you?'*
- **Delusions of reference:** *'Are there ever messages in the newspaper or on the television just for you?'*
- **Delusions of perception:** *'Would you say you see things in the same way as others?'*
- **Grandeur:** *'Do you have any special powers?'*
- **Nihilistic:** *'Do you ever feel like things around you are dying or rotting?'*
- **Passivity:** *'Do you ever feel like you're not in control of your thoughts or actions?'*
- **Test conviction:** *'Is there a chance you might be wrong?'*

Hallucinations

- **Auditory:** *'Have you ever heard things said when there is no-one about and nothing to explain it?', 'Do you recognise the voice?', 'How many different voices do you hear?', 'What do they say?', 'Have they ever told you to harm yourself or others?', 'Do they comment on your actions?', 'Have you ever heard your thoughts being repeated?'*
- **Visual/Olfactory/Gustatory:** *'Have you ever seen anything that you could not explain?', 'Have you ever smelled or tasted something you couldn't explain?'*

Thought interference

- **Thought insertion:** *'Do you ever feel like ideas are being deliberately placed into your head?'*
- **Thought withdrawal:** *'Do you ever feel your thoughts have been taken away?'*
- **Thought broadcast:** *'Can others hear your thoughts without you saying them out loud?'*

Differential Diagnosis

- *Organic syndromes e.g. dementia, brain tumour, temporal lobe epilepsy*
- *Drug-induced e.g. amphetamines, LSD, cocaine*
- *Mood disorder e.g. depression or mania with psychotic features*
- *Schizoaffective disorder*
- *Schizoid personality disorder*
- *Acute psychotic reaction*

General questions

- **Pre-morbid personality:** *'How would you describe yourself growing up?', 'How do you think others would describe you?'* (a schizoid personality sometimes predates a diagnosis of schizophrenia)
- **Psychiatric illness:** *'Does anyone in your family have a history of mental illness?' 'Have you ever had any issues with your mental health?'*
- **Insight:** *'Do you think there is anything wrong?', 'Do you think you need help?'*
- **Social history:** *'What support do you have at home?', 'Do you work?', 'Have you got any stress in your life at the moment?'*
- **Risk:** *'Have you ever had thoughts of (or attempted) harming yourself or others?' 'Have you ever had thoughts of (or attempted) ending your life?'*

Differential Diagnosis

- *'Do you smoke (if so, what do you smoke)?', 'Do you drink?', 'Have you ever taken any recreational drugs?'* If yes, explore further
- *'Do you have any health problems?'*
- **Mood:** *'Have you ever had periods of particularly low or high mood?'*

Schneider's first rank symptoms of schizophrenia are:

1. Thought Interference:

- Thought broadcasting (the experience of thoughts escaping one's head and being heard by all around)
- Thought insertion (the experience of a third party putting a thought into your head)
- Thought withdrawal (the experience of a third party taking a thought out of your head)

2. Auditory Hallucinations:

- Third-person hallucinations
- Voices providing running commentary
- Thought echo (patients hear their thoughts spoken out loud)

3. Delusional Perception:

- A person believes that a normal percept (product of perception) has a special meaning for them e.g. a post box may be a message that the world is about to end

4. Delusions of Control:

- The false belief that another person/group of people/outside force has control over your thoughts, feelings, impulses or behaviour

While suggestive of schizophrenia, first rank symptoms can be seen in other illnesses (e.g. delirium or mania) and are not sufficient for a diagnosis.

What is necessary for a diagnosis of schizophrenia?

ICD-10 states there must be at least one very clear symptom from Group A or two or more from Group B.

Group A:

A) thought echo, insertion, withdrawal or broadcasting

B) delusions of control, influence, or passivity

C) hallucinatory voices

D) persistent delusions of other kinds that are culturally inappropriate and completely impossible

Group B:

A) persistent hallucinations in any modality, when accompanied either by fleeting or half-formed delusions, or by persistent over-valued ideas

B) breaks or interpolations in the train of thought, resulting in incoherence, or irrelevant speech, or neologisms

C) catatonic behaviour

D) "negative" symptoms such as marked apathy, paucity of speech, and blunting or incongruity of emotional responses

Define the following: delusion, hallucination and psychosis.

A **delusion** is a fixed false belief which is not congruent with cultural norms.
A **hallucination** is a perception in the absence of a stimulus.
Psychosis is an umbrella term for a loss of contact with reality. There are many causes of psychosis, one of which is schizophrenia.

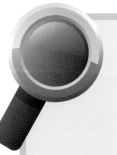

PRESENT YOUR FINDINGS...

'This is a 19-year-old student referred due to his strange behaviour. He describes a persecutory delusion of his classmates wishing to harm him. He also believes he has been sent threatening messages and has confirmed this through his TV. He frequently hears unpleasant voices talking about him and does not feel in control of his thoughts. He describes his classmates stealing his thoughts and often 'leaving him blank'. At the start of university, he describes using cannabis but has no relevant psychiatric or medical history. He denies thoughts of harm to himself or others.

These psychotic features may be associated with recreational cannabis misuse or the onset of psychotic illness such as schizophrenia. I would like to get a collateral history to further my assessment.'

Mrs Bradley has recently separated from her husband, and lost her job. She seems to be very depressed. Please perform a mental state examination on her and present your findings.

Appearance and Behaviour

Appearance

- **Dress:** loose (e.g. anorexia) vs. dishevelled (e.g. psychosis or dementia)? Brightly coloured? (e.g. mania)
- **Evidence of self-harm:** cuts? Bruising?
- **Evidence of physical neglect:** personal hygiene?
- **Evidence of physical illness:** e.g. hyper or hypothyroidism, Cushing's disease

Behaviour

- Quality of rapport and eye contact
- Tearful/anxious/suspicious

Mood (this is mostly from the history of the presenting complaint)

- Subjective and objective
- *'How are you feeling in your spirits?', 'Have you had any episodes of feeling sad or miserable?' 'How bad does it get/has it got?'*
- *'Have you ever felt on top of the world, like you could do anything?'*
- Affect (i.e. reactivity): *'Does your mood vary?', 'Do you find yourself getting tearful?'*
- Suicidal intentions and harming: *'Do you ever feel hopeless/like there's no hope left for the future?'*

Speech

- Tone
- Rhythm
- Rate e.g. pressure of speech
- Volume e.g. loud or quiet

Thoughts

- Thoughts are probably best considered as 'The How' of thinking (the 'mechanics' – or the form of your thinking) and 'The What' (the content or the beliefs you hold). Form is rarely disturbed but is highly significant when it is

Thought Form

- Coherence of conversation

Thought Content

- Ask the patient to describe present worries/preoccupations/obsessional ruminations
- Ask about self harm thoughts
- Ask the patient about abnormal thoughts (i.e. psychosis):
- *'Have you ever felt that people were against you?'*
- *'Have there been times when you felt something strange was going on?'*

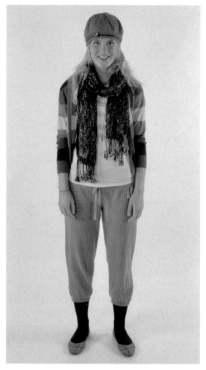

Fig 8.1: Brightly coloured clothes, in keeping with possible mania

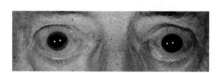

Fig 8.2: Medical disorders that might be noted on 'appearance': for example lid retraction suggestive of hyperthyroidism

> 'The single most important symptom predictor of suicide is hopelessness'
>
> ### David Cunningham-Owens
>
> *Professor of Psychiatry Royal Edinburgh Hospital*

Psychiatry

- 'Have your thoughts been directly interfered with by some outside force or person?'

Perceptions

- 'I'd like to ask you a routine question we ask everyone'
- 'Have you ever had the experience of hearing noises or voices but when you look there's no-one there and nothing to explain it?'

Cognition

- Is the patient orientated in time, place and person? (This is the order that people lose orientation)
- **Concentration:** e.g. serial 7s or list the months in reverse order
- **Other cognitive test function:** e.g. Mini-Mental State Examination (MMSE)

Insight (Into Illness)

- 'Do you think there has been a change in your mental health?'
- 'What do you think may be causing it?'
- 'Do you think you need any treatment?'

'Stick to aspects of orientation always in the same order ... this is the invariable sequence in which these key aspects of cognition are lost — time first, then place, then finally, and far down the road, person. While difficulty with orientation to time may be a source of concern, loss in person represents catastrophic disorder, with place in the middle'

David Cunningham-Owens
Professor of Psychiatry
Royal Edinburgh Hospital

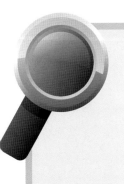

PRESENT YOUR FINDINGS...

'Mrs Bradley is a 56-year-old female who appears well-kempt. She displayed good eye contact throughout the interview and was tearful at times. Her mood was subjectively and objectively low, with a reactive affect. Her thought form is normal and her content centres around the recent separation from her husband, which she believes may be causing her low mood. She denies thoughts of harm to herself or others. She displays no evidence of abnormal perceptions, and is aware she may need treatment. I judge Mrs Bradley to be of reasonable intelligence and she is orientated to time, place and person.

Overall, Mrs Bradley is likely experiencing low mood secondary to adjustment in her life circumstances, namely recent separation from her husband. She has good insight into her condition.'

Mr Ahmed is a 68 year-old man who has been referred because his son has noticed his increasing forgetfulness. The son worries that his father may have some memory problems. Please make an assessment of the father's mental state.

History

- *'Tell me what's been going on?', 'What do you feel the problem is?', 'Do you ever get lost in familiar places?', 'Why are your friends/family concerned?', 'When did you start noticing things were different?', 'Is it getting worse?'*
- *'How is all of this affecting your life?'*
- Take a collateral history if possible, from somebody that knows Mr Jones (and his premorbid personality) well

The Mini-Mental State Examination (give score out of 30)

1. Orientation (/10)

- **Time:** *'What is the date?', 'What is the day?', 'What is the month?', What is the year?', 'What is the season?'* (score out of 5)
- **Place:** *'What country are we in?', 'What county are we in?', 'What town/city are we in?', 'What is the name of the building we are in?', 'On what floor are we?'* (score out of 5)

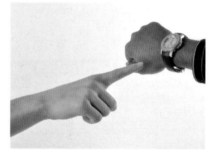

Fig 8.3: 'Can you tell me the name of the following'

2. Registration (/3)

- Say 3 common objects to the patient e.g. lemon, key and ball. *'Can you repeat the words I said?'* (score 1 point per word remembered)
- You can repeat the objects up to 6 times until all 3 are remembered

3. Attention and Calculation (/5)

- Either spell the word "WORLD" backwards (D-L-R-O-W)
  OR
- Keep subtracting 7 from 100. Stop after 5 answers (93, 86, 79, 72, 65)

4. Recall (/3)

- *'What were the 3 objects I told you earlier?'* e.g. lemon, key and ball (score 1 point per word remembered)

5. Language (/3)

- Naming: *'Can you tell me the name of the following?'* Point to watch, then point to pencil. (score out of 2)
- Repeating: Repeat the following after me: *'No ifs, ands or buts'* (score out of 1)

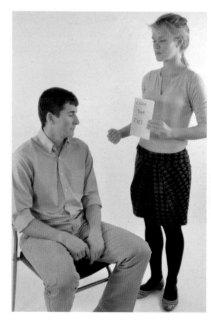

Fig 8.4: 'Close your eyes'

6. Reading and Writing (/2)

- Reading: Show card that says *"CLOSE YOUR EYES"* *'Can you read what is written and do what it says?'* (score out of 1) Do not explain the command on the card
- Writing: *'Can you write down a short sentence for me? It can be about anything'* (score out of 1)

7. Three Stage Command (/3)

- *'Take this paper in your right hand, fold it in half and place it on the floor'.* Do not mime or demonstrate the command

8. Construction (/1)

- *'Try to copy this drawing for me'*
Score 1 if each pentagon has 5 sides and there is a diamond shape in the middle. If there are any errors, then the patient scores 0.

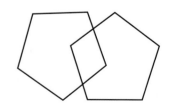

Fig 8.5: Construction

Psychiatry

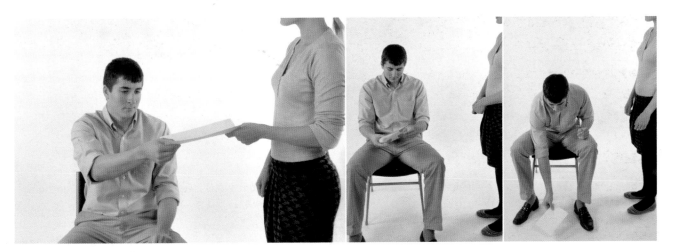

Fig 8.6: Three stage command

What would a normal score be on the MMSE?

The Mini-Mental State Examination is assessed out of a total of 30 points.
The MMSE is not a diagnostic test; instead, it is helpful in monitoring progress over time.

27+   suggests no significant cognitive impairment   **10-20**   suggests possible moderate dementia
24-27   suggests possible mild cognitive impairment   **<10**   suggests possible severe dementia
21-23   suggests possible early dementia

The MMSE does not provide information on executive function and ideally this should be supplemented with further tests such as the Frontal Assessment Battery (FAB) and/or the Addenbrooke's Cognitive Examination-Revised (ACE-R).

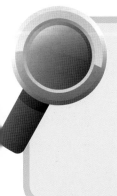

PRESENT YOUR FINDINGS...

'Mr Ahmed is a 68-year-old gentleman presenting with forgetfulness. He scores 15/30 on his mini-mental state examination, with a poor performance across all domains of the test.

This global impairment may be consistent with a diagnosis of dementia of moderate severity. However, a collateral history is required, particularly with respect to long-term cognitive impairment'

Assessing Memory

Immediate

DIGIT SPAN TEST:

- This assesses the ability to recall a list of numbers
- First state 2-3 numbers to the patient, in one second intervals
- Ensure this is done with a monotonous steady delivery
- Ask the patient to repeat the numbers back
- Gradually make the sequence of numbers longer, and repeat the test
- Ensure that the list of numbers is always random, and doesn't follow an obvious pattern e.g. 1-2-3-4, or 2-4-6-8
- The number of digits that can be remembered is the 'digit span'. A normal digit span is considered 7 +/-2

For short term memory, perform 'Recall' of the MMSE test (question 4)

Causes of Dementia

- *Alzheimer's Disease*
- *Vascular Dementia*
- *Lewy Body Dementia*
- *Fronto-Temperal Dementia*
- *Huntington's Disease*

- **Semantic:**
  - Ask the patient to describe a typical every day activity. *'How would you make a cup of tea?'*
- **Episodic:**
  - Autobiographical: *'When were you born?'*, *'Where did you live as a child?'*, *'When did you get married?'*
  - General Knowledge: *'Can you tell me the name of our Prime Minister?'*, *'Can you tell me any important news stories?'*, *'Can you tell me when World War One started?'*

Assessing Frontal Lobe Function

The questions in the MMSE do not adequately cover frontal lobe function. The frontal lobe is important in executive functioning, personality and memory.

Executive Function Tests

This is a loosely defined frontal lobe function. It is the set of brain functions responsible for selecting appropriate information, cognitive flexibility (a context dependant ability to change behavioural response), planning actions, abstract thinking and initiating/inhibiting appropriate actions. Some executive function tests are listed below.

- **FAS Test:** This measures the ability to generate categorical lists, as well as verbal fluency. *'Say as many words as you can in one minute that begin with the letter F'* (normal = 15 in one minute). Repeat this for the letter 'A' and 'S'. A rate of 10 in a minute is acceptable in the elderly
- **Proverb Test:** This measures the patient's ability to think abstractly. Look for reasonable explanations of common proverbs. For example, *'What do you understand by the phrase 'curiosity killed the cat?'* or *'What do you understand by the phrase 'killing two birds with one stone?'*
- **Assess the ability to make 'cognitive estimate':** For example, *'How many giraffes are there in London?'* These questions involve applying common knowledge to a relatively novel question. In this case, knowing that giraffes would only be in zoos, a reasonable answer would be 10-30
- **Association:** *'What do shirts and trousers have in common?'* (any tangible answer would be acceptable i.e. both are items of clothing). As with the above example, this assesses the selection of appropriate information, and abstract thinking

Frontal Assessment Battery

- This is a screening test for frontal lobe dysfunction
- It consists of 6 tasks, each scoring up to 3 points (maximum 18 points)

The test includes the following:

- **Assessment of programming ability:** (fist-palm-edge test) Tell the patient that you are going to demonstrate a series of hand movements to them. Do this (a fist, a palm, and displaying the edge of your hand) five times without verbal prompts and then ask the patient to repeat the series as many times as they can. Score 3 points if six consecutive series are performed, 2 points if 3 consecutive series, and 1 point if the patient requires examiner assistance to perform 3 consecutive series
- **Assessment of conceptualisation:** *'In what way are the following things alike?'* e.g. table, chair, stool, or daisy, tulip, rose. Assess three different categories, one point each
- **Verbal fluency:** This is similar to FAS testing. *'Say as many words (excluding proper nouns) in one minute that begin with 'S''* 3-5 words: 1 point, 6-9 words: 2 points, 9+ words: 3 points
- **Sensitivity to Interference:** This is known as the 'Go-No-Go' test, and assesses the patient's ability to deal with conflicting information. Instruct the patient to tap twice when you tap once. Then perform an example. Instruct the patient to tap once when you tap twice, and again perform an example. Then perform a series of ten single/ double taps (randomised) to assess the patient's ability to follow both commands simultaneously. No errors: 3 points, 1-2 errors: 2 points, 3+ errors: 1 point. 4 consecutive errors: 0 points
- **Inhibitory Control:** Instruct the patient to tap once when you tap once, and not to tap at all when you tap twice. Perform examples of both as before, and then perform a series of ten random single and double taps. No errors: 3 points, 1-2 errors: 2 points, 3 or more errors: 1 point. 4 consecutive errors: 0 points
- **Prehension Test:** This tests the ability to override prehensive (the act of grasping) behaviour by following commands. Instruct the patient *'do not take my hand'*. Place the patient's hand palm up, and then touch the palms of both patient's hands with yours to see if they will take them. Repeat if the patient takes your hand on the first attempt. Patient doesn't take your hand: 3 points, patient hesitates (and then doesn't take your hand): 2 points, patient takes your hand without hesitation (but doesn't the second time): 1 point, patient takes your hand even after repeating the exercise: 0 points

The Adenbrooke's Cognitive Examination-Revised (ACE-R) is a much more sensitive test that provides more information on a wider range of cognitive functions. It is scored out of 100, but takes much more time to compared to an MMSE.

9 Paediatrics and Child Health

The small people of the world have the ability to terrify medical students and doctors alike, particularly during exams. Our aim is to give you a broad framework for paediatric history taking, illustrated through clinically relevant and commonly examined areas. Teaching and demonstration of practical procedures is another important skill we will explore. This applies not only to teaching colleagues, but also to educating patients or parents about conditions, treatments and side effects.

In real practice, vital information can be obtained from asking a verbal child about their presenting problem; should a child be present in your exam, remember to include them, using a 'three way' consultation. You may need to deviate from the generally more structured approach used for adults to develop a rapport and gain the child's trust.

The paediatric OSCE at the medical student level is not a test of your ability to be a paediatrician. It is a test of 3 things:

1) Do you know how to take a paediatric history? This is an important skill because there are elements to the history that differ from an adult history, namely:

   a. The history is indirect, and you have to ask the carer for information, about which they may already have formed an opinion.

   b. The perinatal, immunisation, nutrition and growth, and neurodevelopmental histories are unique to paediatrics.

   c. The family and social history is more particular, given the utter dependence of the child upon these circumstances, the possible importance of congenital factors, and the possibility of child protection issues.

2) Do you know how to conduct a paediatric examination? This means conducting a thorough physical assessment as you would do in any human being, but doing so in a child friendly, age appropriate, opportunistic, but thorough way. Knowledge of what normal is (physiology and development, in particular) is crucial.

3) Do you know some basic facts about paediatric illness – loosely defined as facts that any non-paediatric doctor should know?

If you think about these 3 things, you will realise that just like in trigonometry, showing your working is as important, if not more important, than the answer. The diagnosis often only accounts for a small percentage of the grade compared to how you got there, and leaping to a diagnosis is a great way of selling yourself short – even if it is correct, but particularly if is not.

Remember that it is impossible to know every detail about everything, so when it doubt, do not make something up or guess. Explain that you will find out the answer to the question or you will get someone who knows more about the subject to come back and speak to them. Being aware of your own limitations is one of the most important skills to acquire prior to your first day as a junior doctor. If you are ever in doubt or unsure, the slight dent to your pride from asking for help will always outweigh the deep water you might find yourself in by giving the wrong information or performing procedures with which you are not competent or familiar.

Study Action Plan

- Invite your non-medic friends over and teach them how to use an inhaler, peak flow or spacer device
- Get them to be open and honest with you about your style of teaching and whether they have understood you
- An excellent guide that will tell you whether you have been successful is if your listeners can then subsequently teach another friend the same information
- You can do the same process with counselling about the MMR vaccination, diabetes, cystic fibrosis or Down syndrome

This chapter contains notes on the following systems:

Paediatrics

PAEDIATRIC HISTORY TAKING

- Introduce yourself to the parents and child (if present)
- Establish the name and age of the patient, as well as the source of history (i.e. the relationship of the adult(s) to the child)
- Adapt history taking to the child's developmental age (pregnancy and birth history are more pertinent for a neonate than a 15 year-old)

NOTE: Much of the adult history taking structure can be adapted and used for paediatric history taking

Presenting Complaint

- Start with a broad open question and allow some time for the child or parent to describe the symptoms
- Obtain a chronological description of the mode of presentation, sequence and duration of symptoms, hospital admissions, and management of problem so far including compliance

Remember, your job as a junior doctor is to get the story, and by asking the right questions in the right way, turn that story into a coherent, concise medical story

Past Medical History

- Previous illnesses and hospital admissions in chronological order
- Antenatal problems, gestation and mode of delivery, birth weight, and perinatal problems

Drug History

- Regular and as required medications, generic name, dose, frequency, route and indication
- Known allergies and description of the reaction

Growth and Development

- Appropriate weight, length/height and head circumference for age (plotted in the parent handheld record) – *'May I see your 'red/blue book' please?'*
- Plot on World Health Organisation (WHO) growth chart for hospital notes
- Achievement of developmental milestones: divided into 4 main areas – a) gross motor, b) fine motor and vision, c) hearing, speech and language, d) social

'Remember some children have learning disabilities and their developmental age may be lower than their chronological age — in this case establish their level of understanding'

Catherine Hill
Honorary Consultant Paediatrician
Solent NHS Trust

'Remember, the assessment of neurodevelopment, growth and puberty is all about asking 3 questions for any parameter — is this within the normal range, did they get there at a normal rate, and is it consistent with other parameters I am assessing?'

Ian Rodd
Consultant Paediatrician
Royal Hampshire County Hospital, Winchester

'Always carefully think about how to make the child as comfortable as possible. There are often toys and books available for them. Parents can be really helpful too: simple things like sitting the child in mum's lap can really put them at ease, especially during parts of an examination'

Zeshan Qureshi
Paediatric Trainee
London Deanery

Paediatrics

	Gross Motor	Fine Motor and Vision	Hearing, Speech and Language	Personal and Social
6 weeks	–	Fixes and follows	Coos and startles to noise	Smiles
6 months	–	Palmar	–	Smiles at self in mirror
7 months	Sits without support	–	–	–
9 months	–	–	–	Stranger anxiety
10 months	–	–	Says mama dada ('double babble')	–
12 months	Cruises, 1st step unsupported	Neat pincer grip	–	Plays peek-a-boo
15 months	Broad-based gait	–	–	Uses cup and spoon
18 months	–	Circular scribble	–	–
2 years	–	6 brick towers	20 words in total, and 2 words can be said together	Temper tantrums and can share with/ comfort others
3 years	Tip toes	Copy circle, 9 brick tower	First and last name and knows colours	Make-believe play
4 years	Hops, and climbs up and down stairs 1 foot per step	Build steps and draw a man	Count to 10 or more	Able to undress
5 years	Skips and runs on toes	Copy triangle	Asks 'how' and 'when'	Independent toileting

Developmental milestones up until the age of 5 should be enquired about. If the main focus of the station doesn't appear to be related to developmental problems, it is sufficient to ask 1 or 2 questions pertinent to each of the 4 categories. The ages in the table correspond to **AVERAGE AGE** and are a rough guide. Be aware that a large variation exists for these ages depending on the source of information.

'As a student, I sat down with a Denver Developmental Screening Kit and worked out what 95% of kids were doing at this age, looking for things I could assess easily and followed an obvious progression. That meant I could follow a logical progression from one to the next whilst having an idea of what a child of that age should look like, comparing in my minds eye to the child in front of me.

For example, with gross motor: normal power, tone, symmetry and reflexes > head control > sit > crawl > pull to stand > cruise > walk > run > jump up > jump across > stand on one leg'

Ian Rodd
Consultant Paediatrician
Royal Hampshire County Hospital, Winchester

Nutritional History

- Breast/ bottle-fed, weaning, current dietary and fluid intake
- For each mode of feeding, document what they are taking, whether it seems to be going well or whether there are any concerns

Family History

- Similar illness especially if symptoms infective in nature or symptom complex associated with a familial disease
- Serious illness (genetic, metabolic, allergic, or infectious)
- Asthma, diabetes, eczema, food allergy, epilepsy
- *'Has anyone in the family ever had any similar problems?'*
- *'Are there any problems that run in the family, particularly in childhood?'*

> 'In practice, asking a child about their school, teacher or friends is a good way to establish a rapport and gain trust prior to examining them. Most children will know the name of their teacher, what they look like and whether they are nice or not so this is a much safer bet than asking whether they have seen the latest pixelated Hollywood film!'
>
> **Sebastian Gray**
> *Paediatric Trainee*
> *Wessex Deanary*

Immunisation History

	DTaP	IPV	HiB	PCV	Men C	MMR	HPV
2 months	Yes	Yes	Yes	Yes	X	X	X
3 months	Yes	Yes	Yes	X	Yes	X	X
4 months	Yes	Yes	Yes	Yes	Yes	X	X
12 months	X	X	Yes	X	Yes	X	X
13 months	X	X	X	Yes	X	Yes	X
3-5 years	Yes	Yes	X	X	X	Yes	X
12-13 years	X	X	X	X	X	X	Yes
13-18 years	dT*	Yes	X	X	X	X	X

DTaP: Diphtheria, tetanus, acellular pertussis

IPV: Inactivated polio virus

HiB: Haemophilus influenzae B

PCV: Pneumococcal conjugate vaccine

Men C: Meningococcal C

MMR: Measles, mumps, rubella

HPV: Human papilloma virus

BCG and hepatitis B vaccination is given to newborns in high risk groups

dT*: Diphtheria, tetanus

Social History

- *'Who else is at home?'* – draw a family tree of 1st degree relatives (parents and siblings) with a larger pedigree diagram if there is a genetic condition
- Check blood relationships (important for parental responsibility and thus consent)
- Age, occupation and health of parents and age and health of siblings
- If parents are separated or divorced, establish where the child spends time
- Ask about parental smoking, pets, housing (particularly if respiratory or allergic symptoms)
- Recent travel (if relevant from history)
- Education and school: Impact of illness/problems on school performance and behaviour; is the child in mainstream or special needs school; peer relationships and behaviour

Station 1: A CRYING BABY

Mrs Jones is a 32 year-old mother of Mabel, who is 5 months old. She is consulting her GP today as Mabel will not stop crying. Please take a full history from Mrs Jones about her child.

Presenting Complaint – Crying

- Onset: recent (e.g. trauma or sepsis) or persistent?
- How often? Duration? (normal baby's crying increases in frequency from birth to an average peak of 2.5 hours a day by 2 months)
- Intermittent (e.g. infantile colic/ gastro-oesophageal reflux/cow milk protein intolerance) or constant (e.g. trauma)?
- Character: high-pitched (e.g. meningeal irritation) or distinctive cry (e.g. cat like cry in cri du chat)?
- Any triggering factors? (e.g. recent immunisations, cow's milk introduction)
- Timing in relation to feeds, time of day? (e.g. infantile colic in evenings)
- Has anything helped? What have you tried to soothe her? (e.g. upright posture helps with reflux)
- Has anything made it worse? (e.g. lying flat in reflux)
- Associated symptoms or signs (e.g. fever, drawing up of knees (infantile colic), rashes, stool (frequency, consistency, blood), back-arching (infantile colic or regurgitation))
- Any investigations so far?

Past Medical History

- Systemic enquiry: e.g. stool: loose in gastroenteritis, red currant jelly in intussusceptions, rash, strong smelling urine, cough, coryza
- Take a full paediatric history as described at the beginning of this section
- Ask if there is any other information the parent feels is relevant that hasn't been mentioned or whether they have any questions or specific concerns
- Social situation: family set-up, other siblings, support network, stress or anxiety

Common Causes of Crying

Non-Organic Causes

- Organic causes should never be overlooked and the first priority is to exclude serious organic illness. However, babies are sensitive to their environment and the emotional climate (if parents are stressed, anxious, or irritable)
- This can easily be transmitted to the baby and manifest itself as persistent crying
- Persistent crying can also be a sign of neglect or non-accidental injury
- Mothers can also complain of incessant crying when in fact the baby is crying a normal amount; in these cases, it is important to screen the mother for postnatal depression (can present up to 2 years from the time of birth)

Infantile Colic

- Unlikely at this age – colic normally resolves by 4 months
- The child is completely well but cries paroxysmally and inconsolably with associated drawing up of knees; usually takes place several times a day, especially in the evening
- Such a diagnosis can only be made once all other possible diagnoses have been excluded (usually by no improvement with trial of cow's milk-free diet followed by trial with anti-reflux treatment)

Gastro-Oesophageal Reflux

- Typical symptoms include: crying after feeds, regurgitation/ vomiting of food, arching of the back, and if severe, failure to thrive
- It is common in the first year of life but by 1 year of age, nearly all cases of symptomatic reflux have resolved (due to a combination of maturation of the lower oesophageal sphincter, weaning onto solid food and a more upright posture)

Cow's Milk Protein Allergy

- Quite common (incidence approximately 4%) with 60% of cases non IgE-mediated (IgA)
- Post-infective transient cow's milk protein intolerance can present similarly
- It can present with crying, as well as diarrhoea, vomiting, failure to thrive, acute colitis (with bloody diarrhoea), constipation, or non-GI atopic symptoms (e.g. eczema)
- Treatment is with a cow's milk protein-free diet, using hydrolysed milk formulas (e.g. Pepti or Nutramigen) or an elemental feed (e.g. Neocate)

Causes of a Crying Baby

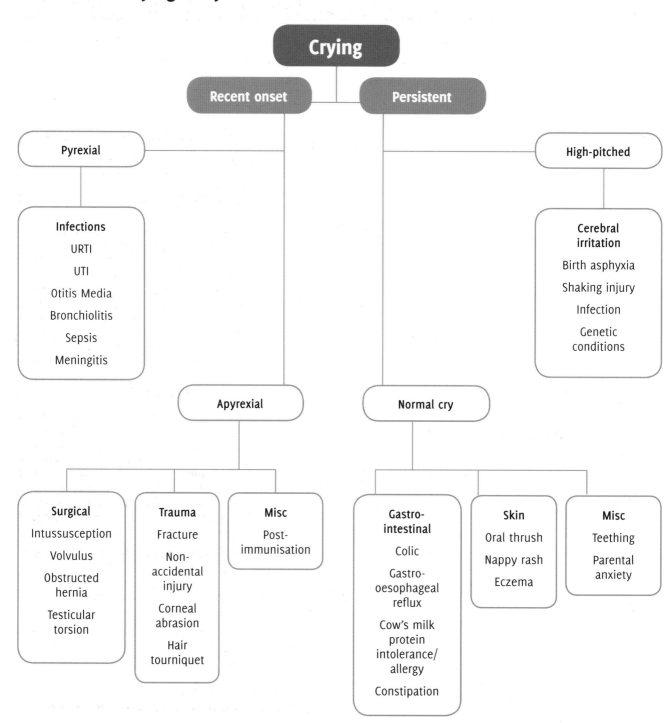

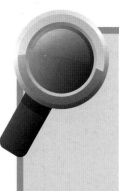

PRESENT YOUR FINDINGS...

'Mabel is a 5 month-old girl who presented with occasional intermittent crying since birth following feeds associated with small vomits, which had been decreasing in frequency. Her mum reports that she is growing along the 50th centile for height and weight. Today, the crying has become more persistent and unrelated to feeds. She has been rubbing her right ear and been coryzal with a low-grade temperature of 37.9°C.

The history is suggestive of an acute viral infection on a background of gastro – oesophageal reflux. I would like to fully examine Mabel and have a period of observation on the paediatric assessment unit.'

Station 2: FEBRILE CONVULSIONS

You are asked to see Fred, a 2 year-old child who has been brought in with his mother. He has presented with a temperature and a fit. You examined the patient and found signs consistent with acute otitis media. Take a history from the mother and arrive at a likely diagnosis.

Presenting Complaint – Convulsions

- *'Was he ill in any way before the fit?' 'Did he have a fever?'*
- *'What immediately preceded the event?'*; consider pain, temper tantrum or breath-holding attack
- *'How long did the fit last?'* (febrile convulsions tend to last less than 2 minutes)
- *'What happened during the fit?'*; *'What areas of the body were involved and in what order?'*; colour changes; stiff or floppy; clonic movements; loss of consciousness; eye-rolling; incontinence (if toilet-trained), injuries sustained
- *'What happened after the fit' 'How long was it before he completely recovered?'* (Children rapidly recover from simple faints, whereas fits are associated with a 'post-ictal' phase)
- *'Did he start acting any differently after the event?'*
- *'Did he appear weaker on one side?' 'Has there been any obvious change in his behaviour?'* (consider space occupying lesion for either of the above)
- *'What do you think this was?'* (useful in terms of framing your feedback in terms of level of prior understanding)

Past Medical History

- *'Does he suffer from epilepsy?'*
- *'Does he suffer from febrile convulsions?'*
- *'Do either of these conditions run in the family?'* (known increased risk of febrile convulsions if positive family history)
- Systemic enquiry: this will particularly focus on identifying a potential source of infection
- Take a full paediatric history as described at the beginning of this section
- Ask if there is any other information the parent feels is relevant that hasn't been mentioned or whether they have any questions

NOTE: Unless the history is consistent with an obvious febrile convulsion secondary to a respiratory tract infection it is always worth at the very least to perform a urinalysis and check the blood sugar

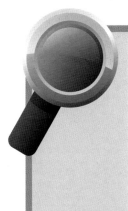

PRESENT YOUR FINDINGS...

Fred is a 2 year-old boy who presented to hospital with a 'fit' today. He has had no medical problems so far, other than one previous 'fit' four months previously. Today's episode lasted 3 minutes. Fred became pale and began to shake all four limbs. He was less responsive after the seizure, but was back to his normal self after a few minutes. He has been suffering from an ear infection for the last 2 days, with a temperature of 38.5C. His older brother and father both suffered from 'febrile convulsions'.

Given that the examination findings are consistent with acute otitis media, this is consistent with a diagnosis of febrile convulsions, but I would check a urine dipstick, and blood glucose. I would reassure Fred's parents about this diagnosis and also give them advice about how to prevent and manage any further febrile convulsions along with a written information sheet.'

What is your differential diagnosis?

I am reassured by the history, and the most likely diagnosis is febrile convulsions. Other diagnoses more generally for convulsions include:

- Epilepsy
- Rigor (associated with infection)
- Infantile Spasm (although the patient in this scenario is too old for this)
- Breath-Holding Attack (hypoxic mechanism)
- Reflex Anoxic Seizure (vaso-vagal mechanism)
- Meningitis
- Head Injury

'In any febrile child it is important to have a thorough search for a focus of infection, including ear and throat examination (which you may not necessarily do in every febrile adult)'

Zeshan Qureshi
Paediatric Trainee, London Deanery

Can you explain the diagnosis to the mother?

- Ask if she has heard of 'febrile convulsions' and if so, what is her understanding of these convulsions
- Infection can lead to a rising temperature which can increase the body's susceptibility to a 'fit'. These fits tend to have two phases, the first where the body goes stiff and muscles tense up, the second, where there is rapid contraction and relaxation of the muscles. The fit is usually brief, and usually symmetrical
- Age range: 6 months to 6 years, less than 6 times, no increased risk of developing epilepsy (if brief, typical febrile convulsion)
- Reassure the mother that there should not be any permanent damage: the child will develop normally and that most children tend to grow out of them
- The best treatment is to prevent the fits from happening in the first place:
  - When pyrexial – don't panic, cool the child down using simple measures (e.g. remove clothing, fan in vicinity but not directly on them), antipyretics (currently debatable – recommended by most paediatricians in practice but not by NICE – more to alleviate symptoms associated with fever than to prevent febrile convulsions, as there is no evidence to support this)
- If fits do occur:
  - Again, don't panic, place the child in the recovery position to protect their airway (ensure that the parent understands this and if not, explain +/ – demonstrate) and ensure the child is safe by removing objects that could result in injury
  - Ring for an ambulance if at all concerned, particularly if the seizure is different in any way or is longer than 5 minutes in duration. The child may need medication to stop the seizure. The ambulance can always be cancelled if the seizure self-resolves

Station 3: WHEEZE

Tommy, a 3 year-old boy, has presented to the Accident and Emergency department with wheeze. Please take a history from Mrs McShire, his mother.

Presenting Complaint

- *'When you say wheeze, what do you mean?'*
- *'When did the wheezing start?'* (gives a time frame of illness, particularly useful in bronchiolitis which gets worse before getting better, and onset is usually before the age of 18 months)
- *'Did it start suddenly or has it gradually come on?'* (e.g. sudden onset with a large foreign body aspiration, although smaller body can cause gradual onset wheeze due to oedema and inflammation)
- *'Is it getting better, worse or staying the same?'* (allows judgement of disease progression, if already improving then only supportive management may be required)
- *'Is the wheezing constant or does it come and go?'* (e.g. intermittent with allergen triggered asthma, constant with inhaled foreign body)
- *'Was he unwell when the wheezing started in any other way?'* (e.g. preceding cough, coryza and low grade pyrexia, typical of viral induced wheeze)
- *'Does he have any other symptoms?'* (e.g. cough, pyrexia, coryza, poor feeding, weight loss, rashes, sweating with feeds)
- *'Can you think of anything that may have triggered this?'* (e.g. inhalation of foreign body, triggers of asthma e.g. exercise, viral infections)
- *'What have you tried so far to help?' 'Did it help?'* (e.g. parents sometimes use medication from older siblings e.g. salbutamol inhaler. Be aware that this is not effective in under 1s due to decreased B receptor sensitivity and different pathophysiology – small airway calibre with increased mucous secretion causing clogging rather than bronchospasm)

Past Medical History

- Birth and neonatal history: more thorough if premature, including respiratory management, days ventilated, days in oxygen, whether home oxygen required
- *'Has he ever been wheezy before?'*
- *'If so, what treatment did he receive?' 'Did it help?'*
- If recurrent admissions, ask about frequency of GP visits, hospital admissions and maximal treatment (IV salbutamol, paediatric intensive care, intubation and ventilation); previous investigations (e.g. imaging, sputum cultures, sweat test, skin prick testing, and lung function tests. Spirometry if an older child)
- Ask about interval symptoms: *'Does he cough at night?'* *'Does he get more breathless when he runs around than other children his age do?'*
- *'Does he suffer from asthma, eczema or hay fever/ allergic rhinitis?'*
- Current medication. Any recent courses of steroids? Are there any issues with compliance (with any medication) or technique with an inhaler? (if the patient is a known asthmatic, a thorough exploration of inhaler use and technique is required)
- Plot on the growth chart and ask to see red/blue hand-held parent record

Paediatrics

Other Questions

- Family History: *'Does anyone in the family suffer from wheeze, asthma, eczema or hay fever?'*
- *'Is he exposed to any pets either at home or where he spends a lot of time?'; 'Do they make him worse?'*
- *'Does anyone at home smoke?' 'If so, where?'*
- Details of housing, type of flooring, furnishing, recent change of address
- Systemic enquiry
- Take a full paediatric history as described previously
- Ask if there is any other information the parent feels is relevant that has not been mentioned or whether they have any questions or concerns

'Parents will often say that because of the child, they now only smoke outside. It is important to tell the parents that this is still harmful for the child (due to smoke particles remaining on their clothes and on their breath), and that they should ideally stop smoking completely'

Zeshan Qureshi
Paediatric Trainee
London Deanery

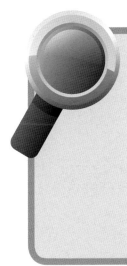

PRESENT YOUR FINDINGS...

'Tommy is a 3 year-old boy who has presented with his first episode of wheeze. He has had cough and coryza for the last two days. His mum gave him his brother's salbutamol inhaler via a spacer which initially helped but as he has become more breathless, it had no further effect. Both parents smoke, they have no pets and they live in a 2 bedroom flat, where Tommy shares a room with his 7 year-old brother, who has asthma. He has no interval symptoms but does suffer from eczema.

The history is consistent with viral-induced wheeze which I would manage in the same way as an acute asthma exacerbation. He has no interval symptoms and therefore does not currently warrant initiating regular preventer inhalers. Given the positive family history and his eczema, there is a strong chance he may develop asthma and I would strongly recommend that the parents stop smoking.'

What is your differential diagnosis of wheeze?

The most likely diagnosis given the above history is viral-induced wheeze. However other diagnoses that I would consider in a wheezy patient include:

- Asthma
- Bronchiolitis (e.g. Respiratory Syncytial Virus, Adenovirus)
- Severe gastro-oesophageal reflux with recurrent aspiration
- Chronic lung disease of prematurity
- Inhaled foreign body
- Cystic fibrosis (or other causes of bronchiectasis)
- Atypical pneumonia (e.g. Mycoplasma pneumoniae)
- Heart failure – 'cardiac wheeze'
- Congenital abnormality of lungs or airways (e.g. distal bronchomalacia)

What factors would you use to assess the severity of an acute asthma attack?

Severe

- Oxygen saturations <92%
- Unable (too breathless) to complete sentences, talk or feed
- Tachypnoea (>40 breaths/min in 2-5 year-olds, >30 breaths/min in over 5's)
- Tachycardia (>140 beats/min in 2-5 year-olds, >125 beats/min in over 5's)
- Peak flow 33-50% predicted or best value

Other Factors

- Use of accessory muscles (intercostals, sternocleidomastoids, diaphragm)
- Nasal flaring, grunting and head bobbing in infants
- Pulsus paradoxus (difficult to measure accurately)

Life-threatening

- Oxygen saturations <92%
- Silent chest
- Poor respiratory effort
- Cyanosis
- Exhaustion
- Hypotension
- Signs of cerebral hypoxia (drowsiness, confusion, agitation, coma)
- Peak flow <33% predicted or best value (unlikely to be measured if this unwell!)

Paediatrics

Zac White is a 14 year-old boy who has been recently diagnosed with diabetes and is about to commence insulin therapy. Please explain the diagnosis, and options for insulin treatment to him. Address any concerns he and his parents may have.

- *'I understand you have been recently diagnosed with diabetes. Would it be OK if I discussed this further with you and your parents?'*
- *'I would like to start by asking you a few questions first to help me understand your lifestyle better?' 'What school do you go to?' 'What year are you in?' 'What interests do you have outside school?' (Ask specifically about sports) 'What is your diet like?'*
- *'How much do you know about diabetes? Do you know anyone with diabetes?'*
- *'We will chat things through today, but before we start, is there anything in particular you are worried about?'*

Note: The approach in paediatrics is very dependent upon the age and maturity of the child or adolescent. Adjust your approach so that the salient points are conferred to the most appropriate person. For example, the management of diabetes in a 6 year-old should primarily be explained to parents as opposed to a mature 16 year-old, who should be given the information directly. Nonetheless it is crucial to involve the child from the outset.

Description of Diabetes

- *'Diabetes is a condition where your body becomes unable to control sugar levels due to a lack of the hormone insulin. Every cell in your body needs sugar to work properly and insulin acts like a key to unlock the door to get sugar from the blood. Without insulin, the sugar stays in the bloodstream and can make you feel unwell. You may experience symptoms like weeing a lot, being very thirsty, losing weight, tummy ache and becoming very drowsy'*
- *'As your body cannot produce its own insulin, it is important we give it in the form of an injection to control the sugar levels'*
- *'Controlling your sugar levels is very important in preventing long-term problems that could affect your eyes, kidneys, heart, blood vessels, skin, nerves and feet'*
- *'We will continue to monitor your diabetes control by performing blood tests, looking at HBA1c levels (which are a measure of more long term sugar control). You will have regular appointments but it also very important that you keep a diary of your sugar levels at home'*
- *'You will be meeting a lot of different people who help look after people with diabetes. These include the diabetes specialist nurses, dieticians, podiatrists, eye specialists as well as your paediatrician and GP'*
- *Check understanding of what has already been discussed before moving on*

Potential Concerns

These can come from either the parent or the child. Adapt the encounter to address the specific concerns that matter to the family. For example:

What is Diabetes? Why did I get this? Have I done anything wrong? How do I find out more about the disease?

What is the Treatment? How do we administer it? Fitting it into, and adapting it to lifestyle. What do I do if I miss a dose? Weight gain with insulin?

What are the Complications? How can we prevent the complications (of disease, and of treatment): Sugar too high? Sugar too low?

Lifestyle Consequences: Change with age: diet, alcohol, exercise, driving, injecting at school, sexual relations

Anxieties from Experience of Disease: Relative/ friend with disease (may be type II diabetes), suffering complications or even death from diabetes

Treatment of Diabetes

- There are various different insulin regimens used to treat diabetes:
  - Basal bolus:
    - **Advantages:** More flexible with greater control over eating pattern, allows self-adjustment of insulin by 'carbohydrate counting', more physiological
    - **Disadvantages:** Increased frequency of injections, children need to inject during school hours (social stigma, requires good adherence)
  - Twice daily:
    - **Advantages:** Fewer injections
    - **Disadvantages:** Requires regular small snacking to prevent hypoglycaemia, stricter meal times
  - Insulin pump:
    - **Advantages:** Precise insulin dosing control
    - **Disadvantages:** Expensive (to set-up and to maintain), attached permanently, infection risk, requires frequent glucose monitoring, increased risk of insulin delivery failure
- *'The diabetes specialist nurse will show you how and where to give the insulin injections'*
- *'It is important to rotate the injection sites to prevent complications and problems with absorbing the insulin'*

- 'We will also put you in touch with a dietician who can give you advice on your diet'
- Good glycaemic control can be particularly challenging during puberty and adolescence due to a number of factors:
  - Increased insulin requirement associated with the pubertal growth spurt
  - Rebellious behaviour and less rigid monitoring
  - Exposure to alcohol (may be unable to see that the short-term gain of drinking does not outweigh the long-term benefit of good glycaemic control)
  - Body image issues and deliberate missing of insulin to lose weight (particularly in adolescent girls)

Potential Complications: Hypoglycaemia

- 'With diabetes, there is an increased risk of your sugar levels dropping dangerously low and it is very important that you can recognise this early and know what you can do to treat it'
- Symptoms can be divided into:
  - **Neuroglycopenic**
    - Headache, irritability, confusion, seizures, coma
  - **Adrenergic**
    - Tremor, tachycardia, sweating, hunger, pallor, visual changes

  Note: Some may be completely asymptomatic – hence stress importance of regular monitoring!

- Treatment:
  - When to treat? → '4 is the floor'
  - Dextrose tablets or 50mls sugary drink (e.g. Coke, Lucozade)
  - Followed by a longer-acting carbohydrate (e.g. bread, banana)
  - If drowsy → HYPOSTOP
  - If unconscious → GLUCAGON
- Check understanding

Diabetes is a huge area and particularly for the newly diagnosed, there is a vast amount of information to take in. It is therefore important to offer written literature and details on advice or support groups. The diabetes specialist nurses provide excellent support and advice and it is well worth spending some time with them during your training. It is also important to remember that children with diabetes will need continuous re-education as they grow up and their level of understanding improves. New issues such as driving may then become important.

Station 5: NON ACCIDENTAL INJURY

Fred, a 5 month-old baby boy, has been brought to the Emergency Department by his mother after he "rolled off the sofa". He has broken his right humerus. You are asked to see his mother in the ED about his injury.

Child abuse is classified into four main areas:

Physical	Causing physical harm Examples: hitting, shaking, poisoning, burning, suffocation
Emotional	Constant neglect or ill treatment, adversely affecting emotional development Examples: making a child feel worthless, inducing fear in a child, deprivation of social activity
Sexual	Enforcing/enticing sexual activity. Includes non-penetrative acts Examples: encouraging sexual behaviour, looking at pornographic material, sexual contact
Neglect	Constant failure to meet basic needs of the child (physical or psychological) Examples: insufficient food, clothing, shelter, or medical care

Parents have also been reported to fabricate or induce illness in their child (Fabricated or Induced Illness; FII). This can lead to harm from unnecessary medical investigations, and by taking time away from normal daily activities such as school.

History

Child abuse is an extremely delicate matter and when suspected, should be handled by the most senior, experienced person available. However, every medical professional that is exposed to children should have the training and awareness to recognise and act upon suspected cases of child abuse. It is a legal duty to do so, and to escalate concerns until you are satisfied that your concerns have been dealt with appropriately.

Paediatrics

General Points

- Ask questions in a calm, non-judgmental manner (e.g. *'what happened?'*) Avoid leading questions (e.g. *'Were you hurt?'* or *'Did mum hit you?'*) Remain calm and open, explaining your reasons for questions if challenged
- Try to speak to the child separately, with an additional professional present who can document the child's account accurately; this can be done without the carer's consent (the reasons must be documented clearly in the notes)
- Never make promises of confidentiality to a child, as you may need to break such promises in order to notify the police or social services
- Speak to all third parties involved
- If interpreters are required, use one from outside the family
- Whilst taking a history of this nature, family members may become very defensive or angry in response to questioning
- Leave if you feel threatened (ensuring the child is safe)

Things to look out for include:

- The child's manner and behaviour while recounting the history – do they look uneasy or worried? Are they looking around for confirmation of their story from their parents?
- Inconsistency between family members or accounts of the history over time
- Does the history match a) the injury sustained? b) the child's developmental age?

Different cultural or social sensibilities are no defence for hurting a child

> 'Remember, you are not a policeman or social worker and are not collecting forensic evidence or building a case. You are simply doing your job; taking a history, assessing red flags and risk factors, forming a differential diagnosis and making a management plan'
>
> **Ian Rodd**
> *Consultant Paediatrician*
> *Royal Hampshire County Hospital, Winchester*

> 'Carefully document, sign and date your history and clinical findings. If a child discloses information to you document their words as accurately as possible, preferably contemporaneously or if this is not appropriate, immediately after seeing the child' (the same applies to parents' accounts)
>
> **Catherine Hill**
> *Honarary Consultant Paediatrician*
> *Solent NHS Trust*

Past Medical History

- Have any previous injuries been sustained? Were any of them suspicious?
- Does the patient suffer from any chronic illnesses? (risk factor for child abuse)
- Predisposing factors to pathological fractures: could there be another explanation to the current presentation? (e.g. Osteogenesis Imperfecta is associated with an increased fracture risk)

Aspects of a presentation that would arouse suspicion include:

- Injuries inconsistent with history
- Delayed presentation
- Multiple admissions
  - In different surgeries, and different hospitals
  - Sometimes life-threatening
  - Witnessed only by one carer
  - No medical explanation

Social History

Family situation:

- Who's at home?
- Are the parents together?
- How are the parents coping? Do they have any troubles (e.g. financial)?
- Are there any domestic abuse issues involving the parents/carers?

Social services involvement:

- Involvement for problems relating to this child
- Involvement for problems involving other children/issues

Risk Factors

Specifically elucidate whether risk factors for abuse are present:

- Previous child abuse in the family (includes child abuse suffered by the suspected offender); this information can normally be acquired from social care records and is likely to be inflammatory if directly asked
- Illness or disability in parents/carers – both physical and mental illness
- Illness or disability in the child/sibling

- Domestic abuse
- Drug/alcohol misuse
- Criminal record
- Parental learning disability
- Single parent families/social isolation
  - Look out for very young parents, especially those with little support

N.B. Some children are vulnerable to being 'lost' by the system and therefore it will be difficult to find out information about their background (e.g. where the families are homeless or asylum seekers)

Examination (unlikely as an OSCE station but important to know about)

- Gain consent: from child (if competent), carer with parental responsibility or if parents refuse to cooperate consult social care and police (police protection order or emergency protection order may be required)
- Examination can be done without explicit consent if it is considered an emergency and in the child's best interest
- Clearly mark examination findings on a body map which should be counter-signed by a second doctor (always sign and date clearly)
- Do not do anything invasive that will need repeating soon or that you are not experienced at doing, in particular genital examination

Observation

- The examination begins by noting the appearance and behaviour of the child and their interaction with carers
- Look for any sign of anxiety or apprehension in the child when examining. Is the child very reluctant to be touched/undress? Is the child excessively clingy? Look for signs of neglect (e.g. clothing and hygiene)
- Some children may be inappropriately friendly and fail to show healthy attachment with the parent(s)
- 'Frozen watchfulness' is a sign of severe abuse; the child looks watchful, carefully tracking other people's movement; they may also have an expression of fear on their face
- Observe the relationship of the parent to the child; do they stop the child from speaking to healthcare professionals alone? Are they hostile to the child?

Establishing Whether the Injury Pattern is Suspicious

- Remember that children are often hurt/marked in places that are thought to be less likely to be seen or found, so be thorough in your examination
- Be as objective as possible and describe your findings without making conclusions or judgements

Bruising, Burns and Scalds

- Describe the location, colour and size (by measuring accurately) of each individual insult
- How many insults are there? multiple bruises are suspicious

- Where are they? Accidental bruises tend to be on bony prominences (e.g. shins); unusual sites for accidental bruises include the ears, neck, abdomen and back
- What shape are they? This can offer a clue as to the cause of the injury, if at all suspicious (e.g. cigarette stub or belt mark)
- Is the insult well demarcated?
- Are the insults symmetrical? Submersion in hot water will give a symmetrical 'glove and stocking' distribution of scalds
- If there are multiple bruises or burns, are they regularly or irregularly distributed? Accidental injuries tend to be irregularly distributed
- Petechiae can be suggestive of shaking or suffocation (suggestive, but not diagnostic – around 10% of 'well' babies will have one or more petechiae)

Fractures

- *Any* fracture in a baby too young to walk or crawl
- Multiple fractures, at different healing stages
- Rib fractures – very suspicious if:
  - In young children
  - Posterior rib fractures
- Sternal fracture
- Long bone fracture
  - Metaphyseal or spiral fractures – spirals imply a twisting action has been applied
  - Subperiosteal haemorrhage – this is often a result of pulling or grabbing (may take around two weeks to show up on x-ray)
- Spinal injuries without confirmed major trauma
- Skull fractures

Head and Eye Injuries

- Can occur from a blow to the head or shaking
- Accidental skull fractures are rare in children under 5 years of age, even after a fall from more than 90cm; question a fall/ roll from a bed or sofa, which is often cited as a cause for such an injury
- Intracranial injury with no major confirmed trauma or medical cause, especially in children under 3 years of age

Internal Injuries

- Intrathoracic or intraabdominal injuries, without confirmed major trauma

'It is important that the student mentions referral to social care is made immediately as they are the lead agency for Child Protection investigations'

Catherine Hill
Honorary Consultant Paediatrician
Solent NHS Trust

Management

- The child's safety and wellbeing is the *single most important thing;* act to ensure that this is maintained at all times, which can include overriding confidentiality and consent, if necessary

- **The role of the student/ junior is not necessarily to diagnose child abuse, but to refer to somebody more experienced in the field**

- Talk to a senior doctor, nurse or child protection lead as soon as possible

- Document your findings without conjecture (useful for assessing consistency of story following subsequent assessments)

- In the case of sexual abuse, to avoid further unnecessary trauma to the child, the examination should be performed only once by the most senior child protection trained doctor available

What investigations might be requested in cases of suspected non-accidental injury?

If child abuse is suspected in a non-ambulant infant, they will need the following 4 investigations:

Bloods – full blood count and clotting screen to exclude bruising/bleeding disorders

Skeletal survey – a series of X-rays that can take up to 1 hour to complete to exclude occult fractures (if any found, to be repeated 2 weeks later to exclude previous subtle fractures)

CT Brain – to exclude intracranial bleeds (may need a subsequent MRI if abnormal)

Ophthalmological assessment – to exclude retinal haemorrhages (seen in shaken babies)

Further investigations are based on the site and nature of injuries and may include:

Ultrasound – for soft tissue injury, such as muscle haematoma

STI screening – if sexual abuse is suspected

Dentist review – to interpret bite marks, even to identify the abuser

Plastic surgery review – to interpret and also guide further management of burns

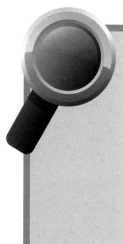

PRESENT YOUR FINDINGS...

'This 5 month-old boy, Fred, sustained a fracture to the right humerus after his mother reported him rolling off the sofa 4 days previously. There are no other injuries found on examination.

His mother, a single parent, has a history of alcohol dependence and says that she has been struggling with life recently. Fred looks very anxious, and is reluctant to be examined. It is of note that his 3 year-old sister has been into A and E on previous occasions with multiple unexplained injuries.

This raises safeguarding issues, which must be referred to social care and investigated further by senior colleagues. I would like to look at an X-ray of the right humerus, and organise a skeletal survey, CT brain, ophthalmology assessment and perform blood tests.'

Station 6: MMR VACCINATION

Mr and Mrs Fletcher have come to your clinic with their son Sandy. They are keen to get the MMR vaccine for him, but have some concerns about what they have heard in the media. Please discuss the pros and cons of getting the MMR vaccine with his parents.

'What have you heard about the MMR vaccination?' 'Would you like me to tell you a bit more about it?'
The MMR vaccine is given at 12-13 months and again at 3-5 years, unless contraindicated or if the parents refuse.

	Rubella	**Measles**	**Mumps**
Presentation	Headaches, general body aches, anorexia, low-grade fever, and nausea. There may also be a discrete rose – pink maculopapular rash ranging from 1-4 mm. Other signs include eye pain on lateral and upward eye movement, conjunctivitis, and tender lymphadenopathy (particularly posterior auricular and suboccipital lymph nodes).	Fever, coryza, cough, lymphadenopathy, and a generalised maculopapular, erythematous rash. Koplik spots are pathognomonic. These are small red spots with a white centre on buccal mucosa.	Fever, malaise, rash, and swelling of parotid glands and cervical lymph nodes.
Complications	The major risk of rubella occurs when it is acquired during pregnancy, resulting in congenital rubella. In childhood, it can cause arthritis, and rarely thrombocytopenia and encephalitis.	Pneumonia, otitis media, haemorrhagic problems, blindness, and subacute sclerosing panencephalitis (SSPE). Potentially lethal in immunosuppressed patients.	May cause unilateral deafness and meningitis. If infected after puberty, epididymo-orchitis and infertility may occur.

Benefits

- Provides protection for the child against measles, mumps and rubella; it is the safest and most effective way to decrease risk
- Also protects the community but only if there is a greater than 95% uptake rate 'herd immunity'. If there is a less than 95% uptake, the risk of MMR re-emerges

Contraindications

- Immunocompromised
- Malignancy
- Another live vaccine given in previous 3 weeks
- Acute febrile illness (defer until recovered)
- Allergies to gelatine or neomycin; egg allergy is not an official contraindication to MMR vaccine (due to miniscule amounts of egg protein)

Risks

- Can develop a fever or rash for a couple of days, usually about 1 week after immunisation
- Liquid paracetamol can be given as analgesia; however, NICE does not currently recommend it as a means to prevent febrile convulsions
- There is <u>NO</u> evidence of any link to autism or inflammatory bowel disease

Potential Concerns

- **General Concerns about Vaccinations:** Do they cause long term side effects? Do they work? Can having lots of vaccinations 'overload' the immune system (by constantly challenging the immune system)?

- **Need for the MMR Vaccination:** What are measles, mumps and rubella? Why give now rather than in a few years? Can my child still get these diseases?

- **Risks of the MMR Vaccination:** Links to autism and inflammatory bowel disease

- **Contraindication to the MMR Vaccination:** Particularly may be concerned about egg allergy. Recent infection

- **Alternatives to MMR Vaccine:** Can we just be very careful, with healthy living, and keeping him clean? What about single vaccinations?

- **Anxiety from the Child:** Will it be painful?

Paediatrics

Alternatives

The MMR vaccine is recommended by the Royal College of Paediatrics and Child Health and the World Health Organisation. Single jabs are not available on the NHS – the patient would need to use private healthcare.

- There is no evidence that these are as effective as, or safer than the combined MMR vaccine
- Single jabs entail 6 injections instead of 2; this is more painful and traumatic for the child

- Single jabs leave the children more vulnerable to the disease for a longer period of time
- Poor compliance is more likely, since the parents might forget to bring the child back for further vaccinations
- Single jabs would mean that the child is not fully immunised until the age of 7
- Advise the parents that the final choice remains with them, but that from a medical perspective, the MMR vaccine is strongly recommended

Station 7:
GENETIC COUNSELLING – CYSTIC FIBROSIS

Mr and Mrs Taylor are pregnant with their first child. They are concerned about cystic fibrosis, since Mrs Taylor's sister recently gave birth to a child with this condition. Please inform the couple about cystic fibrosis and advise them about their available options.

'What do you understand about cystic fibrosis? What concerns do you have at the moment?'

Establish how Mrs Taylor's niece with cystic fibrosis (CF) has affected their perception of the disease

'Would you like me to explain what CF is?'

Introduction to Cystic Fibrosis

- CF is a genetic disease that causes some of the secretions produced by the body to thicken
- The main organs affected are the lungs and the pancreas, which is a gland needed to help digest food
- This can result in children being susceptible to lung infections, having difficulties with absorbing food properly, and general ill health

Genetics

- On average, one out of 25 white European individuals have one copy of the faulty gene but there is a higher 'carrier rate' if there is a family history of the disease
- To have a baby with CF, the baby needs to inherit 2 affected genes, one from each parent; therefore, both parents must be carriers
- If both parents are carriers, there is a 1 in 4 chance of the baby having CF (you could use simple diagrams to represent this if you can do this quickly and clearly)

Testing for Cystic Fibrosis

'The tests available are carrier testing, antenatal testing and neonatal testing'
- Carrier testing: simple mouthwash test can tell if you or your partner carries the gene
- Antenatal testing: if both the parents are carriers, the test can be carried out early in the pregnancy to tell whether baby has CF

Potential Concerns

- **What is Cystic Fibrosis** Why do people get it? How does it affect the body? Can you live to a normal age with it?

- **Living with Cystic Fibrosis** What does it mean to have child with CF? How will life be different? Will we both be able to continue working? What help would we be able to get?

- **Testing for Cystic Fibrosis** What is the chance one of my children would have CF? What are the possible tests? What are the risks of the tests? How certain can you be that my child won't have the disease if the tests are negative? Will the results be kept confidential? Will I be able to terminate the pregnancy if the test is positive?

- Chorionic villus sampling: at 8-10/40 gestation (1% risk of miscarriage)
- Amniocentesis: at 16-20/40 gestation (0.5% risk of miscarriage)
- Neonatal testing: heel-prick test on a Guthrie card – determines the level immunoreactive trypsin (IRT): higher levels of this enzyme make CF more likely (this is now part of the national neonatal screening programme)

Management of Cystic Fibrosis

- If a child is diagnosed with CF, the baby and the parents can be supported in many ways
- Management involves a multi-disciplinary team approach
- There is no known cure, but treatments such as physiotherapy, antibiotics, and enzyme replacement prolong and improve the quality of life

- The available treatment has greatly improved over past 10 years
- Median survival is into the 30's and increasing due to the availability of better treatments; there is potential for leading a nearly normal life
- Termination of pregnancy is an option that can be considered
- Another option is IVF with pre-implantation DNA analysis (not currently offered on the NHS)
- Ask the parent how they would feel about having a baby with CF (may be premature in this scenario but could be discussed if mother is confirmed a carrier)
- Encourage discussion with the partner and family
- Offer further follow up and written information about CF

The 5 Generic Stages of Educating Patients/ Families:

1. Establish what they already know about the subject
2. Explain what you know about the subject
3. Allow opportunity for questions or any concerns and address these
4. Summarise what has been discussed and check understanding
5. Offer written literature or reference to helpful websites and opportunity to meet again

Station 8:
GENETIC COUNSELLING – DOWN SYNDROME

Mr and Mrs Bradley are pregnant with their fourth child. They are concerned about the possibility of Down syndrome due to Mrs Bradley's age (35 years-old). Please advice the couple as to what Down syndrome is and what screening options are available.

- *What do you understand about Down syndrome?'*
- *'Would you like me to go through with you what Down Syndrome is?'*
- Establish understanding, concerns, and specific fears
- *'Our genes that determine our make up are divided across units called 'chromosomes'. Normally we have two copies of each chromosome, but in Down syndrome, there is a third copy of chromosome 21'*

People with Down Syndrome:

- Look different compared to babies without Down (must not compare to 'normal')
- Are slower to develop and will have some degree of learning difficulty
- May develop or be born with heart and bowel problems
- Likely to develop an early onset dementia, similar to Alzheimer's disease

Likelihood of Down Syndrome

- The risk increases with older age of the mother at the time of pregnancy
- Pregnancy at age 35 gives a risk of 1/250

Testing for Down Syndrome

- If you were to become pregnant, we can calculate the specific risk of Down syndrome for that pregnancy
- Triple blood test (alpha fetoprotein, a-FP; beta human chorionic gonadotropin, ß-hCG; oestrogen) and nuchal fold translucency on ultrasound can be performed at 16/40 to elucidate the risk of Down syndrome for that pregnancy
- These investigations give individual risks, which may increase or decrease the relative risk calculated based on age – but this is not an absolute yes or no

Potential Concerns

- **What is Down Syndrome:** Why do people get it? How does it affect the body? Will it affect the heart? Can you live to a normal age with it?

- **Living with Down Syndrome:** What does it mean to have child with Down Syndrome? How will life be different? What help would we be able to get? Will my child have learning difficulties/ need to go to a special school/ have behavioural problems?

- **Testing for Down Syndrome:** What is my risk of having a child with Down syndrome? Are there any possible tests for it? What are the risks of the tests? Will I be able to terminate the pregnancy if the test is positive?

- Based on these results, parents may wish to proceed to a definitive screening test for Down syndrome
- The severity of learning and behaviour difficulties and in many cases the congenital defects (e.g. cardiac) cannot be predicted antenatally

Risks of Investigations

- 2 definitive tests can be done
- At 8-10 weeks of pregnancy, chorionic villous sampling may be carried out; there is a 1% risk of miscarriage and foetal abnormality
- Amniocentesis can be done at 16-20 weeks with a 0.5% risk of miscarriage

Other Issues to Consider

- 'How would you feel if your baby has Down syndrome?'
- 'Would you continue with the pregnancy?'
- 'Parents have often found their lives enriched by children with Down syndrome – they are loving and affectionate'
- Offer to provide written information about Down syndrome (including information about the Down Syndrome Association) and an opportunity for further discussions

'You won't have time to talk about every aspect of Down syndrome. It is important to cover the key facts of the disease, but make sure you identify and address the parent's main concerns: the concerns may not be what you expected them to be'

Zeshan Qureshi
Paediatric Trainee
London Deanery

Station 9: ASTHMA – PEAK FLOW

Mrs Patel has come to your clinic with her 7 year-old son, Sandeep. He has recently been diagnosed with asthma, and has been advised to keep a peak flow diary. Please teach him how to perform a peak flow.

Benefits of Peak Flow

'I understand you have recently been diagnosed with asthma. Asthma can make breathing difficult. Peak flow measures how bad your asthma is at any time, by showing how much air you can breathe out quickly.'

How to Perform Peak Flow

1) 'Stand up'
2) 'Move the dial to 0; when using the device, ensure that your fingers do not touch the scale or markers'
3) 'Put the mouthpiece on – there should be a tight seal around the mouthpiece'
4) 'Inhale and fill your lungs as much as possible'
5) 'Put your lips around the device'
6) 'Lift your chin up, and straighten your back to open airways'
7) 'Breathe out as fast and as hard as you can (as if you are blowing out candles)'
8) 'Check the dial, record the reading and move the dial back to 0'
9) 'Allow a short period to recover and then repeat, doing it a total of 3 times'
10) 'The highest of the 3 readings is your peak flow of that time'

- Language used may need to be adjusted dependent on child's level of understanding (the language above is what would be explained to a young adult/ adult, as children are unlikely to appear in your exam)
- Ask the patient to demonstrate how to perform peak flow
- The patient may be asked to keep a peak flow diary. This is important to establish diurnal variation in peak flow associated with asthma, and in establishing any environmental triggers associated with asthma
- Show the child the peak flow diary, and give them an example of how to record measurements

'Make sure the patient can perform a peak flow independently: after talking them through it, watch them do it completely on their own. And make sure they do it standing up!'

Zeshan Qureshi
Paediatric Trainee
London Deanery

Station 10: ASTHMA – INHALER TECHNIQUE

Mrs Andrews has come to your clinic with her son James, aged 8 years. He has recently been diagnosed with asthma, and has commenced using regular inhalers. Please teach them how to use an inhaler with a spacer.

Background Information

- The *blue* inhaler is a reliever and should be used when symptomatic (e.g. when the patient is wheezy)
  - 'If you use this inhaler more than 3 times/week, make an appointment to see your GP'
- The brown inhaler is a preventer and should be used regularly (e.g. twice daily)
  - 'Remember to rinse your mouth with water (or mouthwash) thoroughly after using it to prevent side effects'

Note: When starting patients on inhalers it is important to highlight that they will feel immediate symptomatic relief after using the reliever inhaler (blue) but the effect of the brown inhaler is longer term. Emphasising this early on should improve adherence.

Technique (Metered Dose Inhaler (MDI) Without Spacer)

1) 'Check the expiration date'
2) 'Shake the inhaler well'
3) 'Sit up straight and lift your chin to open your airways'
4) 'Remove the inhaler cap'
5) 'Empty your lungs as fully as possible'
6) 'Put the inhaler in your mouth'
7) 'Ensure a good seal with lips firmly around the mouthpiece (do not bite it)'
8) 'Take a slow deep breath in while pressing the canister at the same time'
9) 'Once your lungs are full, take the inhaler out of your mouth, hold your breath for 10 seconds, and then breathe out slowly'
10) 'If more than one puff is required, wait 30 seconds, then repeat steps 2 to 9'
11) 'Replace the lid on the inhaler'

- The inhalers last for about 200 puffs
- The inhalers have a use-by-date printed on the side; if this expires, you will need to get another inhaler from your doctor
- Emphasise that if the child needs more than 6 puffs at any one time or is using the inhaler more than 3 times a week, they should see their GP
- Offer to watch the child use the inhaler

Using a Spacer

Depending on age, different systems are used for delivery of inhaled asthma medications:

- Older child/adult: MDI with or without spacer
- 2-10 years old: MDI with spacer
- <2 years old: MDI with spacer and mask

There are different types of spacers. For example:

- Babyhaler: in <2 year-olds (with face mask) – does not have to be upright; listen for 5 clicks
- Volumatic: in >2 year-olds (with or without face mask) – should be seated upright
- Aerochamber with 3 different sized masks for infants, children and adults (now most commonly prescribed spacer in the UK)

Advantages of a Spacer

'You use a spacer because using an inhaler on its own can be tricky even if your technique is really good. Using a spacer makes it easier, so more of the contents of the inhaler will get into your lung, which is where it needs to go to make your breathing easier.'

It can be used approximately 200 times before it needs to be replaced.

Using a Spacer

1) 'Check the expiry date of the inhaler'
2) 'Assemble the spacer: this will depend on the particular design, but is straightforward'
3) 'Shake the inhaler well'
4) 'Remove inhaler cap and slot inhaler into the spacer'
5) 'Place in mouth or if using a mask, put mask over baby's mouth and nose'
6) 'Press canister once to release a dose into the spacer'
7) Get the patient to take 5 normal tidal breaths; in the case of babies, leave it over their face for 10 seconds, ensuring it clicks or the valve in the spacer moves
8) 'Take the device out of the mouth'
9) 'If another puff is required, wait 30 seconds, shake the inhaler well, replace into spacer and press again'
10) 'When finished, remember to put the cap back on the inhaler'

Washing a Spacer

- 'Wash it once a week'
- 'Take it apart and wash in warm, soapy water'
- 'Leave to drip dry – do not wipe dry or put in dishwasher'

- Should also be replaced every 3-6 months

Side Effects of Inhaled Steroids

Inhaled steroids produce fewer side effects than systemic steroids. Side effects are more likely to occur with higher doses and when the inhaler technique is poor. They include:

- *Candida* infection of the mouth
- Hoarseness

Rarer Side Effects

- Adrenal suppression: non-specific symptoms like anorexia, abdominal pain, weight loss, headache, nausea and vomiting
- Skin: easy bruising and thinning of skin
- Weakened immunity: instruct patient that they should inform their doctor if ill
- In comparison with non-asthmatic children, children with asthma may have a later onset of puberty and growth retardation

'Good technique should be reinforced on several occasions, not just one, especially if the asthma is worsening'

Zeshan Qureshi
Paediatric Trainee
London Deanery

9 // Paediatrics and Child Health

10 Practical Prescribing

Prescribing in emergencies can be very daunting for a junior doctor, let alone a medical student given an acute scenario in a prescribing exam! However a sensible, systematic approach to any scenario will ensure that you can prescribe in a safe and competent manner.

Below are some key points that are essential for establishing a systematic and safe approach to prescribing.

Essential Tips to Good Prescribing

- ABCDE (airway, breathing, circulation, disability, exposure) still remains the basic approach for any sick patient
- Write clearly with black ink and use CAPITAL LETTERS
- Each separate page of the prescription chart needs to have the patient's full details clearly documented. This should include name, surname, date of birth and hospital number (and weight in paediatric patients)
- Document clearly any allergies; state the drug and describe the reaction
- Acceptable dose abbreviations include mg (milligrams), g (grams), ml (millilitres). All other units must be written in full (micrograms NOT mcg)
- Insulin prescriptions must have Units written in full (e.g. Lantus 40 units, rather than Lantus 40U)
- Never abbreviate ORAL or INTRATHECAL, other routes of administration may be abbreviated, e.g. IV (intravenous), IM (intramuscular), SC (subcutaneous), PR (per rectum), INH (inhaled), NEB (nebulised)
- When prescribing antibiotics, write the indication and an end or review date
- Oxygen is a drug and needs to be prescribed, with the device to be used (e.g. Hudson mask, venturi mask etc) and target saturations stated (e.g. 94-98%)
- Always consider whether the patient will need prophylaxis for venous thromboembolism
- Always consider whether the patient will benefit from 'as required' medication, such as anti-emetics, analgesia, laxatives, inhalers or GTN
- Correct fluid balance is essential to the management of any medical and surgical emergency, so always check IV fluids are appropriately prescribed on a fluid chart
- Consider which of the patient's routine medication are contraindicated or may have contributed to any given emergency. They may need to be discontinued in the acute setting (if unsure, always speak to a senior doctor)
- Review the usage of intravenous medication: do not give via this route unless necessary
- Your signature must always be accompanied with your name clearly printed, and bleep/ extension number if applicable to your hospital
- Write the date and reason for stopping any medication on the prescription chart (see scenario 5 for an example)

In the scenarios below we will be considering the immediate treatment of common clinical scenarios. This chapter contains the following scenarios:

Study Action Plan

- Practice, practice, practice is the key to learning prescribing
- Try to see patients on the ward/in the medical admission unit and then make an active judgement on what drugs need to be stopped or started. Check your decisions with that of the doctor who subsequently sees the patient
  - It's always easier to remember things if you can relate it to a patient encounter
  - Similarly you'll be able to learn from your mistakes
- Don't worry too much if you can't remember the dose of a drug at the beginning
  - Doses become second nature with practice
  - If you are not sure, always check in the British National Formulary (BNF)
- Try developing new scenarios with friends – this chapter shows you some of the more common medical and surgical emergencies

Prescribing

You are the junior doctor covering a cardiology ward overnight. The nurses fast bleep you to see a 75 year-old man who has become acutely breathless and is coughing up frothy pink sputum. An echo done on this admission showed severe left ventricular dysfunction. He had been written up for IV fluids overnight (1L IV NaCl 0.9% over eight hours) since he was deemed to be dehydrated.

Obs: *Sats 74% (on 2L/min oxygen), RR 30, HR 142, BP 148/86, T 37.6°C*

O/E: *The patient is acutely dyspnoeic and looks panicked. There is frothy pink sputum in the sick bowl next to him. He is tachycardic but has normal capillary refill. You can see a rhythmic "wiggling" of his earlobes. He has loud bilateral crepitations on auscultation and a third heart sound.*

ECG   *Sinus rhythm at 150 beats per minute with ST depression anterolaterally.*

CXR   *Portable CXR shows fluid in both horizontal fissures, upper lobe diversion, "bats wing shadowing" and Kerley B lines.*

Initial Assessment

Airway

- Is the airway obstructed? Is the airway patent?
- Is the patient able to maintain their own airway? Secure the airway if necessary

Breathing

- Assess the respiratory rate and oxygen saturations
- Perform a respiratory exam, especially looking for increased work of breathing (and evidence of tiring) and listening for basal lung crepitations
- Give oxygen if saturations are less than 94%
- Sit the patient up
- Perform an Arterial Blood Gas (ABG), and request an urgent Chest X-ray (CXR)

Circulation

- Assess haemodynamic stability by measuring pulse (rate, rhythm and character), blood pressure, capillary refill time and urine output (if being recorded)
- Perform a cardiovascular exam, looking at the JVP for evidence of right heart failure, listening to the lung bases for evidence of pulmonary oedema, and auscultating the heart looking for evidence of valvular disease (especially mitral regurgitation or aortic stenosis)
- Obtain intravenous access and send blood for urea and electrolytes. Also send full blood count and C-reactive protein (CRP) if concerned about infection, and glucose if concerned about diabetic states
- Perform an ECG if an infarct is suspected, the patient has gone into an abnormal heart rhythm, or the patient is very tachycardic
- Stop intravenous fluids

Disability

- Assess the patient's conscious level, either using AVPU (Is the patient **Alert?** If not, do they respond to **Verbal** or **Painful** stimuli? Or are they **Unresponsive?**) or Glasgow coma score (GCS)
- Check glucose levels. Breathlessness may be Kussmauls respiration in diabetic ketoacidosis (DKA). Acute clinical deterioration can be associated with insulin resistance, and consequently DKA or hyperosmolar non-ketotic diabetic state (HONK)

Exposure

- Expose the patient, and look for further evidence of fluid overload (e.g. pitting peripheral and sacral oedema). Look for evidence of a DVT

> ## Management of LVF: "L,M,N,O,P"
>
> - *Loop Diuretic*
> - *Morphine*
> - *Nitrates*
> - *Oxygen*
> - *Posture*
> - *Regular reassessment*

Initial Investigations

- **ABG:** Assess the degree of hypoxia, and whether this is associated with an acidosis (this will be important in determining whether BiPAP (bilevel positive airway pressure) or CPAP (continuous positive airway pressure) is required). Be careful in patients with renal failure; they may be in type 1 respiratory failure and have an acidosis from a metabolic aetiology as well
- **CXR:** Confirm the diagnosis of pulmonary oedema. Look for potential causes of pulmonary oedema. Heart failure is differentiated from acute respiratory distress syndrome (another cause of pulmonary oedema) by cardiomegaly, and upper lobe blood diversion (since fluid collecting in the alveoli at the base of the lungs increases vascular resistance). Look for other causes of breathlessness (e.g. consolidation or pulmonary embolism). A portable CXR will be required if the patient is too unstable to go to the X-ray department safely
- **ECG:** Look for evidence of a myocardial infarction. Look for arrhythmias such as atrial fibrillation, which may be a cause or a consequence of pulmonary oedema
- **BLOODS:** Look for evidence of infection, assess renal function

Initial Management

Use the acronym "L,M,N,O,P" to help you remember:

- **LOOP DIURETIC:** Furosemide. If currently on a diuretic or in renal failure may require higher doses e.g. 40-100mg IV. May also require a furosemide infusion (given slowly due to ototoxicity risk). Elderly patients, especially with low body weight, might require lower doses
- **MORPHINE:** Titrate to pain 1-10mg IV over 5-10 minutes. It acts a) as an analgesic b) to reduce anxiety and consequent hyperventilation c) as a weak venodilator, directly reducing pulmonary oedema. Prescribe with an appropriate antiemetic
- **NITRATES:** GTN spray in the first instance if systolic blood pressure >100mmHg. If the patient is not responding to furosemide, or sublingual nitrates, and their blood pressure is still holding, consider starting a GTN infusion (starting dose depending on baseline BP between 0.3mg/hr and 1mg/hr)
- **OXYGEN:** High flow oxygen (>60% via Venturi mask). If the patient is in 'type 1 respiratory failure', consider CPAP early for refractory hypoxia
- **POSTURE:** Sit the patient up; gravity can be your friend!
- **CONSIDER EARLY HDU/ITU REFERRAL:** Either for monitoring (central venous pressure, arterial blood pressure) or for treatment (CPAP for type 1 respiratory failure or BiPAP for type 2 respiratory failure)
- Ensure the patient is on **thromboprophylaxis,** and is written up for PRN GTN, morphine, and an antiemetic
- **MONITOR URINE OUTPUT:** This is important to assess whether a good diuresis has occurred. Insert a urinary catheter if not already in place

PRESCRIPTION AND ADMINISTRATION RECORD

Standard Chart

Hospital/Ward: WGH/53	Consultant: CAP	Name of Patient: JOHN SMITH
Weight: 75kg	Height: 1.82m	CHI Number: 1202350034
If re-written, date:		D.O.B.: 12/02/35
DISCHARGE PRESCRIPTION Date completed:-	Completed by:-	(Attach printed label here)

OTHER MEDICINE CHARTS IN USE		PREVIOUS ADVERSE REACTIONS This section must be completed before any medicine is given		Completed by (sign & print)	Date
Date	Type of Chart	None known ☐			
6/9/10	NONE	Medicine/Agent	Description of Reaction		
		PENICILLIN	FACIAL SWELLING AND RASH	M Jones (JONES)	6/9/10

CODES FOR NON-ADMINISTRATION OF PRESCRIBED MEDICINE

If a dose is not administered as prescribed, initial and enter a code in the column with a circle drawn round the code according to the reason as shown below. **Inform the responsible doctor in the appropriate timescale.**

1. Patient refuses
2. Patient not present
3. Medicines not available – CHECK ORDERED
4. Asleep/drowsy
5. Administration route not available – CHECK FOR ALTERNATIVE

6. Vomiting/nausea
7. Time varied on doctor's instructions
8. Once only/ as required medicine given
9. Dose withheld on doctor's instructions
10. Possible adverse reaction/side effect

ONCE ONLY

Date	Time	Medicine (Approved Name)	Dose	Route	Prescriber – Sign + Print	Time Given	Given By
6/9/10	2000	FUROSEMIDE	40MG	IV	M Jones (JONES)		
6/9/10	2000	GTN SPRAY	2 PUFFS	SL	M Jones (JONES)		
6/9/10	2000	MORPHINE (TITRATE TO PAIN)	1-10MG	IV	M Jones (JONES)		
6/9/10	2000	METOCLOPRAMIDE	10MG	IV	M Jones (JONES)		

O X Y G E N		Start		Route		Prescriber – Sign + Print	Administered by	Stop	
	Date	Time	Mask (%)		Prongs (l/min)			Date	Time
	6/9/10	2000	VENTURI (60)			M Jones (JONES)			

24 HOUR FLUID PRESCRIPTION CHART

Hospital/Ward: WGH/53	Consultant: CAP	Name of Patient: JOHN SMITH
Weight: 75 kg	Height: 1.82m	CHI Number: 1202350034
		D.O.B: 12/02/35
		(Attach printed label here)

Date/ Time	FLUID / ADDED DRUGS	VOLUME / DOSE	RATE	PRESCRIBER – SIGN AND PRINT
6/9/10 1700	0.9% SODIUM CHLORIDE	1000ml	OVER 8 HOURS	P Smith (SMITH) STOPPED DUE TO FLUID OVERLOAD 6/9/10 2000 M Jones (JONES)

You are the junior doctor covering the acute receiving unit overnight. The nurses fast bleep you to see a 70 year-old man who has been admitted with acute severe chest pain.

Obs: Sats 90% (on 2L/min oxygen), RR 30, HR 142, BP 148/86, T 37.6°C

O/E: The patient is clutching his chest and is feeling very sweaty and nauseated. He is tachycardic but has normal capillary refill.

ECG   2mm ST elevation throughout anterior leads

CXR   Portable CXR is unremarkable

Patients with ST elevation acute coronary syndrome should be considered for primary percutaneous coronary intervention (PCI) as soon as possible. When primary PCI cannot be provided within 90 minutes of diagnosis, patients with ST elevation acute coronary syndrome should be considered for immediate thrombolytic therapy

Initial Assessment

Airway

- Is the airway obstructed? Is the airway patent?
- Is the patient able to maintain their own airway? Secure the airway if necessary

Breathing

- Assess the respiratory rate, and oxygen saturations
- Give supplementary oxygen to maintain oxygen saturations >94%
- Perform a respiratory exam, particularly listening for basal crepitations which suggest left heart failure
- Request a CXR

Circulation

- Assess haemodynamic stability by looking at pulse, blood pressure, JVP, capillary refill time and urine output
- Perform a cardiovascular exam. Particularly listen for murmurs, and look for signs of heart failure
- Obtain intravenous access and take bloods
- Perform ABG only if likely to affect management: damages arteries, making PCI more difficult, especially if repeated attempts
- Perform an ECG and place on telemetry

Disability

- Assess the patient's conscious level, either using AVPU or GCS. Check glucose

Exposure

- Expose the patient, and perform a full examination focusing on any obvious precipitating factors (haemorrhage, sepsis). Look for evidence of DVT

Initial Management of Acute MI:

ROMANCE:

- **Reassure**
- **Oxygen**
- **Morphine**
- **Aspirin**
- **Nitroglycerine**
- **Clopidogrel**
- **Enoxaparin (or Fondaparinux)**
- **Regular reassessment**

Initial Investigations

- **BLOODS:** Look for evidence of anaemia, infection, electrolyte derangement, renal impairment, myocardial ischaemia. Baseline and 12 hour troponin, full blood count, urea and electrolytes, liver function tests, lipid profile, glucose, thyroid function
- **ABG:** Allows assessment of the metabolic status of the patient as well as the ventilation/oxygenation. May find respiratory acidosis or features of peripheral hypoperfusion giving mixed picture
- **CXR:** Look for evidence of heart failure (pulmonary oedema) secondary to the acute MI. This will need to be a portable CXR if the patient is not stable enough to go to the X-ray department
- **ECG:** Look for evidence of a myocardial infarction and monitor dynamic ECG changes and secondary arrhythmias by performing serial ECGs

Initial Management

- **OXYGEN:** to keep saturations >94%
- **IV ACCESS**
- **ANTI-EMETIC:** Metoclopramide 10mg IV (caution as may precipitate oculogyric crisis, particularly in young women, consider cyclizine 50mg IV as an alternative)
- **MORPHINE:** 2.5-10mg IV initially titrating to pain
- **ASPIRIN:** 300mg to chew and **CLOPIDOGREL** 300mg
- **NITRATES:** sublingual spray, but if chest pain continues, consider a nitrate infusion

- **Consider treatment with Enoxaparin or Fondaparinux**

- **CONTACT:** Cardiology and/or critical care areas (CCU/HDU/ICU) for definitive management of STEMI and further support
- Contraindications to thrombolysis include known or suspected intracranial tumour, aortic dissection or pericarditis, a stroke, gastrointestinal or genitourinary haemorrhage within the last 3 months, major surgery, trauma, biopsy or head injury within the last 6 weeks, puncture of a non compressible vessel, bleeding diathesis, prolonged cardiopulmonary resuscitation (>10 minutes), impaired consciousness following cardiac arrest and pregnancy
- Patients undergoing primary percutaneous coronary intervention, or those with other acute coronary syndrome presentations that are considered high risk, may also be treated with a glycoprotein IIb/IIIa receptor antagonist as well

Note: always consider the overall clinical presentation before administering treatment. For example, myocardial ischaemia may be caused by anaemia, particularly with an acute bleed. In this case, blood transfusion and cessation of bleeding are appropriate and most of the above therapy is contraindicated i.e. heparin, GTN, antiplatelet agents. If renal function is poor, fondaparinux may be contraindicated.

PRESCRIPTION AND ADMINISTRATION RECORD
Standard Chart

Hospital/Ward: WGH/ARU	Consultant: CAP	Name of Patient: JOHN SMITH
Weight: 85kg	Height: 1.75cm	CHI Number: 1284933023
If re-written, date:		D.O.B.: 12/03/40
DISCHARGE PRESCRIPTION Date completed:-	Completed by:-	(Attach printed label here)

OTHER MEDICINE CHARTS IN USE		PREVIOUS ADVERSE REACTIONS This section must be completed before any medicine is given		Completed by (sign & print)	Date
Date	Type of Chart	None known ☐			
		Medicine/Agent	Description of Reaction		
		PENICILLIN	RASH	J Bloggs (BLOGGS)	15/09/10

CODES FOR NON-ADMINISTRATION OF PRESCRIBED MEDICINE

If a dose is not administered as prescribed, initial and enter a code in the column with a circle drawn round the code according to the reason as shown below. **Inform the responsible doctor in the appropriate timescale.**

1. Patient refuses
2. Patient not present
3. Medicines not available – CHECK ORDERED
4. Asleep/drowsy
5. Administration route not available – CHECK FOR ALTERNATIVE

6. Vomiting/nausea
7. Time varied on doctor's instructions
8. Once only/ as required medicine given
9. Dose withheld on doctor's instructions
10. Possible adverse reaction/side effect

ONCE ONLY

Date	Time	Medicine (Approved Name)	Dose	Route	Prescriber – Sign + Print	Time Given	Given By
3/10/10	2200	ASPRIN	300mg	ORAL	J Bloggs (BLOGGS)		
3/10/10	2200	CLOPIDOGREL	300mg	ORAL	J Bloggs (BLOGGS)		
3/10/10	2200	GTN	2 PUFFS	SL	J Bloggs (BLOGGS)		
3/10/10	2200	MORPHINE (TITRATE TO PAIN)	2.5-10mg	IV	J Bloggs (BLOGGS)		
3/10/10	2200	METOCLOPROMIDE	10MG	IV	J Bloggs (BLOGGS)		

		Start		Route		Prescriber – Sign + Print	Administered by	Stop	
	Date	Time	Mask (%)		Prongs (l/min)			Date	Time
O X Y G E N	3/10/10	2200	Venturi (60)			J Bloggs (BLOGGS)			

Prescribing

Station 3: EXACERBATION OF COPD

You are the FY1 working in acute medical admissions and your next patient is an acutely breathless 68 year-old lady with a history of COPD. She normally controls this with inhalers alone and has no home nebulisers or long-term oxygen therapy. She also reports a worsening cough productive of green sputum.

The patient is acutely dyspnoeic with an audible wheeze and some use of accessory muscles. The nurses are concerned about CO_2 retention so have given her oxygen at 2L/min via nasal prongs.

Obs	*Sats 83% (on 2L/min oxygen), RR 28, HR 98, BP 120/82, T 38.2°C*
O/E	*Chest expansion reduced on the right; right lower zone dull to percussion. Widespread expiratory wheeze, with inspiratory crepitations and increased vocal resonance in the right lower zone. The JVP is not raised. Heart sounds are normal.*
ABG (2L/min)	*PaO_2 6.2kPa, $PaCO_2$ 3.2kPa, H^+33nmol/L (pH 7.48), HCO_3^- 26mmol/L*
CXR	*Highly lucent lung fields in an otherwise appropriately penetrated film. The diaphragm appears flat. There is a well circumscribed area of consolidation around the right base, with an air bronchogram. There is no pneumothorax.*
Bloods	*Hb 159, WCC 17.1, Plt 401* *Urea 5.4, Cr 112, Na^+ 138, K^+ 4.2, CRP 132*

Initial Assessment

Airway

- Is the airway obstructed? Is the airway patent?
- Is the patient able to maintain their own airway? Secure the airway if necessary

Breathing

- Assess the respiratory rate and oxygen saturations
- Initially give high flow oxygen to correct hypoxia
- Perform a respiratory exam, especially looking for work of breathing (and evidence of tiring) and listening for wheeze and/or crepitations. Percuss carefully, particularly to exclude pneumothoraces (increased risk in COPD, especially with bullous emphysema)
- Give nebulisers if the presentation is suspicious of an exacerbation of COPD
- Perform an ABG and request an urgent CXR. These are **PRIORITY** investigations. Peak flow is NOT helpful in the acute management of COPD (in contrast to acute asthma)

Circulation

- Assess haemodynamic stability by measuring pulse, blood pressure and capillary refill time. Review urine output
- Perform a cardiovascular exam. Looking at the JVP for evidence of right heart failure, listening to the lung bases for evidence of pulmonary oedema, and auscultating the heart looking for evidence of valvular disease (especially mitral regurgitation or aortic stenosis). All of these can cause dyspnoea
- Obtain intravenous access and take routine bloods (full blood count, urea and electrolytes, C-reactive protein and glucose). Take venous blood cultures if the patient is pyrexial
- Perform an ECG to confirm the heart rhythm and assess for ischaemic damage
- Consider commencing intravenous fluids

Disability

- Assess the patient's conscious level, either using AVPU or GCS. Check glucose

Exposure

- Expose the patient, and perform a full examination looking for sources of infection, and a possible DVT

Management of COPD Exacerbation:

- *Oxygen + ABGs*
- *Bronchodilators*
- *Antibiotics (if indicated)*
- *Steroids*
- *Fluids*

Prescribing

Initial Investigations

- **ABG:** One of the most important investigations in an exacerbation of COPD. It allows assessment of the degree of oxygenation (PaO2) and ventilation (PaCO2). Check within 20 minutes of starting or changing flow of oxygen. Aim for a PaO2 >6.6KPa and H$^+$ <55 (pH>7.25). If this is achieved, increase the oxygen to achieve PaO2>7.5kPa. Aim for sats 88-92%. If possible, compare to a baseline (e.g. clinic ABG result)
- **CXR:** To exclude other causes of dyspnoea, especially a pneumothorax. Look for areas of consolidation. This is a priority investigation and may need to be a portable CXR if the patient is not stable enough to go to the X-ray department
- **ECG:** Look for evidence of a myocardial infarction. Look for arrhythmias such as atrial fibrillation, which may be a consequence of infection
- **BLOODS:** Look for evidence of infection, assess renal function and monitor potassium closely as salbutamol can lead to hypokalaemia

Initial Management

- **HIGH FLOW OXYGEN:** Best delivered by a venturi mask as this allows controlled oxygen delivery regardless of the respiratory pattern/rate. Oxygen is required to treat hypoxia but has to be used carefully in a certain cohort of COPD patients who rely on a hypoxic drive for respiration. However, in the acute setting, the patient will die faster from hypoxia than from hypercapnoea. Titrate oxygen therapy using ABGs as indicated above
- **BRONCHODILATORS:** Nebulised salbutamol 5mg and ipratropium bromide 500 microgram immediately and then 4-6 hourly. Nebulisers can be driven with oxygen or air, depending on the result of ABGs. If the patient is not responding, salbutamol can be given more frequently and the medical (or respiratory) registrar on call should be contacted
- **ANTIBIOTICS:** The choice depends on local policy. One option is amoxicillin 500mg oral tds (three times daily) or clarithromycin 500mg bd (twice daily) if the patient is allergic to penicillin
- **STEROIDS:** Prednisolone 40mg oral od (or hydrocortisone 200mg IV if oral route unavailable) should be given if there are no contraindications to steroids
- **INTRAVENOUS FLUIDS:** Patients with an infection, particularly those who are septic, often require intravenous fluids. If the patient is shocked, use fluid challenges to assess response to fluid resuscitation. It is important to exclude heart failure as the cause of dyspnoea before prescribing fluids. In addition, an acute exacerbation of COPD may itself tip a patient into right heart failure

- Call for help early if the patient is unwell
- Consider early HDU/ITU referral and contact the on call medical (or respiratory) registrar if the patient is not responding to treatment; they may need some form of ventilation (CPAP – type 1 respiratory failure or BiPAP – type 2 respiratory failure) or inotropic support
- Ensure the patient is on appropriate thromboprophylaxis as per local protocol

PRESCRIPTION AND ADMINISTRATION RECORD

Standard Chart

Hospital/Ward: RIE/CAA	**Consultant: COPD**	**Name of Patient: MARY SMITH**
Weight: 65kg	**Height: 1.82m**	**CHI Number: 1205420125**
If re-written, date:		**D.O.B.: 12/05/42**
DISCHARGE PRESCRIPTION **Date completed:-**	**Completed by:-**	(Attach printed label here)

OTHER MEDICINE CHARTS IN USE		PREVIOUS ADVERSE REACTIONS This section must be completed before any medicine is given		Completed by (sign & print)	Date
Date	Type of Chart	None known ☐			
12/9/10	NONE	Medicine/Agent	Description of Reaction		
		IBUPROFEN	PEPTIC ULCER	M Jones (JONES)	12/09/10

CODES FOR NON-ADMINISTRATION OF PRESCRIBED MEDICINE

If a dose is not administered as prescribed, initial and enter a code in the column with a circle drawn round the code according to the reason as shown below. **Inform the responsible doctor in the appropriate timescale.**

1. Patient refuses
2. Patient not present
3. Medicines not available – CHECK ORDERED
4. Asleep/drowsy
5. Administration route not available – CHECK FOR ALTERNATIVE

6. Vomiting/nausea
7. Time varied on doctor's instructions
8. Once only/ as required medicine given
9. Dose withheld on doctor's instructions
10. Possible adverse reaction/side effect

ONCE ONLY

Date	Time	Medicine (Approved Name)	Dose	Route	Prescriber – Sign + Print	Time Given	Given By
12/09/10	1600	SALBUTAMOL	5mg	NEB	M Jones (JONES)		
12/09/10	1600	IPRATROPIUM BROMIDE	500 microgram	NEB	M Jones (JONES)		
12/09/10	1645	AMOXICILLIN	500mg	ORAL	M Jones (JONES)		
12/09/10	1645	PREDNISOLONE	40mg	ORAL	M Jones (JONES)		
12/09/10	1800	ENOXAPARIN	20mg	SC	M Jones (JONES)		

	Start		Route		Prescriber – Sign + Print	Administered by	Stop	
O X Y G E N	Date	Time	Mask (%)	Prongs (l/min)			Date	Time
	12/09/10	1600	VENTURI (60)		M Jones (JONES)			

You are the junior doctor in the medical admissions unit. The nurse asks you to come and see a new admission urgently. The patient is an 18 year-old male who has a background of asthma and has become breathless.

Obs	Sats 84% (on 2L/min oxygen), RR 32, HR 128, BP 148/86, T 36.9°C
O/E	The patient is dyspnoeic and distressed. There is an audible wheeze, he is struggling to speak in sentences and having to use accessory muscles.
ABG (2L/Min)	PaO2 6.8KPa, PaCO2 3.2KPa, H+30nmol/L (pH7.52), HCO3⁻ 26mmol/L
CXR	CXR shows hyper-expanded lungs, clear lung fields. No pneumothoraces.
Bloods	Hb 153, WCC 11.6, Plts 475, Urea 4.2, Creat 102, Na⁺ 136, K⁺ 4.3

Initial Assessment

Airway

- Is the airway obstructed? Is the airway patent?
- Is the patient able to maintain their own airway? Secure the airway if necessary

Breathing

- Assess the respiratory rate and oxygen saturations
- Initially give high flow oxygen
- Perform a respiratory exam, especially looking for increased work of breathing (and evidence of tiring) and listening for wheeze and/or crepitations. Percuss for hyper resonance (associated with hyperinflated asthmatic lungs or pneumothoraces)
- Give nebulisers if the presentation is suspicious for an exacerbation of asthma
- Perform an ABG and request a CXR. These are PRIORITY investigations. Peak flow assessment is less urgent, but is important in assessing the severity of an exacerbation of asthma

Circulation

- Assess haemodynamic stability by measuring pulse, blood pressure and capillary refill time. Review urine output
- Perform a cardiovascular exam, looking at the JVP for evidence of right heart failure, listening to the lung bases for evidence of pulmonary oedema, and auscultating the heart looking for evidence of valvular disease (especially mitral regurgitation or aortic stenosis). All of these can cause dyspnoea but are uncommon in a patient this age
- Obtain intravenous access and take routine bloods (full blood count, urea and electrolytes, C-reactive protein and glucose). Take venous blood cultures if the patient is pyrexial
- Perform an ECG to confirm the heart rhythm and assess for ischaemic damage
- Consider commencing intravenous fluids, particularly if there is evidence of dehydration

Disability

- Assess the patient's conscious level, either using AVPU or GCS. Check glucose

Exposure

- Expose the patient, and perform a full examination looking for sources of infection, and evidence of a DVT

Management of Asthma Exacerbation:

- *Oxygen + ABGs*
- *Bronchodilators*
- *Steroids*
- *Regular reassessment*
- *Antibiotics if indicated*

Prescribing

Initial Investigations

- **BLOODS:** Look for evidence of infection, assess renal function, check glucose
- **ABG:** One of the most important investigations in an exacerbation of asthma. It allows assessment of the severity of the exacerbation. All patients are likely to be hypoxic. Furthermore, as they are hyperventilating, their $PaCO_2$ should be low, giving a respiratory alkalosis (low H+/high pH). As the patient tires, their respiratory rate drops and subsequently the $PaCO_2$ rises. A normal $PaCO_2$ and normal H+/pH can signify a severe episode, whereas a high $PaCO_2$ and H+/low pH signify a life threatening episode. ABGs help assess response to therapy. Note also that as the patient gets better, a low CO2 will go back to normal levels
- **PEAK FLOW:** To assess severity (see table) and response to therapy
- **CXR:** To exclude other causes of dyspnoea, especially a pneumothorax. Look for areas of consolidation. This is a priority investigation and may need to be a portable CXR if the patient is not stable enough to go to the X-ray department
- **ECG:** Look for evidence of a myocardial infarction (though this is very unlikely in an 18 year old). Look for arrhythmias such as atrial fibrillation, which may be a consequence of infection

British Thoracic Society guidelines 2011 for assessing severity of acute asthma

Moderate	Acute Severe	Life Threatening
Increasing symptoms	Any one of:	Acute severe asthma + any one of:
Peak Expiratory flow >50-75% of best or predicted	Peak Expiratory Flow 33-50% of best or predicted	Peak Expiratory Flow <33% of best or predicted
No features of acute severe asthma	Respiratory rate >25/min	Oxygen Saturations <92%
	Heart rate >110/min	PaO2 <8kPa
	Unable to complete sentences in one breath	Normal PaCO2 (4.6-6kPa)
		Silent chest
		Cyanosis
		Poor respiratory effort
		Arrhythmia
		Exhaustion, altered conscious level

Initial Management

- **HIGH FLOW OXYGEN:** Via non re-breath bag or venturi mask, adjusting to ABGs. Aim for oxygen saturations of 94-98%. Note: In contrast to COPD patients, abolishing the hypoxic drive for respiration in asthmatic patients is not usually an issue. However, any severe type 1 respiratory failure can lead to tiring, and subsequent type II respiratory failure
- **BRONCHODILATORS:** Nebulised salbutamol 5mg, repeated every 10 minutes if necessary (back to back). Consider nebulised ipratropium bromide 500 microgram 4-6 hourly in severe or life-threatening episodes
- **STEROIDS:** Prednisolone 40mg oral or hydrocortisone 200mg IV if there are no contraindications to steroids. Remember IV steroids do not work any quicker than oral steroids unless the patient has specific issues such as gastrointestinal problems (impairing absorption)
- **INTRAVENOUS FLUIDS AND ANTIBIOTICS:** May be needed if there is evidence of an infection

- Call for help early if the patient is unwell
- Consider early HDU/ITU referral and contact the on call medical (or respiratory) registrar if the patient is not responding to treatment. They may need some form of ventilation (CPAP – type 1 respiratory failure or BiPAP – type 2 respiratory failure)
- Ensure the patient is on appropriate thromboprophylaxis as per local protocol

Prescribing

PRESCRIPTION AND ADMINISTRATION RECORD

Standard Chart

Hospital/Ward: RIE/CAA	Consultant: MJS	Name of Patient: MARK MACDONALD
Weight: 83kg	Height: 1.86m	CHI Number: 2503920145
If re-written, date:		D.O.B.: 25/03/92
DISCHARGE PRESCRIPTION Date completed:- Completed by:-		(Attach printed label here)

OTHER MEDICINE CHARTS IN USE		PREVIOUS ADVERSE REACTIONS This section must be completed before any medicine is given		Completed by (sign & print)	Date
Date	Type of Chart	None known ☐			
15/9/10	NONE	Medicine/Agent	Description of Reaction		
		PENICILLIN	FACIAL SWELLING, BREATHLESSNESS	J Bloggs (BLOGGS)	15/09/10

CODES FOR NON-ADMINISTRATION OF PRESCRIBED MEDICINE

If a dose is not administered as prescribed, initial and enter a code in the column with a circle drawn round the code according to the reason as shown below. **Inform the responsible doctor in the appropriate timescale.**

1. Patient refuses
2. Patient not present
3. Medicines not available – CHECK ORDERED
4. Asleep/drowsy
5. Administration route not available – CHECK FOR ALTERNATIVE

6. Vomiting/nausea
7. Time varied on doctor's instructions
8. Once only/ as required medicine given
9. Dose withheld on doctor's instructions
10. Possible adverse reaction/side effect

ONCE ONLY

Date	Time	Medicine (Approved Name)	Dose	Route	Prescriber – Sign + Print	Time Given	Given By
15/09/10	1100	SALBUTAMOL	5mg	NEB	J Bloggs (BLOGGS)		
15/09/10	1100	PREDNISOLONE	40mg	ORAL	J Bloggs (BLOGGS)		
15/09/10	1115	SALBUTAMOL	5mg	NEB	J Bloggs (BLOGGS)		

		Start		Route		Prescriber – Sign + Print	Administered by	Stop	
	Date	Time	Mask (%)		Prongs (l/min)			Date	Time
O X Y G E N	15/09/10	1100	NON RE-BREATH MASK	15L/Min		J Bloggs (BLOGGS)			

Prescribing

Station 5: HYPERKALAEMIA

You are the junior doctor in the medical assessment unit. A 72 year-old patient has been admitted from A&E with a 3 day history of vomiting and dehydration. You are asked to chase his bloods and review him overnight. His bloods are:

Hb 130, WCC 11, Platelets 350
Urea 21, Creatinine 192, Sodium 135, Potassium 7.1

You have established that the blood sample was not taken from his drip arm.

The patient's vomiting has settled with IM cyclizine. He feels thirsty. He has a past history of two myocardial infarctions two and ten years ago. His medications are aspirin, ramipril, bisoprolol, co-amilofruse, simvastatin and spironolactone.

Obs	*Sats 99% (on 2L/min oxygen), RR 20, HR 103, BP 110/68, T 36.9°C*
O/E	*He has cool peripheries, dry mucous membranes and his JVP is not visible. Examination is otherwise unremarkable.*
ECG	*Sinus rhythm, 103 bpm, tenting of T waves, no prolongation of the PR interval or QRS complex.*

Initial Assessment

Airway

- Is the airway obstructed? Is the airway patent?
- Is the patient able to maintain their own airway? Secure the airway if necessary

Breathing

- Assess the respiratory rate, and oxygen saturations
- Give supplementary oxygen to maintain oxygen saturations > 94%

Circulation

- Assess haemodynamic stability by measuring pulse, blood pressure, capillary refill time and JVP. Review urine output
- Obtain intravenous access and take urgent repeat sample for urea and electrolytes
- Perform an ECG and an ABG
- Intravenous fluids

Disability

- Assess the patient's conscious level, either using AVPU or GCS. Check glucose

Exposure

- Expose the patient, and perform a full examination looking for causes of hyperkalemia such as burns or trauma (causing rhabdomyolysis)

Management of Hyperkalaemia

- *Cardiac stabilisation*
- *Reduce serum potassium*
- *Eliminate potassium*
- *Regular reassessment*

Prescribing

Initial Investigations

- **BLOODS:** Whilst urgent repeat urea and electrolytes to confirm the hyperkalaemia are important, the patient should be treated on the basis of the first sample (although if the potassium was minimally raised, consider the clinical history and likelihood of a spurious result). This patient will require repeat bloods overnight and during the next day to assess the renal function and hyperkalaemia in response to treatment
- **ABG:** Can allow a rapid measure of potassium (serum K+ is measured in some laboratories) but bear in mind this can be inaccurate. It will also identify a metabolic acidosis which may be the result of hypovolaemia and renal impairment, and might be worsening the hyperkalaemia
- **ECG:** Hyperkalaemia can lead to sudden death from arrhythmias. There may also be evidence of myocardial instability such as flattening of P waves, prolonged PR interval, widening of QRS, ST depression, tented T waves

Initial Management

Cardiac Stabilization

- **CALCIUM CHLORIDE/GLUCONATE:** If there are ECG changes associated with myocardial instability, give IV 10% calcium chloride/gluconate titrated in 1ml aliquots to resolution of ECG changes. If no ECG monitoring is available, give 10mls of calcium chloride/gluconate slowly IV and repeat the ECG. This stabilises the myocardium but does not lower the serum potassium
- *Note that excessive calcium chloride/gluconate can cause cardiac arrest. Therefore, always titrate to the ECG if available*

Reduce Serum Potassium

- **SALBUTAMOL:** Nebulised salbutamol 5mg is quick to administer and will drive some of the extracellular potassium into cells. This can be given whilst the below measures are being instituted and repeated as needed
- **INSULIN:** Bolus IV insulin with dextrose (10 units Actrapid in 50ml 50% dextrose (or equivalent amount of dextrose, e.g. 250mls 10% dextrose)) drives extracellular potassium intracellularly. Blood glucose must be monitored regularly; the patient may need a slow infusion of 10% dextrose 10-50ml/hr to maintain their blood glucose
- **SODIUM BICARBONATE:** This may be required, especially if the patient is acidotic

Eliminate the Potassium

- This is achieved by restoring normal renal function
- **INTRAVENOUS FLUIDS:** This patient is tachycardic (despite being on a β-blocker) and hypotensive, has cool peripheries and a low JVP. He is hypovolaemic secondary to diarrhoea and vomiting. Fluid resuscitation will involve administering fluid challenges, (e.g. 500mls 0.9% sodium chloride over 20 minutes) and assessing the response. This will allow replacement of the fluid deficit and should prevent overloading the patient, which is a potential hazard in patients with a cardiac history. Once the deficit has been replaced, maintenance fluids, incorporating ongoing losses, can be prescribed
- **CATHETER:** Catheterising this patient will help to exclude a post renal cause of the renal impairment, and will allow accurate fluid balance assessment, especially if urine output is poor
- **WITHHOLD NEPHROTOXOIC DRUGS:** Medications such as ramipril, co-amilofruse and spironolactone may impair renal function and should be withheld until renal function is improved. Spironolactone and ramipril will also increase serum potassium
- **HAEMODIALYSIS/HAEMOFILTRATION** may be needed if the above measures are not working
- *Note: Ion exchange resins such as calcium resonium are seldom used in acute situations*

- Ensure the patient is on appropriate thromboprophylaxis as per local protocol. Note that in patients with renal impairment (e.g. eGFR<30ml/min) heparin 5000 units bd is more appropriate than low molecular weight heparin
- Call for help early if the patient is unwell

PRESCRIPTION AND ADMINISTRATION RECORD
Standard Chart

Hospital/Ward: RIE/CAA	Consultant: MJK	Name of Patient: PETER JONES
Weight: 65kg	Height: 1.73m	CHI Number: 2206381254
If re-written, date:		D.O.B.: 22/06/38
DISCHARGE PRESCRIPTION Date completed:-	Completed by:-	(Attach printed label here)

OTHER MEDICINE CHARTS IN USE		PREVIOUS ADVERSE REACTIONS This section must be completed before any medicine is given		Completed by (sign & print)	Date
Date	Type of Chart	None known ☐			
10/9/10	NONE	Medicine/Agent	Description of Reaction		
		ERYTHROMYCIN	RASH	M Jones (JONES)	10/09/10

CODES FOR NON-ADMINISTRATION OF PRESCRIBED MEDICINE

If a dose is not administered as prescribed, initial and enter a code in the column with a circle drawn round the code according to the reason as shown below. **Inform the responsible doctor in the appropriate timescale.**

1. Patient refuses
2. Patient not present
3. Medicines not available – CHECK ORDERED
4. Asleep/drowsy
5. Administration route not available – CHECK FOR ALTERNATIVE
6. Vomiting/nausea
7. Time varied on doctor's instructions
8. Once only/ as required medicine given
9. Dose withheld on doctor's instructions
10. Possible adverse reaction/side effect

ONCE ONLY

Date	Time	Medicine (Approved Name)	Dose	Route	Prescriber – Sign + Print	Time Given	Given By
10/9/10	2040	CALCIUM GLUCONATE 10% (TITRATE ABOVE TO ECG)	1-10mls	IV	M Jones (JONES)		
10/9/10	2050	SALBUTAMOL	5mg	NEB	M Jones (JONES)		
10/9/10	2050	ACTRAPID IN 50MLS OF 50% DEXTROSE	10 UNITS	IV	M Jones (JONES)		

	Start			Route	Prescriber – Sign + Print	Administered by	Stop	
	Date	Time	Mask (%)	Prongs (l/min)			Date	Time
O X Y G E N	10/9/10	2040		2L/MIN	M Jones (JONES)			

Prescribing

Name: PETER JONES
Date of Birth: 22/06/38

REGULAR THERAPY

PRESCRIPTION		Date →	10/9												
		Time ▼													
Medicine (Approved Name) **ASPIRIN**		6													
		(8)													
Dose **75mg**	Route **ORAL**	12													
Notes	Start Date **10/9/10**	14													
		18													
Prescriber – sign + print *S Smith* **(SMITH)**		22													
Medicine (Approved Name) ~~RAMIPRIL~~		6													
		(8)													
Dose **5mg**	Route **ORAL**	12													
Notes	Start Date **10/9/10**	14						STOPPED DUE TO HYPERKALEMIA AND ACUTE KIDNEY INJURY							
		18													
Prescriber – sign + print *S Smith* **(SMITH)**		22						10/9/10 *M Jones* (JONES)							
Medicine (Approved Name) **BISOPROLOL**		6													
		(8)													
Dose **10mg**	Route **ORAL**	12													
Notes	Start Date **10/9/10**	14													
		18													
Prescriber – sign + print *S Smith* **(SMITH)**		22													
Medicine (Approved Name) ~~CO-AMILOFRUSE 5/40~~		6													
		(8)													
Dose **1 TABLET**	Route **ORAL**	12													
Notes	Start Date **10/9/10**	14						STOPPED DUE TO HYPERKALEMIA AND ACUTE KIDNEY INJURY							
		18													
Prescriber – sign + print *S Smith* **(SMITH)**		22						10/9/10 *M Jones* (JONES)							
Medicine (Approved Name) **SIMVASTATIN**		6													
		8													
Dose **40mg**	Route **ORAL**	12													
Notes	Start Date **10/9/10**	14													
		18													
Prescriber – sign + print *S Smith* **(SMITH)**		(22)	*SJ*												
Medicine (Approved Name) ~~SPIRONOLACTONE~~		6													
		(8)													
Dose **25mg**	Route **ORAL**	12													
Notes	Start Date **10/9/10**	14						STOPPED DUE TO HYPERKALEMIA AND ACUTE KIDNEY INJURY							
		18													
Prescriber – sign + print *S Smith* **(SMITH)**		22						10/9/10 *M Jones* (JONES)							

Prescribing

24 HOUR FLUID PRESCRIPTION CHART

Hospital/Ward: RIE/CAA	Consultant: MJK
Weight: 65kg	Height: 1.73m

Name of Patient: PETER JONES

CHI Number: 2206381252

D.O.B: 22/06/38
(Attach printed label here)

Date/ Time	FLUID / ADDED DRUGS	VOLUME / DOSE	RATE	PRESCRIBER – SIGN AND PRINT
10/9/10 2100	0.9% SODIUM CHLORIDE	500mls	20 MINS	*M Jones* (MJ JONES)
	Further fluid prescriptions will be determined by the patient's response to this fluid challenge.			
	Repeat obs are performed after this bag has gone through. There is a transient improvement but his obs return to: Sats 99%, RR 18, HR 98, BP 116/72, T 36.9. His peripheries are cool and the JVP is not visible. He is improving but still hypovolaemic.			
10/9/10 2130	0.9% SODIUM CHLORIDE	500mls	20 MINS	*M Jones* (MJ JONES)
	Further fluid prescriptions will be determined by the patient's response to this fluid challenge. The patient needs reassessed before more fluids can be prescribed.			

Prescribing

Station 6: BOWEL OBSTRUCTION

You are the FY1 working on a general surgical ward and are asked to see a 70 year-old man who has presented with abdominal pain, severe nausea and vomiting. On closer questioning, you discover he has not had a bowel motion for the last five or six days. His past history is remarkable for ischaemic heart disease; he is on aspirin, simvastatin, ramipril and atenolol for a previous MI.

He is an average sized man, is confused and looks dehydrated.

Obs	Sats 93% (on air), RR 18, HR 96, BP 102/86, T 37.4°C
O/E	Cool peripheries, weak pulse. Abdomen distended, with generalised tenderness; no peritonism. Fullness in the right iliac fossa. Loud, "tinkling" bowel sounds. PR examination – no masses.
Bloods	Hb 123, WCC 9.1, Plt 324
	Urea 8.1, Cr 129, Na$^+$ 134, K$^+$ 3.0
	Bil 16, ALT 43, ALP 165, GGT 98
	Amylase/CRP/lactate normal
Plain AXR	Dilated small bowel proximal to the caecum with no gas seen in distal bowel
Erect CXR	Lung fields clear, no pneumoperitoneum

Initial Assessment

Airway

- Is the airway obstructed? Is the airway patent?
- Is the patient able to maintain their own airway? Secure the airway if necessary

Breathing

- Assess the respiratory rate, and oxygen saturations
- Give supplementary oxygen to maintain oxygen saturations >94%
- Perform a respiratory exam, particularly listening for basal crepitations which may indicate aspiration pneumonia
- Request an erect CXR

Circulation

- Assess haemodynamic stability by measuring pulse, blood pressure, capillary refill time and JVP. Review urine output
- Obtain two sites of intravenous access with large-bore cannulae and take bloods
- Perform an ABG, and an ECG
- Commence intravenous fluids

Disability

- Assess the patient's conscious level, either using AVPU or GCS. Check glucose

Exposure

- Expose the patient, and perform a full examination, particularly focusing on the abdomen, looking for evidence of perforation

---

Management of bowel obstruction:

- *NG tube*
- *Nil by mouth*
- *IV fluids*
- *Regular reassessment*

Initial Investigations

- **BLOODS:** Look for electrolyte derangement, renal impairment, pancreatitis and infection. Do venous blood cultures if patient pyrexial
- **ABG:** Allows assessment of the metabolic status of the patient as well as the ventilation/oxygenation
- **ERECT CXR:** Look for free air under the diaphragm suggestive of perforation. There may be evidence of consolidation if the patient has aspirated vomit. This will need to be a portable CXR if the patient is not stable enough to go to the X-ray department
- **AXR:** To assess for obstruction (dilated bowel loops) and perforation
- **ECG:** To assess the rhythm and look for evidence of a myocardial infarction
- **URINE DIPSTICK:** To assess for evidence of a urinary tract infection. β-hCG if a female of childbearing age

Initial Management

- This patient has clinical and plain film evidence of bowel obstruction. The most pressing issue is hypovolaemic shock secondary to the obstruction. It is not necessary to know the cause of the obstruction to be able to treat the hypovolaemic shock
- **DECOMPRESS THE STOMACH:** This patient should be made nil by mouth and a nasogastric tube should be inserted
- **FLUID RESUSCITATE:** This patient is peripherally shut down, has a relative tachycardia (N.B. on atenolol) and is hypotensive with a narrow pulse pressure. He needs aggressive fluid resuscitation to restore organ perfusion
- **TWO LARGE BORE CANNULAE:** Should be inserted. Both crystalloids and colloids can be used in shock. In bowel obstruction, Hartmann's is a good choice as it contains electrolytes which will have been lost into the bowel. Normal saline plus potassium chloride may be needed to replace lost potassium but caution is needed over the speed of IV potassium replacement
- 500mls of Hartmann's given stat via each cannulae, with assessment of his response to the fluid challenge, would be appropriate in the first instance

There are three potential outcomes following a fluid challenge:

Rapid Responder	Transient Responder	Non Responder
These patients respond fully to the challenge and become haemodynamically stable. Their fluid deficit has been replaced. They may still require maintenance IV fluids.	These patients have a brief response to the challenge but return to being haemodynamically unstable. They continue to have a fluid deficit which needs to be replaced.	In these cases there is no response to the fluid challenge. This implies either the fluid deficit is so large that the fluid administered is not sufficient for any correction of haemodynamic instability, or the shock is not hypovolaemic.

- Fluid challenges are a good way to replace acute fluid losses as they incorporate regular reassessment of the patient
- Once the deficit has been replaced, maintenance fluids, including ongoing losses from, for example, the NG tube, can be prescribed
- Given his age and background of ischaemic heart disease, there may be some concern regarding fluid overload. However the fluid deficit is likely to be large for two reasons. 1. The obstruction is likely to have been developing for several days. 2. In addition to obvious fluid losses from vomiting, gastrointestinal secretions collecting proximal to the obstruction (third space losses) will be adding to the fluid deficit. These, combined with his clinical evidence of shock (reduced peripheral perfusion, confusion), mean he is likely to be in a large negative fluid balance. To overload this patient, we would first have to replace the entire fluid deficit and then add enough further fluid to compromise his cardiac output. This would take a substantial amount of fluids in this scenario
- **CATHETER:** A urethral catheter should be inserted to monitor urine output and help assess fluid balance
- **ANALGESIA:** Use the WHO analgesic ladder. Regular paracetamol given IV as the patient is NBM. IV/SC/IM morphine should be titrated to pain. Caution needs to be exercised with opiates as this patient has renal impairment which will result in the reduced clearance of opiate metabolites
- **ANTIEMETIC:** Cyclizine 50mg IV/IM/SC 8 hourly is an appropriate choice. Ondansetron 4mg IV/IM/SC 6 hourly can also be used. Metoclopramide should be avoided as it is a prokinetic, and therefore may exacerbate the symptoms of bowel obstruction
- Ensure the patient is on appropriate thromboprophylaxis as per local protocol and consider any potential operation – liaise with seniors before prescribing anticoagulants in emergency surgical patients
- Withhold ramipril until renal function has improved
- This patient needs early senior review. Once stable the patient will need investigation to identify the cause of the obstruction, and allow potential operative planning

Prescribing

PRESCRIPTION AND ADMINISTRATION RECORD

Standard Chart

Hospital/Ward: WGH/27	Consultant: DNA	Name of Patient: **WILLIAM MACDONALD**
Weight: 70kg	Height: 1.78m	CHI Number: **0706401225**
If re-written, date:		D.O.B.: **07/06/40**
DISCHARGE PRESCRIPTION Date completed:-	Completed by:-	(Attach printed label here)

OTHER MEDICINE CHARTS IN USE		PREVIOUS ADVERSE REACTIONS This section must be completed before any medicine is given		Completed by (sign & print)	Date
Date	Type of Chart	None known ☐			
10/9/10	NONE	Medicine/Agent	Description of Reaction		
		PENICILLIN	RASH	*J Bloggs* (BLOGGS)	10/9/10

CODES FOR NON-ADMINISTRATION OF PRESCRIBED MEDICINE

If a dose is not administered as prescribed, initial and enter a code in the column with a circle drawn round the code according to the reason as shown below. **Inform the responsible doctor in the appropriate timescale.**

1. Patient refuses
2. Patient not present
3. Medicines not available – CHECK ORDERED
4. Asleep/drowsy
5. Administration route not available – CHECK FOR ALTERNATIVE

6. Vomiting/nausea
7. Time varied on doctor's instructions
8. Once only/ as required medicine given
9. Dose withheld on doctor's instructions
10. Possible adverse reaction/side effect

ONCE ONLY

Date	Time	Medicine (Approved Name)	Dose	Route	Prescriber – Sign + Print	Time Given	Given By
10/9/10	1400	MORPHINE (TITRATE TO PAIN)	1-10mg	IV	*J Bloggs* (BLOGGS)		
10/9/10	1400	CYCLIZINE	50mg	IV	*J Bloggs* (BLOGGS)		
10/9/10	1400	PARACETAMOL	1g	IV	*J Bloggs* (BLOGGS)		

	Start		Route		Prescriber – Sign + Print	Administered by	Stop	
O X Y G E N	Date	Time	Mask (%)	Prongs (l/min)			Date	Time
	10/9/10	1400		4 L/MIN	*J Bloggs* (BLOGGS)			

24 HOUR FLUID PRESCRIPTION CHART

Hospital/Ward: WGH/Ward 27   Consultant: DNA

Weight: 70kg   Height: 1.78m

Name of Patient: WILLIAM MACDONALD

CHI Number: 0706401225

D.O.B: 07/06/10
(Attach printed label here)

Date/ Time	FLUID / ADDED DRUGS	VOLUME / DOSE	RATE	PRESCRIBER – SIGN AND PRINT
Venflon 1 10/9/10 1400	HARTMANN'S	500mls	20 Mins	*J BLOGGS* (BLOGGS)
Venflon 2 10/9/10 1400	HARTMANN'S	500mls	20 Mins	*J BLOGGS* (BLOGGS)
Venflon 1 10/9/10 1440	HARTMANN'S	500mls	20 Mins	*J BLOGGS* (BLOGGS)
	Further fluid prescriptions will be determined by the patient's response to this fluid challenge. The patient needs reassessed before more fluids can be prescribed.			

Prescribing

Station 7: ABDOMINAL SEPSIS

You are the FY1 working on a general surgical admissions unit. Your next patient is a 43 year-old woman who has presented with a 3 day history of worsening left iliac fossa pain and vomiting. She has had some loose stools over the last couple of days and has a background of diverticular disease and asthma. Her only medications are Seretide 250 and salbutamol inhalers.

She is clearly in pain.

Obs	Sats 96% (on air), RR 22, HR 96, BP 136/72, T 38.3°C
O/E	Warm peripheries, good volume pulse. The abdomen is tender in the left iliac fossa; no peritonism. Bowel sounds are normal. PR – no masses
Bloods	Hb 143, WCC 18.9, Plt 532 Urea 6.8, Cr 109, Na 135, K 4.0 Bil 8, ALT 43, ALP 120, GGT 65 CRP 286, lactate 4.3, amylase normal, β-HCG negative
Urinalysis	No leukocytes, nitrites or blood. β-HCG negative
Plain AXR	Non-specific bowel gas pattern, no evidence of obstruction or perforation
Erect CXR	Lung fields clear, no pneumoperitoneum

Initial Assessment

Airway

- Is the airway obstructed? Is the airway patent?
- Is the patient able to maintain their own airway? Secure the airway if necessary

Breathing

- Assess the respiratory rate, and oxygen saturations
- Give supplementary oxygen to maintain oxygen saturations >94%
- Perform a respiratory exam, particularly looking for signs of pneumonia
- Request an erect CXR

Circulation

- Assess haemodynamic stability by measuring pulse, blood pressure, capillary refill time and JVP. Review urine output
- Obtain two sites of intravenous access and take bloods
- Perform an ABG, and an ECG
- Commence intravenous fluids

Disability

- Assess the patient's conscious level, either using AVPU or GCS

Exposure

- Expose the patient, and perform a full examination, particularly focusing on the abdomen
- Examine the entire patient looking for sources of infection

Initial Investigations

- **BLOODS:** Provide supporting evidence for problems such as infection, electrolyte derangement, renal impairment and pancreatitis. Check full blood count, urea and electrolytes, liver function tests, amylase, calcium, lactate, C-reactive protein, glucose, and venous blood culture if patient pyrexial
- **URINALYSIS:** Look for evidence of a UTI as a source of sepsis. Pregnancy in women of child bearing age

> ## Management of Abdominal Sepsis:
>
> - *Nil by mouth*
> - *Antibiotics*
> - *IV fluids*
> - *Analgesia*
> - *Regular reassessment*

- **ABG:** Allows assessment of the metabolic status of the patient as well as the ventilation/oxygenation
- **ERECT CXR:** Look for free air under the diaphragm suggestive of a perforation. There may be evidence of consolidation if the source of the sepsis is pneumonia. This will need to be a portable CXR if the patient is not stable enough to go to the X-ray department
- **AXR:** To assess for obstruction (dilated bowel loops) and perforation
- **ECG:** To assess the rhythm and look for evidence of a myocardial infarction

Initial Management

- This patient is probably septic (N.B. Sepsis is an objective term: sepsis = systemic inflammatory response syndrome (SIRS) plus confirmed or suspected source of infection)
- Sepsis is a serious condition with a high mortality rate. Successful outcomes require early diagnosis and early institution of appropriate treatments
- Given the clear CXR, negative urinalysis and normal β-hCG, the clinical picture fits with diverticulitis

- **NIL BY MOUTH:** This patient may require surgical intervention. She should be nil by mouth until the senior review
- **ANTIBIOTICS:** The time between onset of sepsis and delivery of antibiotics is important for prognosis. In this scenario the likely cause is intra-abdominal, mostly likely diverticulitis. Antibiotic choice will be dependent on local antibiotic policies. One option is 4.5g of piperacillin and tazobactam (tazocin) IV tds
- **INTRAVENOUS FLUIDS:** Septic patients require IV fluids as they are relatively hypovolaemic due to peripheral vasodilatation. In addition they have increased insensible losses due to their raised respiratory rate and pyrexia. Furthermore they may be nil by mouth. Therefore they will require maintenance fluids as well as fluids to replace ongoing losses and correct shock
- Fluid challenges should be used to correct shock. Patients with septic shock who are unresponsive to fluid resuscitation should be discussed with the high-dependency unit and considered for inotropic support (e.g. noradrenaline)
- Regular reassessment of the patient and their fluid balance is important
- **CATHETER:** A urethral catheter should be considered to monitor urine output and help assess fluid balance
- **ANALGESIA:** This patient is clearly in pain. Analgesia prescribing should follow the World Health Organisation analgesic ladder, starting at the most appropriate level. An appropriate regimen would be regular paracetamol 1g IV and as required morphine IV/IM/SC 10mg hourly
- **ANTIEMETIC:** Cyclizine 50mg IV/IM/SC 8 hourly is one potential choice

- Ensure the patient is on appropriate thromboprophylaxis as per local protocol. Liaise with seniors before prescribing anticoagulants in emergency surgical patients, especially if surgery is being planned
- This patient needs early senior review to decide further investigations (e.g. CT abdomen/pelvis) and definitive management

SIRS

SIRS is defined by 2 or more of:

a) Pulse greater than 90

b) Respiratory rate greater than 20 or PaCO2 less than 4.3kPa

c) WCC greater than 12x10⁹/l or less than 4x10⁹/l

d) Temperature greater than 38°C or less than 36°C

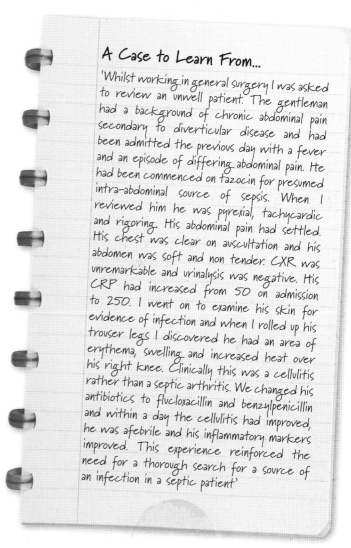

A Case to Learn From...

'Whilst working in general surgery I was asked to review an unwell patient. The gentleman had a background of chronic abdominal pain secondary to diverticular disease and had been admitted the previous day with a fever and an episode of differing abdominal pain. He had been commenced on tazocin for presumed intra-abdominal source of sepsis. When I reviewed him he was pyrexial, tachycardic and rigoring. His abdominal pain had settled. His chest was clear on auscultation and his abdomen was soft and non tender. CXR was unremarkable and urinalysis was negative. His CRP had increased from 50 on admission to 250. I went on to examine his skin for evidence of infection and when I rolled up his trouser legs I discovered he had an area of erythema, swelling and increased heat over his right knee. Clinically this was a cellulitis rather than a septic arthritis. We changed his antibiotics to flucloxacillin and benzylpenicillin and within a day the cellulitis had improved, he was afebrile and his inflammatory markers improved. This experience reinforced the need for a thorough search for a source of an infection in a septic patient'

Prescribing

PRESCRIPTION AND ADMINISTRATION RECORD
Standard Chart

Hospital/Ward: WGH/27	Consultant: MHSC	Name of Patient: JENNIFER WILLIAMS
Weight: 70kg	Height: 1.62m	CHI Number: 1205670125
If re-written, date:		D.O.B.: 12/05/67
DISCHARGE PRESCRIPTION Date completed:-	Completed by:-	*(Attach printed label here)*

OTHER MEDICINE CHARTS IN USE		PREVIOUS ADVERSE REACTIONS This section must be completed before any medicine is given		Completed by (sign & print)	Date
Date	Type of Chart	None known ☐			
20/9/10	NONE	Medicine/Agent	Description of Reaction		
		ERYTHROMYCIN	RASH	M Jones (JONES)	20/9/10

CODES FOR NON-ADMINISTRATION OF PRESCRIBED MEDICINE

If a dose is not administered as prescribed, initial and enter a code in the column with a circle drawn round the code according to the reason as shown below. **Inform the responsible doctor in the appropriate timescale.**

1. Patient refuses
2. Patient not present
3. Medicines not available – CHECK ORDERED
4. Asleep/drowsy
5. Administration route not available – CHECK FOR ALTERNATIVE

6. Vomiting/nausea
7. Time varied on doctor's instructions
8. Once only/ as required medicine given
9. Dose withheld on doctor's instructions
10. Possible adverse reaction/side effect

ONCE ONLY

Date	Time	Medicine (Approved Name)	Dose	Route	Prescriber – Sign + Print	Time Given	Given By
20/9/10	1430	MORPHINE (TITRATE TO PAIN)	1-10mg	IV	M Jones (JONES)		
20/9/10	1430	CYCLIZINE	50mg	IV	M Jones (JONES)		
20/9/10	1430	PIPERACILLIN AND TAZOBACTAM	4.5g	IV	M Jones (JONES)		
20/9/10	1430	PARACETAMOL	1g	IV	M Jones (JONES)		

		Start		Route		Prescriber – Sign + Print	Administered by	Stop	
	Date	Time	Mask (%)		Prongs (l/min)			Date	Time
O X Y G E N									

You are the FY1 cross covering GI medicine one evening. You are paged: a patient on the ward is having haematemesis. He was admitted directly from the medical outpatient clinic yesterday as he "was yellow" and had a scan of his abdomen yesterday. He has never vomited blood before and he does not get indigestion. On arriving at the ward, you are shown into a side room where a dishevelled man is vomiting frank blood into a sick bowl. He is alert, but is slurring his speech. He has blood on his hospital gown and there is blood on the floor around him. He tells you that he was sitting in bed when he vomited 30 minutes ago. He has vomited repeatedly since then.

Obs	*Sats 96% (on room air), RR 25, HR 120, BP 78/40, T 37.8°C*
O/E	*He is unkempt. His hands are cold to his elbows. He is covered in crusted and fresh blood. His abdomen is soft and non-tender. Bowel sounds are present.* *PR – no masses. GCS E4/V4/M6=14*
Erect CXR	*Lung fields clear, no pneumoperitoneum.*

Initial Assessment

Airway

- Is the airway obstructed? Is the airway patent?
- Is the patient able to maintain their own airway? Secure the airway if necessary

Breathing

- Assess the respiratory rate, and oxygen saturations
- Give supplementary oxygen to maintain oxygen saturations >94%
- Perform a respiratory exam, particularly listening for crepitations which may suggest aspiration pneumonia
- Request an erect CXR

Circulation

- Assess haemodynamic stability by measuring pulse, blood pressure, capillary refill time and JVP. Review urine output
- Obtain two sites of intravenous access and take bloods
- Perform an ABG, and ECG
- Commence intravenous fluids

Disability

- Assess the patient's conscious level, either using AVPU or GCS. Check glucose

Exposure

- Expose the patient, and perform a full examination, particularly focusing on the abdomen. Is there evidence of perforation (e.g. peritonism)?
- Examine the entire patient, looking for sources of bleeding

> ## Management of Massive Upper GI Bleed:
>
> - *Major haemorrhage protocol (or equivalent at your hospital)*
> - *Cross match*
> - *Oxygen*
> - *IV fluids*

Prescribing

Initial Investigations

- **BLOODS:** Look for evidence of anaemia, infection, electrolyte derangement (raised urea suggestive of upper GI bleed), coagulation disorders, renal impairment. Cross-match 6 units, full blood count, urea and electrolytes, liver function tests, coagulation screen, amylase, calcium, lactate, C-reactive protein, and glucose. Take venous blood cultures if the patient is pyrexial

- **ABG:** Allows assessment of the metabolic status of the patient as well as the ventilation/oxygenation. Also gives an immediate haemoglobin

- **ERECT CXR:** Look for free air under the diaphragm suggestive of a perforation, for example from a GI ulcer. There may be evidence of consolidation (aspiration pneumonia). This will need to be a portable CXR if the patient is not stable enough to go to the X-ray department

- **ECG:** Especially in the elderly, if there is a history of cardiac disease or if there is massive blood loss. Cardiac ischemia may develop secondary to blood loss

Initial Management for all Severe UGI bleeds

- Upper GI bleed is a common emergency with a 10% mortality rate
- Common aetiologies: Peptic ulcer (50%), Varices (5-10%), Oesophagitis (10%), Mallory Weiss tear (5%), Vascular malformation (5%), Gastritis (15%)
- This patient shows features of a severe bleed (tachypnoea, tachycardia >100 bpm, hypotension SBP <100 mmHg supine or postural drop at any stage, clammy cold and peripherally shut down, reduced conscious level, history of syncope, and likely variceal bleed)
- The modified Rockall Score is a means of assessing risk of re-bleed and mortality following non-variceal upper GI bleeding. This score incorporates prognostic factors including age, shock, and co-morbidity. (The Rockall Score (non modified) incorporates endoscopy findings)
- **ACTIVATE MAJOR HAEMORRHAGE PROTOCOL** (or equivalent)
- **NIL BY MOUTH:** This patient may require surgical intervention. He should be nil by mouth until the senior review. Note any previous history of peptic ulcer, use of NSAID's or anticoagulants, liver disease or dyspeptic symptoms. Look for evidence of chronic liver disease such as jaundice or spider naevi. If present, refer to the GI registrar and continue to stabilise the patient
- **OXYGEN:** Maintain oxygen saturations >94%
- **SECURE IV ACCESS:** 2 large bore cannulae (16G or bigger)
- **INTRAVENOUS FLUIDS:** Rapid IV fluid resuscitation is required since patient is hypovolaemic. 0.9% saline (less favourable in liver disease) or colloid can be used in the first instance until blood is available. If features of circulatory compromise persist after initial bolus of fluids, commence blood transfusion. If available, use type specific or cross-matched blood. If not, use O negative blood. Use O negative blood if patient is exsanguinating or unable to keep BP above 100mgHg systolic, after more than 1 litre colloid given. Coagulopathy should be corrected using appropriate blood products, such as fresh frozen plasma or platelets after consultation with haematology
- **CATHETER:** A urethral catheter should be considered to monitor urine output and help assess fluid balance
- **CONTACT:** GI registrar and critical care areas (HDU/ICU) for definitive management of bleed and further support. Early endoscopy should be performed for all large bleeds and suspected varices, but the patient must be adequately resuscitated first
- Adequate resuscitation remains the cornerstone of management but early endoscopy should be performed for all large bleeds and suspected varices as soon as the patient is in a safe environment and adequately resuscitated

Additional Management for Variceal Bleeding

- This patient has possible variceal bleeding secondary to chronic liver disease
- **CONTACT:** GI Registrar referral immediately
- **FLUID RESUSCITATION:** Avoid saline as these patients will have advanced liver disease with resultant sodium retention. Use colloid, IV dextrose 5% and FFP as required
- **CONTINUOUS MONITORING:** Cardiac rate and rhythm, BP and oxygen saturation
- **TERLIPRESSIN:** 2mg IV then 1-2mg IV every 6 hours until bleeding is controlled, for up to 72 hours. Caution in ischaemic heart disease, peripheral vascular disease and unresuscitated patients
- **SENGSTAKEN – BLAKEMORE TUBE:** Only in dire situations
- **ANTIBIOTICS:** Antibiotic choice will depend on local antibiotic policies. Ceftriaxone 1G OD IV as per British Society of Gastroenterology guidelines. One other option is 4.5g of piperacillin and tazobactam (Tazocin) IV tds
- **FURTHER INTERVENTIONS:** e.g. Transjugular intrahepatic portosystemic shunt (TIPSS) may be considered if endoscopic treatment fails

24 HOUR FLUID PRESCRIPTION CHART

Hospital/Ward: RIE/CAA	Consultant: MJK	Name of Patient: STEVE SMITH
Weight: 65kg	Height: 1.73m	CHI Number: 2206381252
		D.O.B: 01/03/55
		(Attach printed label here)

Date/ Time	FLUID	VOLUME	RATE	PRESCRIBER – SIGN AND PRINT
	ADDED DRUGS	DOSE		
VENFLON 1 10/9/10 2100	GELOFUSINE	500ML	15 MINS	*M Jones* (MJ JONES)
VENFLON 2 10/9/10 2100	GELOFUSINE	500ML	15 MINS	*M Jones* (MJ JONES)

> After 1l of gelofusine, the patient begins to develop central chest pain and ischaemic changes on ECG. HR 110bpm, BP 95/50. This implies significant bleeding, and associated cardiac ischemia: red cells should be prescribed as below:

Date/ Time	FLUID	VOLUME	RATE	PRESCRIBER – SIGN AND PRINT
VENFLON 1 10/9/10 2100	RED CELL CONCENTRATE	1 UNIT	15 MINS	*M Jones* (MJ JONES)
VENFLON 2 10/9/10 2100	RED CELL CONCENTRATE	1 UNIT	15 MINS	*M Jones* (MJ JONES)

> Further fluid prescriptions will be determined by the patient's response to this fluid challenge. The patient needs to be reassessed before more fluids can be prescribed

Prescribing

Station 9: DIABETIC KETOACIDOSIS (DKA)

You are the FY1 on the medical admission unit, and are seeing a 19 year-old girl who has come in with shortness of breath, abdominal pain and vomiting. She is too confused to give you much history, but her mother tells you she has recently been unwell with diarrhoea, and has been passing large amounts of urine.

Obs	Sats 99% (on room air), RR 30, HR 128, BP 104/68, T 38.2°C
O/E	She looks dehydrated and is taking rapid breaths. There is an unusual smell on her breath. (GCS E/4, V/4, M/6= 14)
Urinalysis	Ketones +++, glucosuria ++++, no leukocytes or nitrites
ABG	PaO2 18, PaCO2 3.9, H+ 52nmol/L (pH 7.28), HCO3⁻ 14.2mmol/L, BE– 6.2
Bloods	Hb 143, WCC 13.4 (neutrophils 11), Plt 324, Urea 5.4, Cr 101, Na 136, K 5.0, LFTS and amylase normal. CRP 29
ECG	Sinus tachycardia

Initial Assessment

Airway

- Is the airway obstructed? Is the airway patent?
- Is the patient able to maintain their own airway? Secure the airway if necessary

Breathing

- Assess the respiratory rate and oxygen saturations
- Auscultate the chest, looking for evidence of infection
- Give supplementary oxygen to maintain oxygen saturations › 94%

Circulation

- Assess haemodynamic stability by measuring pulse, blood pressure, capillary refill time and JVP. Review urine output
- Obtain intravenous access and take urgent repeat sample for urea and electrolytes and glucose
- Perform an ABG and ECG
- Intravenous fluids

Disability

- Assess the patient's conscious level, either using AVPU or GCS

Exposure

- Expose the patient. Look for evidence of infection

> ## Management of DKA:
>
> - *IV Fluids*
> - *Insulin sliding scale*
> - *DVT prophylaxis*
> - *Regular reassessment*
> - *Monitor glucose and U&Es*

Initial Investigations

- **BLOODS:** Urgent repeat urea and electrolytes. Full blood count, liver function tests, blood glucose, venous lactate. This patient will require regular blood tests to assess for any electrolyte abnormalities, in particular hypokalaemia
- **ABG:** Can allow a rapid measure of potassium (serum K+ is measured in some laboratories). It will also identify a metabolic acidosis
- **ECG:** Look of evidence of arrhythmias secondary to electrolyte abnormalities
- **CXR:** Evidence of infection precipitating DKA
- **URINALYSIS:** Assess for ketones and for signs of a urinary tract infection
- **STOOL SAMPLE:** For culture and sensitivity

Initial Management

- **OXYGEN:** Correct hypoxia (Sats > 94%)
- **IV ACCESS:** 2 cannulae required for insulin sliding scale
- **NG TUBE:** If impaired consciousness or protracted vomiting

Monitoring

- Respiratory rate, ECG, oxygen saturations, pulse rate, BP, respiratory rate, conscious level and fluid balance
- **ECG:** Monitoring for any arrhythmias since patient may have severe electrolyte abnormalities (hypokalaemia-hyperkalaemia) With hyperkalemia: flattening of P waves, prolonged PR interval, widening of QRS, ST depression, tented T waves
- **BLOODS:** Hourly laboratory glucose required initially, and monitor potassium
- **CATHETER:** If patient is oliguric for monitoring fluid balance

Insulin

- Aim to ensure a gradual reduction in blood glucose over the first 12-24 hours
- Target blood glucose for the end of the first 24 hour period: 9-14 mmol/L
- Make up an infusion of 50 units of soluble insulin (e.g. Actrapid) in 50mls 0.9% NaCl (1unit/ml) and infuse using a syringe driver. Use 6 units/hr initially, and 3 units/hr when blood glucose is less than 13 mmol/L
- Add dextrose 5% at 100ml/hr when blood glucose is <14mmol/L
- If glucose falls <10mmol/L, reduce insulin infusion to 2 units/hr

Fluid and Electrolytes

- **FLUID REPLACEMENT:** Commence fluid therapy with 0.9% NaCl, 1000mls over 1 hour. Following regular reassessment proceed with aggressive fluid resuscitation. Infusion rates will vary between patients; remember the risk of cardiac failure in elderly patients (although DKA is fortunately much less common in the elderly)
- A possible regimen could be 1000mls 0.9% NaCl over 2nd hour, 500mls 0.9% NaCl over 3rd hour, 500mls 0.9% NaCl over 4th hour
- **ELECTROLYTE REPLACEMENT:** Potassium will fall following commencement of insulin; expect to have to give plenty of potassium following acute fluid resuscitation. Severe hypokalaemia complicating treatment of DKA is potentially fatal but is avoidable. Target concentration 4.0-5.0mmol/l

Correction of Acidosis

- Volume resuscitation and insulin infusion will correct metabolic acidosis in the majority
- Intravenous sodium bicarbonate should not be used routinely and certainly not without discussing with a senior doctor

Identification of Precipitating Factors

- Full blood count, CXR, ECG, urine dipstick, and blood cultures. Others, such as infection screen investigations may be required
- **THROMBOPROPHYLAXIS:** As per local protocol e.g. ENOXAPARIN 40mg subcutaneously OD
- **CONTACTS:** Diabetes registrar and/or senior medical staff. Contact critical care areas if organ support and close monitoring (e.g. via central line) required

Prescribing

PRESCRIPTION AND ADMINISTRATION RECORD
Standard Chart

Hospital/Ward: WGH/53	Consultant: CAP	Name of Patient: JANETSMITH
Weight: 65kg	Height: 1.70m	CHI Number: 0103920045
If re-written, date:		D.O.B.: 01/03/92
DISCHARGE PRESCRIPTION Date completed:-	Completed by:-	(Attach printed label here)

OTHER MEDICINE CHARTS IN USE		PREVIOUS ADVERSE REACTIONS This section must be completed before any medicine is given		Completed by (sign & print)	Date
Date	Type of Chart	None known ☐			
6/9/10	NONE	Medicine/Agent	Description of Reaction		
		PENICILLIN	RASH	M Jones (JONES)	6/9/10

CODES FOR NON-ADMINISTRATION OF PRESCRIBED MEDICINE

If a dose is not administered as prescribed, initial and enter a code in the column with a circle drawn round the code according to the reason as shown below. **Inform the responsible doctor in the appropriate timescale.**

1. Patient refuses
2. Patient not present
3. Medicines not available – CHECK ORDERED
4. Asleep/drowsy
5. Administration route not available – CHECK FOR ALTERNATIVE

6. Vomiting/nausea
7. Time varied on doctor's instructions
8. Once only/ as required medicine given
9. Dose withheld on doctor's instructions
10. Possible adverse reaction/side effect

ONCE ONLY

Date	Time	Medicine (Approved Name)	Dose	Route	Prescriber – Sign + Print	Time Given	Given By
6/9/10	2000	50 UNITS ACTRAPID IN 50ML 0.9% NaCl	AS SLIDING SCALE BELOW	IV INFUSION	M Jones (JONES)		

BLOOD GLUCOSE (mmol/l)	INSULIN INFUSION (UNIT ACTRAPID/HOUR =ML/HR)
>16	6
13-15.9	4
10-12.9	3
7-9.9	2
5-6.9	1
4-4.9	0.5
<4	0 (CALL DOCTOR)

OXYGEN

Date		top Time

24 HOUR FLUID PRESCRIPTION CHART

Hospital/Ward: WGH/53	Consultant: CAP	Name of Patient: JANET SMITH
Weight: 65 kg	Height: 1.70m	CHI Number: 0103920045
		D.O.B: 01/03/92
		(Attach printed label here)

Date/ Time	FLUID / ADDED DRUGS	VOLUME / DOSE	RATE	PRESCRIBER – SIGN AND PRINT
Venflon 1 8/10/10 2200	0.9% SODIUM CHLORIDE	500ml	OVER 30 MINUTES	M Jones (JONES)
Venflon 2 8/10/10 2200	0.9% SODIUM CHLORIDE	500ml	OVER 30 MINUTES	M Jones (JONES)
	Reassess fluid status; heart rate, blood pressure, urine output. If patient still fluid deplete continue rehydration (fluid prescribed as below)			
Venflon 1 8/10/10 2300	0.9% SODIUM CHLORIDE	1000ml	OVER 60 MINUTES	M Jones (JONES)
	Reassess fluid status; heart rate, blood pressure, urine output. If patient still fluid deplete continue rehydration (fluid prescribed as below)			
Venflon 1 9/10/10 0000	0.9% SODIUM CHLORIDE	500ml	OVER 60 MINUTES	M Jones (JONES)
	Add dextrose 5% at 100ml/hr once blood glucose ‹14, as shown below. Otherwise run sliding scale with NaCl 0.9% at 100ml/hr. Consider electrolyte replacement following rehydration phase.			
Venflon 2 9/10/10	5% Dextrose	500ml	OVER 5 HOURS	M Jones (JONES)

Prescribing

Station 10: DISCHARGE PRESCRIBING

Mr Smith is a 50 year-old gentleman who was admitted to your hospital recently with a right lower lobe pneumonia. He is now fit for discharge but requires 'to take out' (TTO) prescriptions of his medications. Please complete the TTO form below using Mr Smith's drug chart and the BNF if necessary.

- It is possible to pass this station and do very well if you are methodical in your approach and know the specific information that is required for certain drugs
- The best source of information is the BNF, which also has information on the prescribing of controlled drugs
- You should practice this station before the real OSCE and familiarise yourself with prescribing common drugs

Part 1: Prescribing Regular Medications

- Look at the regular medications section of the drug chart. The patient will need to continue the majority of these drugs once they leave hospital
- Do not continue drugs such as enoxaparin (unless specifically indicated and arrangements have been made for it to be given in the community)
- Antibiotics should only be given for the prescribed course (e.g. for 3 more days). If you do have to prescribe antibiotics on a TTO, you should know how long they need to be continued, and if unsure check with a senior colleague

Examples of regular medications prescribed on a TTO are shown below:

Drug	Dose & Frequency	Number of Days	Pharmacy
Aspirin	75mg OD	28	
Omeprazole	40mg OD	28	
Levothyroxine	125 microgram OD	28	
Ramipril	5mg OD	28	

Do not fill in the pharmacy box on the right. This is for the pharmacy staff to fill in when they dispense the drug.

Part 2: Prescribing PRN (As Required) Medication

- Often a patient will only need to be sent home with PRN analgesia
- It is your job to decide which of these drugs the patient needs to be sent home with
- PRN medication is usually prescribed for 7-14 days after discharge (as opposed to 28 days for regular medications)
- In order to decide which medications to prescribe, you need to determine how many times these drugs have been prescribed in the time leading up to discharge and use your common sense
- If the drug has not been given for a number of days, you may not even need to prescribe it

Example

- *Mr AC has been requiring 20-30mg of oramorph every day as breakthrough analgesia*
- *Assuming his pain is improving, you would want to send him home with, for example, 7 days worth of 20 mg oramorph per day. Oramorph is distributed as 10mg/5ml strength (of morphine sulphate) in 100 and 300ml bottles. (Concentrated forms are also available (100mg/5ml))*
- *The daily dose of 20 mg = 10 ml*
- *7 days x 10 ml = 70 ml*
- *Therefore, you would prescribe a 100-ml bottle, which would leave slightly extra in case this patient needs more analgesia*
- *These types of calculations are mostly done on the basis of common sense, with some help from the BNF. Oramorph is a controlled drug and therefore has a couple of extra issues with its prescription, which are covered in more detail in the next section*

The way to prescribe the above example is shown below:

Drug	Dose & Frequency	Number of Days	Pharmacy
Oramorph oral solution. Morphine sulphate 10mg/5ml. Supply 100ml (One hundred millilitres)	20mg 2 hourly as required	7	

Part 3: Prescribing Controlled Drugs

These drugs often cause the most confusion, but if you follow the simple rules below and are sensible, you shouldn't go wrong!

When prescribing controlled drugs, the prescription must state:

- The name and address of the patient
- The form and strength of the drug (as appropriate)
- Either the total quantity or the number of dosage units of drug written in **both words and figures**
- The dose of the drug

The prescription must then be signed, dated, and also contain the prescriber's hospital address. Without such information, the pharmacy will not prescribe the controlled drug.

Example

If a patient has been receiving morphine sulphate MR (modified release) 5 mg bd in the hospital, you would prescribe it on the TTO as shown:

Drug	Dose & Frequency	Number of Days	Pharmacy
Morphine Sulphate Modified Release 5 mg tablets. Oral. Supply 56 (fifty-six) tablets.	5 mg BD	28	

Station 11: ANALGESIA

Mr Smith is a surgical inpatient who has been diagnosed with appendicitis and is awaiting theatre. He has severe right iliac fossa pain and has not yet received any analgesia. Please prescribe appropriate medication, and indicate how you might proceed if the pain were to persist despite initial treatment.

Pain can be difficult to manage. Furthermore, the side effects of analgesics can be more damaging than the pain itself. A simple, structured approach to analgesia will help address these issues in the majority of cases.

Analgesia should be prescribed using the World Health Organisation (WHO) analgesic ladder as a guide.

Two general rules to note when using the WHO analgesic ladder are:

1) Start at the step most appropriate for the patient's pain (e.g. if the patient has suffered a fractured femur and is complaining of a lot of pain, you should move straight to step 3, rather than trying step 1 and awaiting to see if the pain settles).

2) If the pain is not controlled, avoid changing one drug for another of equal potency in the same class (e.g. do not change codeine to dihydrocodeine). Instead move up the ladder until adequate analgesia is reached.

WHO analgesic ladder

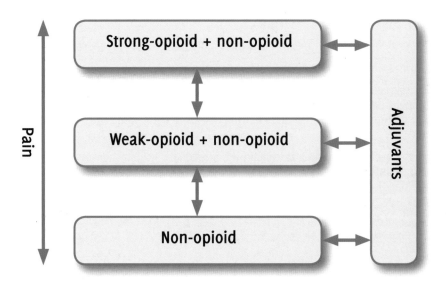

1. **Non-Opioids**

   Paracetamol (1g qds oral/IV) is an effect pain killer, and should (invariably) be prescribed regularly to every patient who has pain.

2. **Weak-Opioids**

   If the pain is not controlled with regular paracetamol alone, a weak opioid should be added. Options include codeine phosphate (30-60mg up to 4 hourly oral, max 240mg/24 hours) and dihydrocodeine (30mg up to 4 hourly oral/SC/IM).

3. **Strong-Opioids**

   If pain continues despite maximum doses of non – and weak opioids, the weak opioid should be stopped and a trial of strong opioids (morphine) commenced. Morphine has serious side effects and needs to be prescribed with care (see below).

4. **Adjuvants**

   They include non-steroidal anti-inflammatory drugs (for bony metastases, liver pain), corticosteroids (for nerve compression, liver pain, raised intracranial pressure), gabapentin and amitriptyline (for neuropathic pain). The nature of the pain will determine which adjuvant is appropriate and these should be considered with any step in the analgesic ladder. It is best to discuss the use of these drugs with a senior and/or the pain team.

Prescribing Morphine

- Morphine can either be immediate release (i.e. short acting) or controlled release (i.e. long acting)
- It can be administered orally, IV, IM, SC or topically
- In most acute scenarios, the oral route is the most appropriate. If this is not available other routes such as IM, IV, SC can be considered
- One should be aware of the dosing differences when using these different routes (see below)

- Most patients with continuous, acute, severe pain should initially be prescribed short acting morphine (Oramorph/Sevredol, Oxynorm)
- This takes about 20 minutes to work and lasts approximately 4 hours
- It is difficult to know how much morphine a patient will need. Therefore, it is best to prescribe it initially as an 'as required' medication (e.g. Morphine, 5mg prn, maximum frequency 4 hourly, oral)
- The dose and frequency of the morphine can be adjusted according to the pain and degree of side effects (e.g. increasing to 5mg prn, maximum frequency 2 hourly, oral if the patient continues to be in pain)

- Long acting morphine (MST Continus/Zomorph/Morphgesic SR, oxycontin) takes longer to have an effect but lasts 12 hours
- It is prescribed twice a day, after titration with short acting morphine has achieved adequate analgesia
- The dose of long acting morphine is calculated by taking the total amount of short acting morphine used in 24 hours and dividing by 2
- 'Break through' short acting morphine will also be required and is one sixth of the total amount of short acting morphine used in 24 hours

For example, if a patient had used 6x10mg prn doses of Oramorph in 24 hours (i.e. 60mg), 30mg (60/2 = 30) of long acting morphine, such as MST, could be prescribed bd as well as Oramorph 10mg prn 4 hourly (60/6 = 10)

It should be noted that MST should be used when Oramorph is the prn opioid, whereas oxycontin should be prescribed when oxynorm is the 'break through' opioid.

Equivalent Doses of Opioids

Oral Morphine 5mg
= oral codeine 60mg
= oral dihydrocodeine 60mg
= SC morphine 2.5mg
= oral oxycodone 2.5mg

Side effects and cautions of commonly prescribed analgesics

Drug	Side Effects	Cautions
Paracetamol	Rare but may include: Rashes Thrombocytopenia Neutropenia	Hepatic impairment – avoid large doses Renal impairment – max rate 6 hourly if Creatine Clearance (CrCl) <30ml/min
Codeine Phosphate, Dihydrocodeine, Morphine, Oxycodone hydrochloride	Nausea and vomiting Constipation Respiratory depression Dry mouth Difficulty micturating Sedation	Hepatic or renal impairment – reduce dose Respiratory depression, asthma attack Prostatic hypertrophy Elderly

In those with renal impairment, instead of morphine or oxycodone, consider alternatives such as alfentanil, or fentanyl.

For the majority of patients, the WHO analgesic ladder will provide sufficient analgesia. However it will not be possible to control every patient's pain with the above strategy. In these cases discussion with your seniors and the pain team would be a useful next step.

Prescribing

11 Critical Appraisal

C ritical appraisal is a difficult skill to master. The key to doing well is developing a simple structure that works for you. Many different people produce excellent answers using different approaches, and reaching very different conclusions. Make sure that you provide evidence for any conclusion that is made, and that you discuss both sides of the argument. It is important to practise as many papers as possible. This is the best way to develop the ability to quickly and accurately apply your system for analysing papers.

This chapter contains notes on the following:

11.1 Writing an Abstract

11.2 The Manuscript

11.3 Application of Results to the Patient

Study Action Plan

- Prepare a rubric that makes sense to you and that you can follow for systematically reviewing each paper

- If you have the opportunity to attend conferences during the year, try and attend a 'late breaking trail' or big research paper presentation. Insight into what is important in analysing papers can be gained from the discussions led by experts passionate about the topic

- Attend and even present at journal clubs within your department: where papers are discussed and appraised (and often a free lunch is given!)

- If applicable, review past papers, answer questions, and compare your answers to the mark scheme. If not, just practice appraising articles in any medical journal (pick an area you're interested in) and get a friend to look at the same article, so you can compare answers

WRITING AN ABSTRACT

Study Background

Why is this study being done? What is the problem?

Objective

What is the specific question being answered by the study?

Design

How is the study designed? Major trials will often be a multi-centre, randomised controlled trial (RCT).

Study Population

State the group being studied, plus the most important characteristics of them. There is no need to list every inclusion and exclusion criteria.

Setting

Where is the study being done? For example, it could be *'rural GP clinics in Germany'*.

Intervention

What is being done? This can be stated very broadly.

Outcome Measures

State the main outcome measures, and any particularly important secondary outcomes.

Results

What was the result as measured by the main outcome? State the confidence intervals (if present) and p-values. Some secondary outcome data may also be stated if it yields important information.

Conclusion

Summarise what can be drawn from the study. In *[group A]*, *[intervention x]* is more effective at improving *[outcome]*, as measured by *[outcome measure]*, than *[intervention y]*. Make a comment on any likely consequences of the study findings. What research is now required? How can the study findings be applied to real life practise?

THE MANUSCRIPT

Study Background

- Was the trial well justified and the purpose/hypothesis clear?
- Is there a gap in research for a clinically important problem?
- Does the purpose of the trial clearly address this problem?
- Can the intervention and the results in principle be applied to the local population (and to the individual in front of you)?

Sample Selection

- What is the source of the patients? Rural clinics vs. urban clinic. Hospital vs. GP practice
- What are the inclusion and exclusion criteria?
- Is there a rationale given for each of the criteria or do they appear arbitrary?

'The first thing I always ask myself when looking at a paper is simply 'why has this research been done?' Have a clear idea in your head what question is being asked, whether a clinically important problem has been clearly identified, and if the question being asked can potentially fix this problem'

Zeshan Qureshi

Paediatrics Trainee, London Deanery

From this information, you should decide whether the trial is *'tightly defined'* (many criteria) or *'loosely defined'* (few criteria). There is often no right answer for this, so just ensure you justify your response.

If the sample is tightly defined, there may be a selection bias. This means the results will apply very specifically to people that meet all of the extensive inclusion criteria of the trial. It is a *'non-differential'* selection bias since both the control and treatment groups will be affected equally.

A tightly defined sample increases the probability of a positive result (because the patients are highly selected to those the study organisers think the treatment will work in, and because the variance is less), but since few people are likely to meet all the criteria, the results are less generalisable.

Generalisability is also supported by a small drop-off rate from invitation. Preferably more than 50% of invited subjects should enter the trial.

Randomisation

The Advantage of Randomisation

Randomisation balances unknown confounding factors (things not measured in the study population). It also produces the highest grade of evidence.

How Was Randomisation Done?

This should be explicitly stated in the paper. Ideally, a phone/central randomisation line should be employed since this reduces the possibility of bias. Conflicts of interest should be avoided. Numbered sealed envelopes dispensed in GP consultations, for example, would be more prone to bias.

1. *Simple Randomisation:* The most common and basic method of randomisation. It is based on a single randomly generated sequence. For example, using a coin: heads could equate to allocation to the treatment group and tails allocation to the control group.

- Advantage: Simple and easy
- Disadvantage: Problematic in small trials since it may result in unbalanced groups: it could result in 10 heads and 1 tails! There may also be a significant difference in the baseline characteristics between the 2 groups

2. *Block Randomisation:* Small 'blocks' with equal treatment and control 'units' are generated to ensure the number of participants in each group is approximately equal. For example, a block size of 4 could be chosen. If the T 'unit' indicates treatment and the C 'unit' indicates control, every possible combination of 4 units, with 2 'T's and 2 'C's (i.e. equal T and C) is calculated. In this case, it would be TTCC, TCCT, CTTC, CTCT, TCTC, and TCTC. Each set of 4 is one block. Participants are then randomised into these blocks, with each subsequent block being randomly selected from the group of possible blocks.

- Advantage: Results in approximately balanced groups
- Disadvantage: Even with this method, there is still the problem of groups being unequal not in numbers but in characteristics e.g. one group may have more diabetic patients

3. *Stratified Randomisation:* The details of this are complicated, but this can be used to balance baseline characteristics, e.g. having an equal number of men and women in both groups, but still randomise participants.

- Advantage: Results in groups of similar numbers, and similar baseline characteristics
- Disadvantage: Can be difficult to generate the model

Potential for Subversion

There should be separation of generator and executor: whoever conducts the randomisation should be blinded to the groups (and thus their ability to subvert the randomisation is limited). There may be other possibilities of subversion. For example, if a GP is deciding on groups he may know the patient and want to put them in the treatment group. In a sealed envelope allocation, he could therefore select the envelopes until one with *'treatment'* comes up, and reseal the others.

Did the Randomisation Work?

- Is there a baseline characteristics table?
- Are all relevant baseline characteristics included?
- Are the groups similar? Are p values shown to assess significance of differences in baseline characteristics?

If there are significant group differences, this is a *'differential'* selection bias, since it affects the 2 groups differently.

If there is a differential selection bias, the next question to ask is how did the authors deal with possible confounding factors in the trial population? There are several possible options. The authors could use multivariate analysis (which essentially accounts for any effect of a confounding factor). Alternatively, they could demonstrate that the potential confounder was not related to the outcome.

The Intervention

Description of Intervention

- Was the intervention described in sufficient detail to replicate it? E.g. staff (experience, cost, training) and resource requirements?
- With regards to what is actually done, either:

  - The intervention could be standardised, to ensure all therapists act in a similar manner. For example, a specific manual could be used, or regular observation of therapists by experts could be employed. This results in reduced internal performance bias (all therapists act similarly). Therefore the result of the trial is a greater reflection of the specific effect of the therapy. However, it has the disadvantage of not replicating real-world behaviour

  - The alternative is no standardisation to the intervention. This results in a performance bias between therapists (therapists may act in a different manner to each other) and therefore trial participants may perform well/poorly because of the arbitrary allocation of therapist to them. However, this method has the advantage of mimicking real-world behaviour

It is also important to establish whether there are multiple facets to the intervention (the components of the 'black box'). If there are, then it is helpful for the authors to demonstrate which particular components of the intervention are important. An intervention that involves both leaflets and one-on-one-therapy may have a positive effect purely due to leafleting. Therefore, including one-on-one therapy in the intervention is an unnecessary cost. You cannot tell if this is the case if the trial does not separate the effect of different facets.

Control Group

- Were the controls given standard therapy? This is more useful clinically than comparison with no therapy though it is less likely to show a positive result
- Apart from the intervention, were the 2 groups treated equally? For example, was there an *attention bias*: did the therapy group gets considerably more time with healthcare professionals?
- Was an attention control used if relevant? This controls for an attention bias by ensuring equal time with healthcare professionals for both groups (good for demonstrating efficacy and teasing out specific effects of the intervention, but not so good for estimating the overall effect, including 'attention' of an intervention)
- Was a normal care control used? (most useful for economic analysis, and the best way of demonstrating overall effect)

Outcomes

Put simply, were all clinically important outcomes included and measured properly?

Choice of Measures

- Are there multiple outcome measures? This has the advantage of looking at the effect of treatment in contrasting manners. The disadvantage is it increases the likelihood of a positive result purely due to chance (type I error)
- Are they surrogate or direct measures of outcome? Direct measures are more accurate, and both easier to explain and more relevant to patients
- Are the measures validated or not validated? Validated measures have been tested to verify that they measure what they are intended to measure. This may be included as a reference in the paper
- Is there any analysis of the harms of the intervention? This is often excluded
- Is there a specific quality of life measure? E.g. quality-adjusted life years (QALYs). This is often very important for patients
- Are the outcome measures important for patients? Can you explain it to the patient in language they can understand?

Analysis of Outcome

- Are the same outcome measures used in both groups?
- Are they measured at the same time point in both groups?
- Is the analysis of outcomes blinded? The use of an independent researcher to analyse outcome is desirable but not always possible (e.g. self-reporting for studies of pain is almost inevitable, and self-reporting versus self-reporting to an 'independent' researcher is not a helpful distinction)

Self-reported outcome measures are perhaps prone to more bias if the participants are not blinded. For example, consider a trial looking at the management of depression, and a questionnaire based outcome measure. The participants may have already prejudged the old treatment as ineffective. This prejudgement, if the participant knows which group they are in, may be reflected in their subjective answers to the questionnaire.

Intention to Treat Analysis

In an intention to treat analysis, patients are analysed in the randomised groups regardless of whether they complied with treatment. Where possible those that drop out of the study have data carried forward as opposed to having all their data excluded. Intention to treat analysis mimics real-world patient decisions, and real-world treatment effects including stopping medication due to reasons such as serious side effects.

Per Protocol Analysis

For real-world treatment decisions, this is not as good, but it should ideally be included as well since it gives an alternative perspective. Per protocol analysis only considers those that remain compliant with therapy. It therefore gives an idea as to what will happen to a patient if they are adherent with treatment for the entire duration of the follow-up. The disadvantage of per protocol analysis is that it in effect undermines the original randomisation groups. If different population samples drop out of each group, like is no longer being compared with like. In addition those that stop taking a drug for example may do so because it isn't working, or it is giving unbearable side effects.

Follow-Up

Is the duration long enough for meaningful clinical decision making? Is the follow-up equal in both groups? The duration is often not long enough: depression for example is a lifelong disease; aspirin therapy is usually taken for life. It is therefore useful to know the effect on chronic disease 5 or 10 years down the line.

Were all the patients accounted for? Was there high loss to follow-up? It is important that a CONSORT diagram (see next page) is included for this purpose: it includes this information. Up to 20% loss to follow-up is considered reasonable. Figures higher than 20% reduces the generalisability of the results.

If participants drop out, it is important that the reason for this is stated. Adverse reaction/lost motivation/death: these may all relate to the outcome! It is also useful to look at the characteristics of those that dropped out: are they different to those that did not drop out? If so, there may be a response bias: for example, young men are often more likely to drop out. This influences application of treatment, as in this scenario you would need to know if demographics relate to treatment efficacy.

Consort Flow Diagram

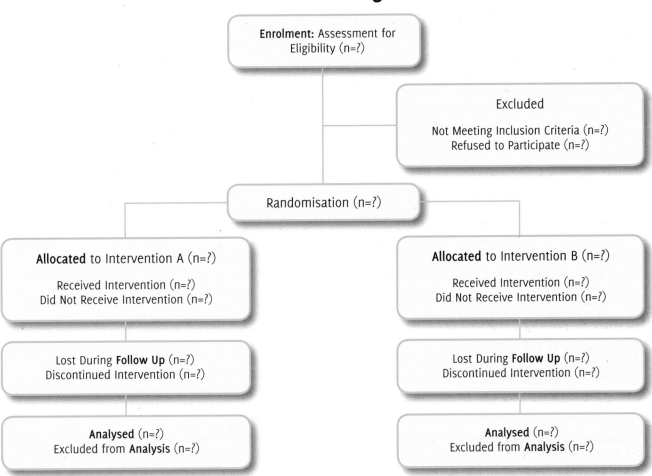

Statistics

Chance

Is there a type I error or a false-positive result? This is a positive result that has occurred due to chance. Simply put, is the primary outcome, measured at the primary time point a statistically significant effect with $p < 0.05$?

Other factors than can also be taken into consideration:

- A type I error is more likely to occur if there are multiple outcome variables, and it happens that only 1 or 2 yield significant results. Since $p = 0.05$ means there is a 1/20 chance that a result has been obtained by chance, if there are 20 different outcome variables being measured, one borderline significant result would probably carry little weight
- A type I error is also more likely if a significant result is found only in secondary analysis or in a new analysis not stated in methods
- Type I errors are less likely if there are multiple significant outcomes, and if the primary outcome is strongly significant

Power

Is there a type II error or a false-negative result? This is a negative result purely due to small sample size.

- To assess this, the power calculation must be looked at. If the power is <80%, the study is underpowered, i.e. there were not enough participants in the study to be able to detect an effect
- If the proposed effect size detailed in the power calculations is larger than a clinically important effect (i.e. the study was trying to find too large an effect), the effect size should be justified. If the power calculation is looking for a 10% change in the depression score, what is the clinical significance of a 10% change in depression score?

Confidence Intervals

- A 95% confident interval of between 1 and 3 implies that there is a 95% chance that the true answer for whatever is being measured is somewhere between 1 and 3. This is equivalent to a 5% chance the result is either above 1 or below 3
- To be significant, the 95% confidence interval should not overlap with the null line (no effect). This means that the upper and lower boundaries of the confidence interval should both show the same effect (either positive or negative)

- If the confidence interval overlaps with the null e.g. upper boundary is a positive effect, but lower boundary is a negative effect, the result is not significant. This is equivalent to p>0.05 (since there is less than a 95% chance that the true answer is definitely a significant effect (either positive or negative)
- Also ask, is the confidence interval wide or narrow? Look at the extremes. At both ends of the CI, is there still a clinically relevant effect?

Clinical Importance of Results

A number needed to treat (NNT) and a number needed to harm (NNH) should be calculated, ideally for a primary outcome.

$$\text{NNT} = \frac{100}{\text{Percentage Difference Between Groups}}$$

For example, if the incidence of death is 2/200 (for the new treatment) and 22/200 (for the old treatment)

This is equivalent to 1% deaths vs. 11% deaths, a difference of 10%.
The NNT to prevent 1 death is therefore 100/10 =10.

- To estimate a meaningful NNT, dichotomous data is necessary (i.e. 2 groups, e.g. alive/dead, off antidepressants/on antidepressants, suicidal thoughts/no suicidal thoughts), and a statistically significant result
- For continuous data (e.g. BP, i.e. not 2 groups): what does the measured difference mean clinically? For surrogate markers like BP, the relationship between the surrogate and important clinical endpoints (e.g. death and MI) should be understood
- For questionnaires: how is it scored? What do the results mean? For continuous questionnaire outcomes (e.g. self scoring pain) it can be helpful to think of the percentage change in the mean relative to the control group (so if the control group mean was 5/10 and the intervention group was 3/10, this would be a 2/10 or 20% improvement)

Conclusions

- Is there new information from the trial?
- Were limitations acknowledged and appropriate conclusions drawn?
- Were the study results related to other evidence (reviews or other trials)?
- How does the study intervention compare with other alternatives?
- Is the trial cost-effective? Is there an estimate of cost given?
- Are there multiple conflicts of interests from the authors?
- Can the intervention and the results in principle be applied to the local population (and to the individual in front of you)?

'The conclusions of a paper should make clear to you what the practical implications of the results are. How does this study change the way a doctor should approach the assessment or management of a patient? How do the results impact on quality of patient care?'

Zeshan Qureshi
Paediatrics Trainee
London Deanery

Biases

Here is a summary of some biases that can be included in the analysis of a trial.

1. *PERFORMANCE BIAS:* Is this how the therapists will act in real-life practice? Standardised instructions may mean performance is less reflective of day-to-day practise.

2. *ATTENTION BIAS:* Giving extra attention to participants may improve outcome even if the intervention itself does not have any direct effect.

3. *ANALYSIS BIAS:* Data is not analysed at the same time interval or by the same method in the 2 groups. An effect may be masked by analysing data at an earlier point in one group compared to the other.

4. *SELECTION BIAS:*
   - **Non-Differential:** Affects both groups equally, e.g. all individuals included in the study are over 60. This biases the result of the entire study to the demographic of patients aged over 60
   - **Differential:** Affects 1 group more than the other, e.g. having more diabetic patients in the control (no intervention) group as compared to the intervention group. The control group may have an artificially greater mortality rate purely due to diabetes-related illnesses, regardless of any effect of intervention

5. *LEAD TIME BIAS:* Conditions are diagnosed earlier, e.g. if the patient sees a therapist very regularly or is in more regular contact with other sufferers of the disease, they may have problems pointed out at an earlier stage, and therefore report them earlier. This is not developing the problem earlier.

6. *HAWTHORN EFFECT:* Just by participating in a trial, the results are different. People may work harder, and are more compliant with advice because they know they are being analysed.

Patient Factors

- Do they have the time and money to do the intervention? Especially relevant if the treatment is not available on NHS.
- What is the current treatment that the patient is on? How does the treatment offered compare to this? Has the patient tried the intervention before?
- Does the patient want to do it?

Trial Factors

- Internal validity: are there any crucial problems with the trial?
- External validity: does the trial group apply to the patient in front of you?

Local Factors

- Trust resources: does the trust have the expertise, funding, staff, facilities, and medication available for this programme?
- What are the views of the local community/local GPs/patient community on using the resource?
- Opportunity cost: is it a cost-effective use of resources? Is it better than other options for using NHS resources?

12 Medical Letters

Writing a hospital letter requires an in-depth understanding of an inpatient episode and the ability to summarise the clinically relevant information, pertinent investigations, results and follow-up.

This is often an area in which students have little experience before finals and before becoming a junior doctor.

Study Action Plan

- Prepare a basic structure that makes sense to you and that you can follow for writing each type of letter
- Practice summarising cases succinctly. Write drafts for both transfer letters and referral letters on the wards, which can then be edited by junior doctors or registrars. Most doctors will be very grateful for this: it will be helping them out! See and try to understand any changes they make to your letter
- Get experience in interpreting letters: whilst on a GP placement, read through discharge letters with your GP. Likewise whilst in clinic or on the wards, read through transfer/referral letters with the doctor who is about to see the patient. This is a great way to learn what relevant information is commonly missed in these kinds letters

This chapter contains the notes on the following:

TRANSFER LETTER

[Insert address of receiving hospital]

[Insert address of doctor sending letter]

[Insert date of letter]

Dear: [Insert doctor's name]
Re: [Insert name and identification details of patient]

Admission Date: Transfer Date:
Ward:
Consultant:

Diagnosis:

- List the diagnosis that the patient has been given
- This can include previous diagnosis given before this hospital admission, but the new conditions should be listed first, and in order of clinical importance
- The conditions should be as specific as possible. *"Left lower lobe pneumonia"* is better than *"chest infection"*

Reason for Transfer:

- State clearly what is expected of the unit receiving the patient
- Does the patient require rehabilitation? Do they require an operation at a specialist centre? Do they require optimisation of medical management post surgery?
- Do any additional investigations need to be performed?

Progress:

- What were the symptoms that the patient presented with, and what diagnosis were they given?
- What was the mode of admission? Emergency or elective?
- What treatment did the patient receive?
- After initial treatment, did the patient develop any complications?
- What services has the patient seen? This could include services such as liaison psychiatry, social work, and cardiac rehabilitation nurses

State the current medical condition of the patient. Is the patient clinically stable?

The skill here is to pick out key pieces of information that the receiving doctor needs to know without repeating the entire contents of the notes verbatim. Depending on the case, it may be relevant to include here elements of past medical and social history.

Key Investigations:

- It isn't necessary to include every blood test, but include the clinically relevant results, and the date that the tests were performed. Recent blood tests are likely to be relevant particularly if abnormal. You need to make a judgement about what is important for continuing care
- Include the results of major scans like CT and MRI
- Note any tests that have been performed but are awaiting results

Drugs on Transfer:

Include here the drugs that will be continued at transfer. Include the following key points:

- Generic name of drug
- Dose
- Frequency of administration
- Route of administration
- Length of treatment

Don't forget to include information about allergies or adverse reactions to drugs. With certain drugs like gentamicin or warfarin, do blood tests need to be done? If so, when?

Also, depending on the reason for transfer, the patient may still be quite unwell, such as in the case of an ITU patient being transferred to a specialist centre for surgery. They may be receiving infusions – these should also be noted. The patient may also be receiving respiratory support – this would also need to be detailed.

Follow Up:

- Has an appointment been made to return to clinic?
- When is the appointment, and who is it with? Is it in the organising hospital, or is the expectation that further follow-up will happen at the destination unit?
- Are other services like psychiatry, physiotherapy, dietician, etc. following the patient up as well?

Information Given to Patient/ Family:

Has the patient/family been counselled about their current problem, the reason for the transfer, and any further follow-up or contact with the referring unit?

It is polite to finish by stating something like *'If you have any further questions, please do not hesitate to contact me or another member of [insert consultant's name] team.'*

Sign off the letter with your details, and a contact number.

Yours sincerely,

[Insert name of referring doctor]

[Insert designation of referring doctor and consultant e.g. FY1 to Dr Jones]
[Insert contact details of referring doctor]

REFERRAL LETTER

[Insert address of corresponding hospital]   [Insert address of doctor sending letter]

[Insert date of letter]

Dear: [Insert doctor's name]
Re: [Insert name and identification details of patient]

Diagnosis:

As with the discharge letter, list the major health conditions attributed to the patient.

Make it clear what you think is the likely problem. At the point of referral, a symptom complex may be all that is known, but the referring GP should make what needs to be assessed clear. The diagnosis may simply be *'breast lump for further investigation'*.

It is nice to start with a polite introduction. For example *'I would be grateful if you could review **[insert name of the patient]** regarding her **[insert name of condition]**'*

Current Problem:

- Describe the issue for which the patient has presented today as you have seen them in your clinic
- What relevant symptoms do they have? Is there a known cause?
- Then relate this to how the disease has developed since first presentation
- When did it start? Is it getting worse? Have new symptoms been developing?

Key Investigations:

Only the most relevant investigations need to be put down. Include the date of the investigations. Note any tests with pending results.

Treatment to Date:

- How has the problem been managed to date?

After this, it is worth documenting other relevant history that is not directly linked to the current problem.

Current Medication:

Medications and allergies should be noted
Include the following key points:
- Generic name of drug
- Dose
- Frequency of administration
- Route of administration
- Length of treatment

Social History:

- Smoking status and alcohol intake (if relevant)
- What is the patient's home and work circumstances?
- How is the disease affecting them?
- What does the patient think about their current situation?
- What has been explained to the patient about the current situation so far?
- Is there any important information (such as a cancer diagnosis) that they are unaware of?

It is important to add specifically what you want from this consultation. *'I would like your opinion with regard to the most likely diagnosis'* or *'I would like advise on further management options for this patient's emphysema'*. It is good to end with something like *'If you would like any more information, do not hesitate to contact me. I look forward to hearing from you.'*

Yours sincerely,

[Insert name of referring doctor]

[Insert designation of referring doctor and senior doctor if relevant]
[Insert contact details of referring doctor]

DISCHARGE LETTER

[Insert address and name of receiving GP]   [Insert address of hospital and ward]

                                                   [Insert date of letter]

Dear: [Insert doctor's name]
Re: [Insert name and identification details of patient]

Admission Date: Discharge Date:
Ward:
Consultant:

Diagnosis:

- List the diagnosis that the patient has been given
- This can include previous diagnosis given before this hospital admission, but the new conditions should be listed first, and in order of clinical importance
- The conditions should be as specific as possible e.g. *'anterior ST elevation myocardial infarction'* is better than *'heart attack'*

Progress:

- Admitted on [date] as an [elective/emergency] with [symptoms]
- What main treatments or procedures did the patient receive?
- What services did the patient see? For example, liaison psychiatry, social work
- Depending on the case it may be relevant to include here key factors in past medical history and social history. For example, if the patient is admitted in neutropenic sepsis, mention if applicable recent chemotherapy. Key excluded diagnosis e.g. no pulmonary embolism was seen on CTPA scan
- What is the state of the patient on discharge? Is the patient now well? If the patient is now very frail and expected to die at home, not only should this be stated, but the GP should be contacted directly as well

The skill here is to pick out key pieces of information that the GP needs to know without repeating the entire contents of the hospital notes verbatim.

Key Investigations:

- It is not necessary to include every blood test, but include clinically relevant results. Also include significant investigations undertaken such as CT and MRI scans (even if the results are unremarkable – an ECG showing normal sinus rhythm is significant if the patient was initially referred querying fast atrial fibrillation)

Letters

Drugs on Discharge:

Include here the drugs that will be continued on discharge. Include the following key points:
- Generic name of drug
- Dose
- Frequency of administration
- Route of administration
- Length of treatment

Don't forget to include information about allergies or adverse reactions to drugs. With certain drugs like warfarin, when is the next drug level due?

Changes to Medication:

Include here which drugs have been discontinued, why they have been discontinued, and whether it is expected that they might be restarted
- e.g. 1 simvastatin has been permanently discontinued due to proximal myopathy
- e.g. 2 lisinopril was discontinued due to renal failure; please consider restarting when renal function is appropriate

Also state which drugs have been added, their indication, the duration of therapy, and whether they need to be reviewed.
- e.g. for 7 day course of oral co-amoxiclav for a lower respiratory tract infection

Changes Made to Care Arrangements:

Changes made to community care. For example, district nurses to administer low molecular weight heparin injection, or social work arranging a package of care in the community.

Outstanding Tests/Results:

List the investigations which are still to be done and those where results are currently awaited. State whether these are being chased by the hospital team or are to be chased by the GP.

Follow Up:

Has an appointment been made to return to clinic in the originating hospital or is the expectation that further follow-up will happen in a more local hospital? Have any follow up investigations been arranged?

It is important to be clear what is expected of the GP (e.g. please could the GP practice arrange for Mrs X to have repeat urea and electrolytes checked in 1-2 weeks) and what is being arranged by the hospital (e.g. Dr Smith's team will arrange for a follow up Chest X-ray in 4-6 weeks time). Are other services like psychiatry, physiotherapy, or the dieticians following the patient up as well?

GP to please consider the following...

Include information that is particularly important for the GP to be aware of with regard to the patient's ongoing care. For example, has the patient gone home with a Do Not Attempt Cardio-Pulmonary Resuscitation (DNA CPR) form? What criteria might require more urgent reassessment – e.g. on discharge from a cardiology ward *'should [patient x] have any further angina, please re-refer her for consideration of further percutaneous coronary intervention to her right coronary artery'*.

Information given to Patient and Family...

Has the patient/family been counselled about their current problem, reason for discharge and any further follow-up or contact with the admitting unit?

Yours sincerely,

[Insert name of referring doctor]

[Insert designation of referring doctor and senior doctor if relevant]

[Insert contact details of referring doctor]

It is also helpful to state the contact details of the consultant or registrar looking after the patient, especially if you are frequently rotating through different units. Ideally, include the contact details of any other services (e.g. community palliative care) that might be involved.